Acupuncture and Related Techniques in Physical Therapy

For Churchill Livingstone:

Commissioning editor: Inta Ozols
Project manager: Valerie Burgess
Project development editor: Valerie Bain
Design direction: Judith Wright
Project controller: Pat Miller
Illustrator: Peter Cox
Copy editor: Christine Wyard
Indexer: Tarrant Ranger Indexing Agency
Sales promotion executive: Hilary Brown

Acupuncture and Related Techniques in Physical therapy

Edited by

Val Hopwood MSc SRP DipAc(Nanjing) MCSP

Senior Physiotherapist, Hythe Hospital, Southampton;
Senior Lecturer, Acupuncture Association of Chartered
Physiotherapists, Nottingham, UK

Maureen Lovesey ONC MBAcC SRP MCSP

Private Practitioner, Berkhamsted, UK;
Chairman, International Acupuncture Association of
Physical Therapists, UK

Sara Mokone BSc (RAND)Physiotherapy

BSc(SocSci) LicAc DipCounselling Skills RSATeaching Cert
Part-time Community Physiotherapist, North Middlesex
Hospital Trust, St Anne's Hospital, North London, UK

Foreword by

George Lewith MA DM MRCP MRCGP

Honorary Clinical Senior Lecturer, School of Medicine,
University of Southampton, Southampton, UK

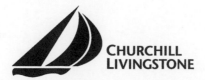

CHURCHILL
LIVINGSTONE

EDINBURGH LONDON NEW YORK OXFORD PHILADELPHIA ST LOUIS SYDNEY TORONTO 1997

Churchill Livingstone
An imprint of Elsevier Science Limited

First published 1997
Transferred to digital printing 2003

ISBN 0 443 05593 9

British Library of Cataloguing in Publication Data
A catalogue record for this book is available from the British
Library.

Library of Congress Cataloging in Publication Data
A catalog record for this book is available from the Library
of Congress.

Note
Medical knowledge is constantly changing. As new
information becomes available, changes in treatment,
procedures, equipment and the use of drugs become
necessary. The authors and publishers have, as far as it
is possible, taken care to ensure that the information
given in this text is accurate and up to date. However,
readers are strongly advised to confirm that the
information, especially with regard to drug usage,
complies with latest legislation and standards of practice.

ELSEVIER
SCIENCE

your source for books,
journals and multimedia
in the health sciences
www.elsevierhealth.com

The
publisher's
policy is to use
**paper manufactured
from sustainable forests**

Produced by Longman Singapore Publishers (Pte) Ltd.
Printed in UK by Antony Rowe Ltd, Eastbourne

Contents

Foreword

It is a great privilege to be asked to write a foreword to this superb text. Ever since I first became interested in acupuncture in the mid 1970s, it was quite apparent to me that physiotherapists would be the ideal people to deliver high quality acupuncture to patients within the National Health Service. Their training in musculoskeletal medicine, allied with the techniques commonly used in physiotherapy and the conditions frequently treated by physiotherapists, argues clearly that they are the most appropriate professional group to take this particular therapeutic technique forward and integrate it into conventional medicine.

Dr Julian Kenyon and I began to teach physiotherapists in early 1980s, and it is a great pleasure now to see that acupuncture has become an accepted part of normal physiotherapy practice. The development of any 'new' technique within physiotherapy necessitates quite specific training, along with the development of appropriate textbooks and teaching methods. It is a matter of great personal satisfaction to know that physiotherapists have now taken ownership of both acupuncture training and the production of appropriate and much needed textbooks that can relate the necessary clinical techniques within acupuncture, to the specific needs of the physiotherapy profession.

I hope that this textbook will be the first of many, and that we will eventually see the development of a truly integrated physiotherapy profession encompassing both acupuncture and many of the other techniques that are currently thought of as alternative or complementary.

1996   G. L.

Preface

Acupuncture is becoming increasingly popular with patients and medical professionals. This book has been designed to be a comprehensive introduction for physical therapists interested in integrating acupuncture into their practice and it should be a helpful adjunct to a practical training programme (Acupuncture is a practical skill and should not be taught from books: nothing replaces structured practical training.) It will also be of interest to individuals, managers or governments who are considering introducing acupuncture into a clinic, hospital or country.

This book's international format, with contributions from all over the world, is unique. It includes contributions from world-renowned researchers and recognized educators in acupuncture, who are either members or friends of the International Acupuncture Association of Physical Therapists (IAAPT), the moving force behind this collection of acupuncture material. IAAPT aims to develop the integration of acupuncture into the practice of physical therapy worldwide. The need to set up international standards of practice and training programmes is acknowledged by the membership.

This book starts with an introduction to Traditional Chinese Medicine and progresses rapidly to the field of research, where the latest physiological theories are clearly described and explained by the Honorary President of IAAPT, Professor Sven Andersson. Interestingly, many of the empirical observations made by the Chinese are now being scientifically validated, although, of course, much more research is needed.

Each of the member countries has contributed their specialized knowledge in acupuncture and allied techniques. The book contains chapters on the main channels, the points for pain relief, safe needling and hygiene procedures. Non-invasive techniques, such as acupressure, moxibustion, cupping, TENS and laser, are included with acupuncture techniques like electroacupuncture, ear acupuncture and use of trigger points. Examples of cases are included at the end of each chapter. Placebo effect and some problems in initiating valid research are also tackled.

Physical therapists are using acupuncture more frequently and finding that it complements other modes of treatment. Several contributors describe how they have integrated acupuncture into different areas of clinical practice and how it was accepted. Acupuncture was first incorporated into physical therapy practice by one or two enthusiasts and often had a bias towards a particular speciality in the early stages. In countries where it has been in use for some time, it is used for a number of conditions and utilizes many variants on the basic techniques.

The last section of the book is geared to self-study and includes a range of case studies that are classified into three different levels of complexity. In addition, three cases are used to highlight differing approaches to treatment. These cases were presented at a recent international conference, 'Advancing Horizons in Acupuncture', as part of the 1995 World Congress of Physical Therapists (WCPT) meeting in Washington DC. This interest group meeting was organized by the Swedish group, SALS. All the case studies assume a level of basic physical therapy knowledge, therefore some common professional terms are not explained.

A list of recommended books is given to stimulate further reading. A small section at the end of the book includes optional questions to aid in the process of learning.

The IAAPT was formed in 1991, at a meeting organized by the Acupuncture Association of Chartered Physiotherapists (UK) held at the 11th World Congress of Physical Therapists in London. The aims of the organization are to provide a network for members and to promote the use of acupuncture by physical therapists to individuals, professional associations and governments. It also seeks to promote international standards in practice, training and research. In March 1996, there were members in 17 countries and six of these had group membership: Canada, New Zealand, South Africa,

Zimbabwe, Sweden and the UK. Membership of these groups varies from a newly formed group of 13 in Canada to 1600 in SALS, the well-established Swedish group. IAAPT maintains a high profile at many international physical therapy conferences and is growing rapidly.

The editors wish to thank all the contributors for the hard work that they have put into the production of this book. This book is only a beginning. As more research is completed, we come closer to understanding the fascinating mystery of acupuncture, and better at incorporating it into clinical practice.

1996   V. H., M. L., S. M.

Contributors

AACP : *Acupuncture Association of Chartered Physiotherapists*

AASASP: *Acupuncture Association of the South African Society of Physiotherapy*

AFC : *Special interest group for doctors, dentists and physiotherapists in Canada*

IAAPT : *International Acupuncture Association of Physical Therapy*

PAPMA : *Physiotherapy and Pain Modulation Association*

SALS : *Svensk Akupunkturförening för Leg. Sjukgymnaster (Swedish Acupuncture Association for Registered Physiotherapists)*

Michael Anderson BSc MBChB DipObst DipAvMed DipIH MRNZCGP
Occupational Health Physician in private practice; part-time physician at Chronic Pain Relief Clinic, Dunedin Public Hospital, Dunedin, New Zealand

Sven Andersson MD PhD
Professor, Department of Physiology, University of Gothenburg, Sweden; Honorary President of IAAPT

David Baxter TD BSc DPhil MCSP
Professor of Rehabilitation Sciences and Director, Centre for Health and Social Research, University of Ulster, Jordonstown, Northern Ireland; Research officer IAAPT

Ana Maria Carballo
Faculty member at the School of Medicine, University of Buenos Aires; Director of the yearly graduate Program of Acupunctural Reflexotherapy at the Hospital de Clinicas; Private Practitioner, Buenos Aires, Argentina; member of IAAPT Committee

Alan Clements JP DipPhysio RegPhysioAcup
PAPMA Tutor/Education Officer; Private Physiotherapist/Acupuncturist, Tauranga, New Zealand

John Cross
Director, Tyringham Clinic, The White House, Tyringham, Buckinghamshire, UK

Sue Czartoryski SRP MCSP
Superintendent Physiotherapist, Tolwarth Hospital, Tolwarth, Surrey, UK; AACP member

Nadia Ellis MSc MCSP
Senior Physiotherapist, Bonsecours Hospital, Beaconsfield, UK; Chair of AACP

Edwin H. Groll BSc PTAP
Physical Therapist, Manor Pines Convalescent Center, and Acupuncturist, Acupuncture Associates, Wilton Manors, Florida, USA

Eva Haker PhD RPT
Lecturer at Department of Physical Therapy, Karolinska Institute, Stockholm, Sweden; Chair of the Swedish Acupuncture Association for Registered Physiotherapists (SALS); Vice Chair of IAAPT

Val Hopwood MSc SRP DipAc(Nanjing) MCSP
Senior Physiotherapist, Hythe Hospital, Southampton, UK; Senior Lecturer on AACP Diploma Acupuncture Course and Chair of AACP Education Committee, Nottingham, UK; member of Education Committee of IAAPT

Sara Jeevanjee SRP DipAc MCSP
Private Practitioner, Shirley, Southampton, UK;
AACP member

Tanya Lee-McCracken BSc(PT) MCPA CMAc CAFCI
President, board member, teacher and examiner at
British Columbia chapter of Acupuncture
Foundation of Canada Institute; private practitioner,
Victoria, British Columbia, Canada

Colette Lehody BSc(PT) CMAc CAFC RAc
Chair, Advisory Committee for Certificate
Programme in Medical Acupuncture, Faculty of
Extension, University of Alberta, Edmonton, Alberta,
Canada

Charles Liggins MCSP GradDipPhysio DipTP
Acupuncture Section, Frank Martin Pain
Management Clinic, Addington Hospital, Durban,
South Africa; Journal Editor of IAAPT

Maureen Lovesey ONC MBAcC SRP MCSP
Private Practitioner, Berkhamsted, UK; Chair of
IAAPT

Thomas Lundeberg MD PhD DipAc
Associate Professor, Department of Physiology and
Pharmacology, Department of Surgery and
Rehabilitation, Karolinska Institute, Karolinska
Hospital, Stockholm, Sweden

Helen Madzokere CertHSM MCSP
Occupational Physiotherapist for National Railway
of Zimbabwe, Bulawayo, Zimbabwe

Val Marston MCSP
Editor of AACP Journal, Riseley, Bedford, UK

Sara Mokone BSc(RAND)Physiotherapy BSc(SocSci) LicAc
DipCounsellingSkills RSATeachingCert
Part-time Community Physiotherapist, North
Middlesex Hospital Trust, St Anne's Hospital, North
London, UK; Secretary/Treasurer of IAAPT

Passion Nhekairo-Musa MSc(RehabStudies) DipTP CertEd
ONC MCSP
Partner, Private Practitioner and Consultant for
Urban Community-based Rehabilitation, Bulawayo,
Zimbabwe

Jan Naslund RPT
Private Practitioner and Vice Chair of SALS,
Eldarevagen, Kristianstad, Sweden; member of
Education Committee of IAAPT

Kim L. T. Ong BA MBAcC MCSP
Private Practitioner, Croydon, UK

Jane Parkinson DipRG DipRT LicAc MCSP
Private Practitioner and Senior Physiotherapist,
Pontefract Infirmary, Pontefract Health Trust, West
Yorkshire, UK

Linda Rapson MD CAFC
Executive President, Senior Lecturer and Examiner,
Acupuncture Foundation of Canada Institute;
Executive President AFC Toronto, Ontario, Canada;
Medical Director, Rapson Pain and Acupuncture
Clinic, Toronto, Canada

Lorrene Soellner MCPA CMAc CAFC
Physiotherapist, Saanich Peninsula Hospital,
Saanichton, British Columbia, Canada

Carol Taylor MCPA CMAc CAFC MCSP
Physiotherapist, Private Practice, Duncan, British
Columbia, Canada

Moolamanil Thomas MBBS PhD
Research Associate, Department of Physiology and
Pharmacology, Karolinska Institute, Stockholm,
Sweden

Diana Turnbull DipPhysio MNZSP
Private Practitioner, Dunedin, New Zealand; Chair of
PAPMA; Education officer at IAAPT

Deirdre M. Walsh BPhysiotherapy DPhil MISCP MCSP
Lecturer in Physiotherapy, School of Health Sciences,
University of Ulster, Jordanstown, Northern Ireland

Joseph Yao DipAc PT
Salem, SC, USA

List of abbreviations used for meridians

LU   Lung
LI   Large Intestine
ST   Stomach
SP   Spleen
HE   Heart
SI   Small Intestine
B   Bladder
KI   Kidney
PE   Pericardium
TE   Triple Energiser
GB   Gall Bladder
LIV   Liver
GV   Governor Vessel
CV   Conception Vessel

Basic acupuncture concepts and procedures

1

Introduction to Traditional Chinese Medicine theory

Val Hopwood

Why should a 20th century physiotherapist be concerned with philosophies and beliefs arising from another culture over 3000 years ago?

The simple answer to that question is that there is no reason at all. We can call what we do "sensory stimulation" or we can call it "acupuncture"; it matters little to the patient. A physiotherapist conceiving an interest in the art of acupuncture could go on to practice and achieve some good results without bothering with Yin, Yang and the rest of the cultural baggage. However, that physiotherapist would miss out on a great deal. The richness of the Chinese experience would be lost and the meticulous recording of results over thousands of years would be wasted.

A Western-trained medical professional experiences considerable intellectual distress when first confronting the traditional theories. This is in part intellectual arrogance, as we suppose what we were taught, what we went to great pains to commit to memory, was the only valid way of looking at the body. Discovering that there is a logical scheme of thinking outside the Western experience can come as a shock. Once across this mental gulf, however, the study becomes quite fascinating, some aspects of the functioning of the body take on a new meaning, and new explanations do sometimes clarify the view.

Interestingly, this interaction has happened before. In the 17th century a Dutchman, Willem ten Rhijne (1647–1700), was employed by the Dutch East India Company in the Far East. He observed the Japanese practising their form of Chinese acupuncture, obtained a few charts showing the channels, made the assumption that they were blood vessels, and proceeded to inform the West of the

techniques. His teaching was rather confused, however, since he learned from the Japanese through a Chinese interpreter and subsequently had to translate it into Latin, the universal scientific language of the time. The reader is referred to the excellent history of acupuncture in Dr Baldry's book (1989) for more details.

Problems with translation are not confined to the 17th century; there are still many misunderstandings and variations in semantics giving rise to a great variety of lesser theories. The most surprising thing about Chinese medicine as it is taught in the West is its coherence; there are still clear threads of logic running through it despite the variations. It is also not necessary to abandon Western knowledge when studying Chinese medicine; the student of acupuncture will find that the two paradigms can coexist quite comfortably, the one enriching the other.

The natural desire to understand the underlying physiological changes produced by needling should be encouraged in all physiotherapy/acupuncture training, as it is no longer enough to accept the traditional teaching unquestioningly. However the purpose of this chapter is to explain some of the ideas underpinning the traditional view, since most acupuncture books giving advice on treatment will still tend to explain the choice of points in these terms. If a serious attempt at research is to be made, a lot of acupuncture needs to be viewed within the traditional framework before it is taken apart and analysed. Quite a lot of research has been marred by the uniformity and simplicity imposed on the art of acupuncture prescription.

In this chapter I shall explain the major traditional

theories briefly and link them to physiotherapy practice as far as possible. The physiology and pathology as conceived by the ancient Chinese will serve as useful hooks upon which we can hang the diagnosis and treatment without losing sight of the scientifically proven medical knowledge that we already have.

Qi

Qi is a basic concept of Chinese medicine; it has no direct equivalent in Western medicine. It is often translated in English as the 'life force' and is present throughout the body. It manifests in the skin, in the organs and permeates every living tissue. It accumulates in the organs and flows primarily in the energy channels, or 'meridians'. This conceived circulatory system for Qi is distinct from the vascular or nervous systems of the body. It is often the most difficult concept for the orthodox medical practitioner to accept. Traditional Chinese Medicine (TCM) has found many ways to explain it, giving different names to each perceived subdivision. For instance, the Qi inherited by the fetus from the two parents is known as the Original Qi, Congenital Qi, Ancestral Qi or Preheaven Qi. In addition there are many other forms, including Postheaven Qi (or Nutritive Qi) produced by the body from the air breathed in and the food digested. It is not possible to describe Qi and the body fluids fully in this short chapter, but one of its important functions is that of defence of the body; this will be mentioned later when discussing the TCM physiology of the lungs. Qi is given many names that indicate its site of origin, composition and density. TCM claims that acupuncture can both influence the flow of Qi within the meridians, and change the balance of Qi within the organs.

Yin and Yang

The fundamental theory of Yin and Yang is not too difficult to assimilate, following on from the basic theories of electricity. It is easy to visualize all aspects

Table 1.1 *Yin and Yang*

Yin	Yang
Wet	Dry
Cold	Hot
Slow	Fast
Internal	External
Dark	Light
Night	Day
Ache	Stabbing pain
Turgid	Volatile
Nutritive	Mobilizing

of the body, and indeed the universe, as either positive or negative. When we see that the Chinese theorists teach that things are never truly either Yin or Yang, but always contain a small amount of the opposite characteristic, then it becomes easier still; for instance, day would be considered Yang in character, while night would be Yin – however, night is always in the process of becoming day and vice versa. Table 1.1 gives an idea of how this global view can be applied.

This list of ideas, by no means exhaustive, can be extended to the practice of medicine. Table 1.2, compiled by Loo (1985), gives interesting examples of two ways of thinking; it is interesting to note that the left side, corresponding to Western medicine, contains words referring to visibility while those on the right, referring to acupuncture, tend to be invisible. This table underlines the duality of medicine, Western medicine inclining to the Yang where Eastern medicine inclines to the Yin. It would

Table 1.2 *Western medicine and Eastern medicine (from Loo 1985)*

Western medicine	Eastern medicine
Objective	Subjective
Visible	Invisible
Seeing	Feeling
Physical	Spiritual
Structural	Physiological
Materialistic	Philosophical
Outer consciousness	Subconscious
Intellectual	Intuitive
Reasoning	Awareness
Organic	Functional
Signs	Symptoms

be unwise to ascribe the listed characteristics exclusively to one side or the other but the comparison is a useful one and also encapsulates some of the thinking about Yin and Yang.

Disease in TCM can be broadly classified into that affecting the channels, that affecting the internal organs (the Zang Fu system), and that affecting both.

The Eight Principles

The eight principles: Yin/Yang, Hot/Cold, Excess/Deficiency and Internal/External, comprise a form of diagnostic logic that enabled the ancient Chinese to codify their observations about the patient. Any form of medicine is:

■ *dependent on philosophical concepts, accepted and utilized by the society in which that model of medicine is practised. Assumptions concerning the nature of disease entities, canons of possible explanations, and the modes of proper treatment are merely extensions of the paradigm that dominates a particular medical system. The characteristics of a given system of medicine can ultimately be traced to the notions held by the then current society as a whole.* MOROZ 1994

Yin/Yang

Yin and Yang have already been discussed in their broader sense but their application to the individual organs of the body and the situations inherent in some medical conditions means that it is useful to remember the imperative of balance between them when treating with acupuncture or Chinese herbal medicine. TCM believes that this delicate balance can be affected by acupuncture treatment and more specifically by technique. No concrete proof exists either way because the concept itself is hardly amenable to verification. However, it would be foolish to discount the centuries of empirical evidence accumulated by the Chinese. The treatment

rationales selected have been shown to be effective in certain conditions and where the traditional explanation involves the balancing of Yin with Yang then Western medical thinking must produce a good physiological explanation before dismissing the points thus selected.

Hot/Cold

Most preindustrial societies have observed that some conditions seem to be predominantly hot, with the patient exhibiting fever symptoms, a raised temperature, flushed skin and an increased heart rate, while others involve cold, pallor, a lack of energy and a slowing down of vital processes. Medical thought in the same societies has then gone on to postulate that the application of cold to bring down a temperature is beneficial, as is the application of heat to a cold condition.

TCM is no different but has been particularly ingenious in the application of heat. Burning moxa punk (see Chapter 8) applied directly to needles or over the skin surface is a simple and effective method of introducing heat into the tissues. Needling can conversely be used to cool the body or a limb (see Chapter 4). The physiological explanations lie elsewhere in this book (see Chapter 2) but the phenomenon itself is easily observable.

Cupping is a technique that increases local superficial circulation by creating a vacuum under the cup; it can lead to a sensation of warming in the affected area although the subsequent stagnation in the superficial vessels needs to be dispersed. This technique was adopted by the Eastern Mediterranean peoples and is still commonly used to this day. Cupping was in vogue in the United Kingdom in Victorian times, and sets of glass cups can still be found in museums, but has been largely forgotten now. The vacuum was traditionally created by use of a naked flame, but the suction cups for an interferential unit can be used to similar effect since the heat arises from the change in circulation not the means of producing the vacuum to adhere the cups.

Excess/Deficiency

The idea of Excess and Deficiency is applied principally to the energy or Qi present within the system or body. Obviously if there is an optimum level for circulating Qi, then there can also be either too much or too little. Deficiency, or Xu, conditions arise when either the body's ability to manufacture new or acquired Qi is diminished or use of existing energy has been immoderate. Most of the problems of old age are due to a deficiency somewhere within the system. This kind of deficiency is not always possible to remedy – even in Chinese medicine there is no cure for old age! However, specific needling techniques can boost the level of energy in specific organs and there is also a technique whereby the reservoirs of Qi said to exist in the extraordinary meridians, or 'extra vessels', can be tapped and utilized.

Excess is defined as Shi in TCM and is characterized by an excessive amount of Qi or Blood in organs and channels. Typical symptoms are acute pain, cramps, increased muscle tone and hypertension. There may also be redness of the face, a loud voice and a strong pulse. Overexcitement, nervousness, restlessness, aimless activity and insomnia are sometimes seen in Excess conditions. An acute flare-up of an arthritic joint can be seen as Shi on an underlying Xu situation.

From a Western viewpoint, some acupuncture points seem to have a tonic effect on the metabolism and are used to stimulate many areas of physiological activity in the Chinese sense. This is also hard to prove but we can surmise from a knowledge of the effects of the various chemoreceptors shown to be susceptible to this form of stimulus that increases or decreases in some activities are certainly possible.

Internal/External

The concept of External/Internal conditions is quite sophisticated. Diseases of the system are perceived as mostly arising from the action of external agents but progressing to a deeper level within the body. When this has occurred the syndrome can be identified by the cumulative effects on the different organ systems, the Zang Fu balance. Acute problems are thought not to have penetrated far into the organism but chronic problems have a deeper origin; they may have arisen externally and not been treated or they may have arisen from fundamental imbalances of energy

within the body. Chinese medicine distinguishes between these situations and different types of treatment are recommended accordingly.

A good example of this exterior to interior progression is a head cold starting in the nose and sinuses and becoming gradually more serious as it passes into the lungs to become a chest cold with associated bronchitis, etc.

Pathogenesis of disease

A combination of the above ideas is evident in the TCM theory concerning the treatment of joint problems, osteoarthritis and rheumatoid arthritis in particular. Pathogenic factors that are thought to cause disease can be External, such as abnormal weather conditions, or Internal, such as emotions. A brief description of these factors and their relative importance follows.

Exogenous pathogens

These refer to six relatively abnormal weather conditions.

Wind

Wind is characterized by mobility in the symptoms produced: a pain that cannot easily be localized or changes site frequently can be caused by Wind. The clinical manifestations of abnormal limb movement such as spasm or twitching are common. The symptoms may vary in intensity and often include a dislike of wind, fever, headache and sweating.

Cold

Invasion of Cold is a common occurrence in the colder countries and is often blamed for painful conditions in folklore. To "catch a cold" or "take a chill" are common sayings. The Cold causes contraction of the channels and blood vessels, and consequently a decreased circulation of Qi and Blood. The symptoms are those of a slight fever, a dislike of cold, headache, muscular aching and occasionally a dark and painful area in the local muscles and skin. A "frozen shoulder" is a good example of a Cold pathogenic invasion, as is Bell's palsy.

Summer Heat

This condition occurs only in the summer and tends to damage the Yin aspect of the body. It may progress to affect the level of consciousness. A good example of this is heatstroke. The symptoms are excessive body heat, profuse sweating, thirst, dry skin, a dry mouth and, in serious cases, delirium. Summer Heat can combine with Damp to produce dizziness or nausea.

Damp

Damp is characterized by diseases that are sticky or greasy and that tend to be due to stagnation. It causes a generalized feeling of malaise, a heavy feeling, dizziness and a stuffy sensation in the chest. There may be abdominal distension or swelling.

Dryness

Tuberculosis is an example of pathogenic Dryness. The typical symptoms are a dry, sore feeling in the nose, mouth and throat, a coarseness of the skin or a tight dry cough, possibly with haemoptysis. Dryness consumes Yin fluids.

Heat

Heat can vary in intensity from mild to severe, Fire being the most severe. In TCM acute infections are thought to be due to the invasion of the pathogen Heat. There is an abrupt onset, high fever, chill, thirst, restlessness, irritability and profuse sweating. In severe cases the patient may lapse into a coma accompanied by convulsions.

Mental pathogens

These are all normal emotions but taken to excess. TCM defines them as Joy, Anger, Anxiety,

Overthinking, Grief, Fear and Fright. They are all capable of inflicting damage on the internal organs. Chinese medicine also holds that many of the mental functions lie under the control or influence of the internal organs (since the ancient Chinese had no concept of the brain): Fear, Fright or Joy are said to damage the Heart; Anger damages the Liver causing, among other things, depression and irritability; Grief, Anxiety or Overthinking can damage the Spleen and Stomach. Excessive grief can also damage the Lung, while Grief, Anxiety and Anger can also affect the circulation of the Qi and Blood causing stagnation and, possibly, lumps and tumours.

Miscellaneous pathogens

Traumatic injuries are understood as in Western medicine and classified in this group.

Chinese medicine holds that irregular feeding can be very damaging to the system. It is important to eat at regular intervals, and skipping meals is never a good idea. Too much raw or uncooked food can affect the delicate energy balance within the body since it requires too much Spleen or Stomach energy or Qi to digest it. Too little food is, naturally, also damaging, reducing the production of Qi and Blood.

Excessive alcohol, and strongly spiced or fatty food is bad for the Liver.

Too little or too much physical labour are both thought to have a detrimental effect on the body systems.

Bi syndromes

The practical application of these approaches to the disease process can be seen best in the definition of the various types of arthritis. All types of arthritis are classified in TCM as diseases of Bi. "Bi" means a blocked or obstructed channel. This blockage may be due to the invasion of a channel by a pathogen such as Cold or direct damage to the channel as in traumatic injury.

Wandering, hot Bi

This is often seen in acute rheumatoid arthritis. The patient complains of fever and there are red, painful, swollen joints. There may also be limitation of joint movement, excessive sweating and irritability. If a single joint is hot and the pain is not mobile then it may be a septic arthritis.

This is due to obstruction of the channel by Wind and Heat.

Painful, heavy Bi

This is characterized by chronic arthritis of either the osteo- or rheumatoid type. There can be slight swelling and the joints are painful with the soreness becoming more intense on cloudy or wet days. There may be chronic malaise and a numb feeling in the joints and the surrounding muscles, with eventual muscle weakness.

This is due to invasion by Cold and Damp.

Painful Bi

This is mostly seen in joint trauma, caused by the disruption of the channels. Usually only one joint is affected. The invading pathogen is usually Cold but it is only superficial and not indicative of a generalized pathogenic state within the body.

Treatment is usually aimed at ridding the body of the invading pathogenic factor and unblocking the channels for the free passage of Qi and Blood. Some good examples of this can be seen in the case histories in Chapter 15.

Zang Fu organ theory

The Zang Fu classification of the major internal organs is the most fascinating part of traditional Chinese theory. The ancient Chinese were never in fact encouraged to perform autopsies and so never discovered the aspects of neuroanatomy so familiar to us in the West. They did, however, observe the role of the heart in the circulation of blood and had a clear idea of the functions of the digestive tract. They did not realize the importance of the brain and, recognizing that it was composed of similar material to bone marrow, decided it was just a large space filled with that substance. The functions that we understand that the brain performs were therefore ascribed to other organs.

Table 1.3 *The Zang Fu organ classification*

Zang organs (Yin)	Fu organs (Yang)
Heart *Xin*	Small intestine *Xiao Chang*
Lungs *Fei*	Large intestine *Da Chang*
Liver *Gan*	Gall bladder *Dan*
Spleen *Pi*	Stomach *Wei*
Kidney *Shen*	Urinary Bladder *Pang Guan*
Pericardium *Xin Bao*	Sanjiao
(Extra: Uterus)	(Extra: Brain)

The following is a very brief description of some of the salient points of Zang Fu physiology. If each organ is referred to by the Chinese name it serves to distinguish it from the same organ in Western medical theory. They are usually listed as six Yang or Fu organs, said to be hollow in nature, and five Yin or Zang organs, said to be solid (Table 1.3). The Pericardium is usually also listed as a Fu organ. The Zang organs are generally thought to be more important and are involved in the processing of substances. The Fu organs are principally involved in storage; they are thought to interact directly with the channels.

Functions of the Zang organs

Heart (Xin)

- governs all the other organs
- regulates the flow of Blood and Qi
- stores and rules the mind, controls consciousness (Shen)
- opens to the tongue
- controls sweat, influenced by Heat
- influences sleep and dreams
- can be injured by excess Joy or agitation

Governs the other organs The Heart is considered to be the most important organ in the body and in Chinese medicine is given considerable control over all the other organs.

Regulates the flow of Blood and Qi The Heart governs the Blood in two ways:

1. The transformation of food Qi into Blood takes place in the Heart.
2. It is responsible for the circulation of Blood as understood in Western medicine.

The relationship between the Heart and Blood is important and determines the strength of constitution of an individual. A generally weak constitution can sometimes be seen as a crack down the centre of the tongue, together with a weak pulse on both the Heart and Kidney positions at the wrist.

The state of the blood vessels reflects the strength of the Heart Qi, or internal energy. This is also manifest in the strength of the Heart pulse.

Since the Heart controls the blood vessels and circulation then a "rosy and lustrous" complexion is a sign of health. A pale or bright white complexion means a deficiency. Stagnant Blood gives a bluish-purple complexion, as in heart failure. Heat in the Heart leads to a red complexion.

Houses the mind and controls consciousness As mentioned earlier, the Heart is said in TCM to house the mind or Shen.

This can be described as comprising five particular functions:

- mental activity (including emotions)
- consciousness
- memory
- thinking
- sleep.

The term 'Shen' can also sometimes used to indicate vitality. Ascribing these functions to the Heart may seem a little odd, in spite of the folk theory in Western medicine that it is possible to die of a broken heart, but when mental illness is tackled in Chinese medicine the Heart points are among the most effective. Treatment of insomnia and depression will always include the use of the powerful point Shenmen, or Heart point 7 (H-7); interestingly, Shenmen translates as "Gateway to the Spirit".

Opens into the tongue All Zang Fu organs have particular sense organs where their general condition is said to be detectable. The tongue is considered to be an extension of the Heart. The Heart has ultimate control of form and colour. A red tip signifies Heat in the Heart; it can be dry and dark red and also can be swollen. Ulcers may appear, indicating that there is an imbalance of energy or Qi in the Heart.

The condition of the Heart also affects speech, stuttering, aphasia, etc. A disharmony of the Heart is said to cause a person to talk incessantly and to laugh inappropriately, as in mania.

Controls sweat, influenced by Heat Since the Blood and Body Fluids have a common origin, sweat is considered to be controlled by the Heart. It is said to come from the space between the skin and muscles. Deficiency of Heart Qi may cause spontaneous sweating and Deficiency of Heart Yin may cause night sweating. Whatever the physiological reason, Heart points work better at controlling these symptoms than others.

The Heart is damaged by Heat, also the Pericardium can be invaded by exterior Heat, which, in the rather picturesque translations from the Chinese, can "cloud the orifices of the heart" leading to dementia, coma or aphasia. A strong connection with the ability to speak eloquently is found in the ancient literature.

Influences sleep and dreams Since the Heart stores the mind it is closely concerned with sleep. If the Heart is weak the mind is said to have no residence and it will float at night, causing disturbed sleep or excessive dreaming, should sleep come at all.

Since the Heart is said to control the mind and hence the emotions, it follows that an excess, i.e. joy or extreme anxiety, will damage the balance of Qi in this Zang Fu organ. Symptoms of a "broken heart" are really a possibility in Chinese medicine.

Lung (Fei)

- controls respiration and is responsible for the intake of clear Qi
- governs the surface of the body, hair and skin
- opens into the nose
- most external organ
- can be injured by Grief

Controls respiration The Lungs are responsible for the intake of clean air, which they convert into "Clear Qi". Together with the Qi produced from substances that are eaten and drunk this goes to make up the Postheaven or renewable Qi within the body. The Qi from the Lungs passes down and is linked with that of the Kidneys, which should rise, effectively controlling the water circulation within the body.

Controls hair and skin The Lungs influence the condition of the skin and also the state of the pores. If the skin is in poor condition the pores may be more open than usual and allow the invasion of exogenous pathogens. The Lung is also said to control the Wei Qi or Defensive Qi in the body. Since it is linked to the Kidney and the water circulation the Lung is also said to control sweating and excessive sweating, hyperhidrosis, can be controlled using Lung points.

Opens into the nose, most external organ Since the Lung opens into the nose and it is the most external organ, it is vulnerable to the external pathogens, Wind and Cold.

Injured by emotion The Lung can be injured by emotions, because it is said to house the Corporeal Soul. It is particularly sensitive to Grief or sadness and treatment of LU-7 Lieque can have a powerful release effect in constrained emotional conditions, like bereavement.

Kidney (Shen)

- stores Jing or Essence, controls the Yang aspect of sexual potency
- controls birth, growth and reproduction
- Kidney energy is lost in old age
- nourishes bones, joints and teeth
- controls mental activity
- rules Water and controls excretion of impurities
- opens into the ear

The Kidneys are said to be the Root of life. They are responsible for storing the Essence, which is partly derived from the parents and established at conception.

The Yin and Yang of the Kidneys are the foundation for the rest of the body, that is, the primary Yin and Yang. Kidney Yin is the fundamental substance for birth, growth and reproduction while Kidney Yang is the motive force for all physiological processes. Although according to the five Elements they belong to Water, they are also said to be the source of Fire in the body. This is called Fire of the Gate of Vitality.

Stores essence The Kidneys store Preheaven Essence or Qi. This determines constitutional strength, vitality, etc. It is also the basis of sexual life. Impotence and infertility can be linked to it. The Kidneys store Postheaven Qi or Essence, the refined essence extracted from food through the transforming power of the internal organs.

Governs birth, growth and reproduction, and ageing The various developmental stages of life are under control of the Kidney: birth, puberty, menopause and death. Ageing itself is due to the decline of Essence during life. There is said to be a 7 year cycle for women and an 8 year cycle for men. The state of Kidney health is also said to be detectable from the state of the hair, white hair is not thought to be a good sign!

Production of marrow "Marrow" in TCM is defined as the common matrix of bones, bone marrow and the spinal cord. If Kidney Essence is strong it will nourish the brain and memory and concentration, thinking, memory and sight will all be keen. The Kidneys have other functions connected with the mental health of the person. In particular they are said to house the willpower.

The bones will also be strong and the teeth firm. If Kidney Essence is weak then the bones will be brittle and the teeth will tend to be loose. A weak Essence in children causes poor bone development, "pigeon chest", etc. The Kidney determines both the physical and mental strength of an individual.

Rules Water and the excretion of impurities
According to Five Element theory, the Kidneys, not unreasonably, belong to Water and they govern the transformation and transportation of Body Fluids in many ways. They act like a gate which opens and closes to control the flow of Body Fluids in the lower Jiao or lower third of the body cavity. Disease or imbalance between Kidney Yin and Yang will cause malfunctioning of the gate and there will be too much or too little urine. Because the Kidneys are in the lower Jiao, often referred to as the Drainage Ditch, they are concerned with the excretion of impure body fluids. They are also responsible for the energy required by the Urinary Bladder to enable it to store urine.

Opens into the ear The Kidneys are said to open into the ear, making Kidney points useful for the treatment of deafness and tinnitus.

(As with all Zang Fu diagnosis, none of these signs and manifestations necessarily mean kidney disease in the Western sense.)

Spleen (Pi)

- governs transformation and transportation
- controls the Blood
- controls the muscles and four limbs
- opens into the mouth and manifests in the lips
- controls the rising Qi
- houses thought

Governs transformation and transportation The Spleen is the main digestive organ in TCM and is responsible for the transformation or breaking down of ingested food and drink and its subsequent transportation. This is intimately concerned with the fluid balance in the body and the Spleen is influential in treating oedema, particularly in the lower limbs.

Controls the blood The Spleen keeps the Blood in the blood vessels and prevents bleeding. Superficial bruising with no apparent cause is thought to be due to a fault within the Spleen energy balance.

Influences muscle bulk/flesh The transformation and transportation of food substances ensures the maintenance of muscle health and bulk. Spleen points can be used to treat muscle wasting. The Spleen is said to like Dryness and is adversely affected by the Western habit of excessive consumption of uncooked foods and icy drinks.

Opens into the mouth The Spleen opens into the mouth and the general state of the Spleen is indicated by the lips, which should be a healthy red colour.

Controls Rising Qi The control over Rising Qi means that the Spleen can influence all types of prolapse; it is, in fact, said to hold organs in their place in the body. Spleen points are effective in the treatment of haemorrhoids.

Houses thought The Spleen is associated with thinking and if the balance is wrong then excessive worrying will be the sign, with general lassitude and lack of energy as a result.

The Spleen influences our capacity for thinking, studying, concentrating, focusing and memorizing.

Note: Excessive studying, mental work and concentration for sustained periods can weaken the Spleen. Heart and Kidneys also have an influence on memory and thought, but in slightly different ways.

Liver (Gan)

- responsible for the movement of the body fluids
- stores Blood and has a direct influence on the menstrual cycle
- nourishes the muscles and tendons
- influences the condition of fingernails
- closely linked with the eye
- said to influence the ability to plan one's life

Controls movement of body fluids The fluids involved are Blood, and Bile chiefly. This involves the Liver in the digestive process, ensuring the free flow of Blood and Qi throughout the body.

Stores Blood When menstruation begins the Liver releases blood in order for it to occur. If it fails to store the blood or fails to release it in sufficient quantities, dysmenorrhoea or amenorrhoea can occur. It is important that Liver Qi is in balance for the normal cycle to happen.

Nourishes the muscles and tendons The Liver controls the muscle tone in the body. If this function is disturbed there will be muscle twitching or spasm or even convulsions. This is said to be due to an "insufficiency of the Yin and Blood in the Liver" resulting in malnutrition of the tissues.

Manifests in the fingernails In Chinese medicine the fingernails are thought to be extensions of the tendons in the body; nails that are broken, flaking or ridged are all signs of imbalance within the Liver.

Closely linked with the eye The Liver is said to open through the eye and is connected to the vision and also movement of the eyeball. "Stirring of the inner Wind of the Liver" can cause poor vision, night blindness and abnormal movements of the eye.

Influences planning This is dependent on the Gall Bladder's ability to make decisions!

Pericardium (Xin Bao)

- no real function other than to protect the Heart
- can be used as a gentle form of therapy for Heart or for sedation

---

The Pericardium is closely related to the Heart; in fact traditionally it is thought to form a protective outer covering for the Heart, protecting it from the invasion of External pathogenic factors, hence the other common name for it: Heart Protector. In some Chinese texts it is not included among the Zang Fu organs at all. The Pericardium is of lesser importance than the Heart but displays many of the same functions. It governs Blood and houses the mind also. The points on the channel are often used to treat emotional problems and used for sedation.

Functions of the Fu organs

Stomach (Wei)

- controls the ripening and rotting of food
- controls the transportation of food Essence
- controls Descending Qi
- origin of fluids
- influence on mental states

The Stomach is the most important of the Yang organs. Together with the Spleen it is known as the Root of Postheaven Qi.

Controls the ripening and rotting of food The Stomach is said to be the site of the Middle Burner or Middle Jiao (see Sanjiao, p. 14). Digestion was understood as a rotting or fermentation process, in which the Stomach was the "maceration chamber". This prepares the way for the action of the Spleen in separating and extracting the refined Essence from food and drink. (It is also compared to a bubbling cauldron!)

After transformation in the Stomach the food passes down to the Small Intestine for further breakdown and absorption. The Stomach is always thought to be the true origin of the Qi of the body and it is vital that it functions well for a healthy situation. It is often necessary to tonify Stomach Qi when there is any disease process present. Zusanli ST-36 is the acupoint most commonly used for this form of tonification.

Controls the transportation of food essences The Stomach has a similar role to that of the Spleen in transporting the Food Qi to all the tissues, most particularly the limbs. Weak muscles and fatigue mean a lack of Stomach Qi. Incidentally the state of the Stomach can be seen quite clearly in the tongue coating, which is formed as a by-product of the rotting process. A thin white coating is normal. Absence of a coating implies impaired function. A yellow coating indicates Heat in the Stomach.

Controls Descending Qi The Stomach sends transformed food down to the Small Intestine, hence the descending function. If this is absent the food stagnates, leading to fullness, distension, sour regurgitation, belching, hiccup, nausea, vomiting, etc. Under normal conditions the Liver Qi helps with this so the two organs need to be considered for treatment together.

Origin of fluids To rot and ripen food the Stomach needs a great deal of fluid to dissolve the valuable parts of the food. Since it is itself a source of fluid the Stomach likes damp, unlike the Spleen. Eating large meals late at night depletes the fluids of the Stomach.

Mental influence The Stomach is susceptible to Excess patterns, such as Fire or Phlegm Fire (linked with mental states similar to mania). Mild cases can suffer from confusion and severe anxiety. Table 1.4 highlights the differences between the two linked organs, the Stomach and Spleen. Some of these variations can be quite subtle.

This sort of comparison is essential to Chinese medicine when differentiating the many combinations of symptoms or syndromes, and the table is taken from Ross (1985). It is not possible to discuss syndromes within the scope of this book but some excellent works have been written to enable

Table 1.4 *Wei and Pi*

Wei	Pi
Yang	Yin
Fu	Zang
Hollow	Solid
Receives food and drink	Transforms food and drink
Wei Qi descends	Pi Qi ascends
Ascent results in vomiting	Descent results in diarrhoea
Likes Damp	Likes Dryness
Tends to deficient Yin and signs of Heat	Tends to deficient Yang and signs of Cold

analysis of the different factors involved. Particularly good are: *Zang Fu, the Organ Systems of Traditional Chinese Medicine* (Ross 1985) and *The Practice of Chinese Medicine* (Maciocia 1994).

Large Intestine (Dachang)

- removes food and drink from the Small Intestine
- reabsorbs a proportion of the fluids and excretes the stools

---

Digestive function This does not vary from what is understood in Western medicine. Many of the normal functions of the Large Intestine are also ascribed to the Spleen in Chinese medicine.

Fluid balance The Large Intestine is linked to the Lung interiorly and exteriorly via the meridians. Stagnation of food in the Large Intestine may give rise to a degree of breathlessness.

Small Intestine (Xiaochang)

- controls receiving and transforming
- separates fluids
- effect on dreams
- relationship with Heart

Controls receiving and transforming, separates fluids The Small Intestine receives food and drink from the Stomach, and separates the clean or reusable fraction from that which is dirty. The clean part is then transported by the Spleen to all parts of the body. The dirty part is transmitted to the Large Intestine for excretion as stools and to the Bladder to form the urine. Hence the Small Intestine has a direct functional relationship with the Bladder and it influences urinary function.

The Small Intestine thus plays a minor part in the Jin Ye or Body Water circulation.

Effect on dreams The effect on dreams is due to the connection with the Heart which has a much stronger effect.

Relationship with the Heart The traditional pairing with Heart is rather tenuous, and only evident when heat from fire in Xin Heart shifts downwards into Xiaochang or the Small Intestine and disturbs the lower Jiao. This relationship is only relevant in the psychological sense. The Small Intestine is said to have an influence on judgement, making the best choices, etc.

Gall Bladder (Gan)

- connected with the Liver, stores Bile
- psychological influence over dreams and decision making

Connection with the Liver The Gall Bladder receives Bile from the Liver, which it stores, ready to release when needed for digestion.

Psychological influence Besides controlling decision making, the Gall Bladder is said to give an individual courage and increase their drive and vitality.

Urinary Bladder (Pang Guang)

- secretes and stores urine
- close relationship with the Kidneys
- transformation of fluids

Secretion and storage of urine, close relationship with Kidneys Fluids already separated by the Small Intestine are passed on to the Bladder, which then transforms them into urine. The energy to do this is derived from the Kidney.

Transformation of fluids The Urinary Bladder is assisted in this transformation by the Lower Jiao or

Burner, which ensures that the water passages in this area are kept open for free circulation.

> *Triple Burner (San Jiao)*
> • control of the water circulation within the body

There is no place in a simple summary like this to go into the finer details of the Triple Burner. It is a uniquely Chinese concept and has been the subject of controversy for many years, hence the wide variation in names, such as Triple Burner, Triple Heater, Triple Energiser, Three Heater, etc. It is easier to refer to it by the Chinese name, Sanjiao, since that sums up exactly what it is: "San" means "three" and "Jiao" means "spaces". The Three Jiaos are the Upper, the Middle and the Lower spaces.

Upper Jiao This is said to contain the Lungs and the Heart and is known as the "Chamber of Mist". It consists of the body cavity above the diaphragm.

Middle Jiao This contains the Spleen and Stomach. The region is therefore particularly concerned with the digestion and absorption of food. It is known as the "Chamber of Maceration" or, more graphically, of "ripening and rotting".

Lower Jiao Basically this area contains everything else, but the Kidney and Bladder are the most influential Zang Fu organs in this space and these give the region its name the "Drainage Ditch" and control the storage and excretion of water.

The Sanjiao taken as a single entity is concerned primarily with water circulation within the body and many words have been written on the subject. Since it is mostly conjectural, from a practical point of view, it is worth remembering that points on this meridian can be very influential in other regions of the body.

Acupuncture prescription

The selection of acupuncture points is both the easiest and most difficult aspect of the art. It is possible to get very good results from doing what purists would regard as very bad acupuncture. This leads to most of the controversy over training programmes. It is undeniable that physiotherapists have a head start over many of their medical colleagues in that their knowledge of anatomy is both detailed and generally in daily use and it is relatively easy to superimpose the maps of acupuncture points over what is known. A basic selection of points is straightforward and requires no great skill other than a safe needling technique. Greater knowledge and skill are required to select the relevant supporting points and visualize and treat the likely imbalances.

If treating musculoskeletal pain, as a physiotherapist often is, then selection is quite simple. The first choice will be local points on channels that pass over or near the painful point or area. Then distal points should be included; these points lie at the ends of those channels already involved. Each channel has a distal point that is commonly employed; for example, that of the Small Intestine channel is Houxi SI-3.

In addition to this basic selection the Ah Shi points should be used. These are those points in the area that elicit a sharp response or "ouch" from the patient when they are palpated. These points are rarely on channels and may vary from treatment to treatment, appearing and vanishing at random. (They are not quite the same as trigger points.)

Points are further selected according to specific symptoms. TCM defines these points and ascribes specific actions to them. The indications for the use of such points can often be confusing, and also contradictory, one point being recommended for both diarrhoea and constipation. This is because the prescription depends upon the perceived state of the internal balance and the system takes the necessary stimulus from the needling. This is problematic for the Western practitioner who takes refuge in the belief that a different kind of needling will produce a different result. This may actually be so but the scientific proof is not yet available.

Combinations of points are often indicated, the sum often being greater than the parts. A well-used combination is that of Hegu LI-4, and Quchi LI-11, for lowering blood pressure. Used individually the points do not appear to have this action but it can easily be demonstrated when they are used in combination.

Back Shu and Front Mu points are used in diagnosis as they are said to be tender when there is an imbalance in the corresponding organ or channel. The Back Shu points are particularly useful when used to tonify a system or Zang Fu organ. A link between the Back Shu point and the organ or meridian has yet to be demonstrated conclusively but some interesting work was done by Kenyon et al (1992).

The use of Antique or Transport points is a fascinating elaboration on TCM theory. These points are all situated around or below the knee and elbow joints, and were frequently used in early forms of treatment, particularly for women because strangers, even doctors, were not supposed to see the female body unclothed. A forearm or lower leg could easily be examined and treated with a curtain discreetly drawn over the rest of the body. These points are defined in terms of Qi or energy flow, with those at the tips of the digits being referred to as the Jing Well points, progressing to Ying Spring, Shu Stream, Jing River and, finally, He Sea at the knee or elbow where the total Qi within the channel could be accessed and influenced. These points are still very frequently used in painful musculoskeletal problems where the stagnation or blockage of the flow of Qi gives rise to the pain. The Spring or Well points are most often used in acute problems, while those further up, particularly the He Sea points, have an influence on the whole system and can be used in the treatment of chronic or systemic problems.

Tonification or "Mother" points and Sedation or "Son" points are designated according to Five Element theory and many Chinese publications give tables showing these and will further explain their use for the interested student.

Accumulation or Cleft points are used when a reservoir of Qi is required to treat a problem in the channel or linked organ; the Energy is thought to accumulate at these points and be available for release.

Luo or linking points connect one or more channels and are thought to have an extended influence because of this.

Influential points are a group of eight points said to have a particular influence, as in Table 1.5. They are frequently included in prescriptions.

All acupuncture practitioners have their favourite

Table 1.5 *The eight influential points*

Tissue	Influential point
Zang organs	Zhangmen LIV-13
Fu organs	Zhongwan CV-12
Respiratory Qi	Shanzhong CV-17
Blood	Geshu B-17
Tendon	Yanglingquan GB-34
Pulse, vessels	Taiyuan LU-9
Bone	Dashu B-11
Marrow	Xuanzhong GB-39

points but those in the rhyme below have been considered to be very important since the Ming Dynasty.

Four Dominant points (Ming Dynasty rhyme)

■ *The Stomach and Abdomen belong to Zusanli the back is Weizhong's territory For the head and neck, Lieque should be sought after and for the face and mouth to Hegu refer.*

Pulse diagnosis

This method is still used quite widely in China where it is carefully taught. Western practitioners have more difficulty in believing that the state of balance between the Zang Fu organs can be read from the pulses at the wrist, but some training schools teach and practise it very well. It is a difficult art and needs many years of practice before the variously described types of pulse can be distinguished. Where used skilfully it provides another good hook to hang a TCM diagnosis on.

Five Element theory

This theory will not be dealt with in detail in this text. Some acupuncture practitioners use it a great deal, believing that it enriches their understanding of the symptoms and syndromes in diagnosis, while others manage without ever referring to it. It tends not to be generally used in China these days. Stated

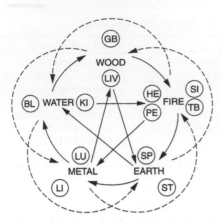

Fig. 1.1 *The Five Phases, or Elements, are Wood, Fire, Earth, Metal and Water. These are intimately interlinked in such a way that they stimulate but also inhibit or control, each being controlled by another, while itself simultaneously controlling a third Element.*

simply, the Five Elements are Water, Earth, Fire, Metal and Wood. These do not exist independently of one another but in a cyclic relationship (Fig. 1.1). When the circular diagram is considered it can be seen that the arrows linking one Element to another form a complex network of influences. They are believed to influence all the body processes.

The application of the Five Element theory in TCM is in classifying into different categories not only the tissues and organs of the body, but also human emotions and natural phenomena external to the body, seasons, climatic conditions, etc. It can be appreciated that this will give a highly complex and subtle form of diagnosis, but is also obvious that randomized, controlled clinical trials are not going to be very successful in proving that it works. Some acupuncture practitioners are quite happy to accept the thousands of years of empirical evidence and base their treatment rationale on these theories, but rather more are accepting them merely as an interesting stage in the history of acupuncture practice.

Tongue diagnosis

In TCM the tongue can be used as an integral part of diagnosis. Considerable information can be obtained about the balance between the Zang Fu organs but it is relevant mainly to the differentiation of chronic or long-standing syndromes. When treating pain, the practitioner will not need to know tongue diagnosis in great detail but the additional information obtained can be useful on the occasions when a quick response is not obtained and the therapist wishes to look deeper.

The tongue is considered as two areas: the tongue proper, or body, and the tongue coating. A normal tongue has a pink body and there is a white, clear coating over the surface. Chronic changes may be seen in the tongue body while acute problems may manifest in the coating; however, any very recent situation change or acute painful problem is unlikely to be evident. Changes in the colour or texture of the tongue coating can indicate invasion by the External pathogens, like Cold or Damp. Changes that are chronic or have progressed deeper within the body lead to more extreme changes in the normal colouring together with those in the shape or colour of the tongue body.

The most common and easily read sign is that of a tooth-marked tongue. Broadly speaking if the tongue is swollen there is Deficiency within the Spleen and if of normal dimensions the Deficiency lies within the Kidney. This is the most common state to be seen among a normal outpatient clientele and occurs frequently in long-standing cases of osteoarthritis. If the reader wishes to become acquainted with tongue diagnosis in detail the definitive work is: Tongue diagnosis in Chinese medicine (Maciocia 1987).

Summary

TCM is an exciting paradox to a medical worker. The ancient writings make statements that our intellects forbid us to believe, yet centuries of empirical evidence are there to support their success. It is evident as more and more research is undertaken that the technique of acupuncture has great value. We are beginning to understand some of the changes that it promotes within the body and physiological research is constantly producing new evidence.

It may be that we shall have to reclassify diseases. Loo (1985) suggests the following: "medical science must recognise at least three kinds of illnesses: physical (treatable by Western medicine), mental (treatable by psychologists or psychiatrists), and physiological (treatable by acupuncture)".

While we cannot accept the old explanations at face value, understanding the logical framework for them does help in the selection of effective points. Until we have a clear, scientific explanation for all these reported actions, we should accept some of this fascinating old logic and let it guide our practice meanwhile.

References

Baldry P 1989 Acupuncture trigger points and musculoskeletal pain, 2nd edn. Churchill Livingstone, Edinburgh

Jessel Kenyon J, Cheng Ni, Blott B, Hopwood V 1992 Studies with acupuncture using a SQUID bio-magnetometer: a preliminary report. Complementary Medical Research 6(3): 142–151

Loo C W 1985 Comparison of Western and Eastern medicine: the important role of acupuncture. American Journal of Acupuncture 13(2): 105–135

Maciocia G 1987 Tongue diagnosis in Chinese medicine. Churchill Livingstone, Edinburgh

Maciocia G 1994 The practice of Chinese medicine. Churchill Livingstone, Edinburgh

Moroz A 1994 East–West medicine: irreconcilably complementary. American Journal of Acupuncture 22(4): 369–374

Ross J 1985 Zang Fu, the organ systems of Traditional Chinese Medicine, 2nd edn. Churchill Livingstone, Edinburgh

2

Physiological mechanisms in acupuncture

Sven Andersson

Introduction

Acupuncture is one of many treatment modalities that are included in Traditional Chinese Medicine (TCM). It is based on empirical findings and intuition; specific diagnoses based on pathology of individual organs are not used. The theoretical basis of TCM is difficult to accept from the viewpoint of biological medicine. In the Western scientific community, acupuncture is often looked upon with scepticism or even considered as quackery and rejected by the Western medical profession. An important reason for this scepticism is the limitation or lack of scientific documentation to prove or disprove the therapeutic effects that are claimed by the supporters of acupuncture. A review of the acupuncture literature shows a large number of publications, but their quality is often poor.

During recent decades, acupuncture has become increasingly popular and partly accepted in many Western countries, mainly as a pain-relieving method. Several factors have contributed to this popularity, such as the many reports of relief of acute and chronic pain following acupuncture, understanding of some mechanisms of action and the interest in Far Eastern cultures with their mysticism. The treatment is also without serious side-effects and is inexpensive. Most important for its partial acceptance in the medical profession has been the accumulating results of the application of scientific methods in the evaluation of its effects. This started in 1950s in China with studies of the analgesia during surgery. Reports about surgery under acupuncture analgesia reached the Western

world in the late 1960s. Visitors to China, both scientists and laymen, observed major surgical interventions during acupuncture analgesia but were unable to believe that the analgetic effect was due solely to acupuncture. Speculations such as analgesic effects due to hypnosis, indoctrination, ethnic background or secretly given analgesic drugs were given as explanations. This scepticism is understandable owing to the limited knowledge of endogenous pain inhibitory systems at that time. Pain alleviation with psychological methods such as hypnosis was, however, well documented, as were the effects of opiates; consequently, it was believed that such methods were used in secret to obtain the analgesic effect.

The description of spinal gate mechanisms by Melzack & Wall (1965) showed that somatic stimulation could induce pain inhibition. Another cornerstone in the understanding of acupuncture analgesia was the discovery of opioid receptors and the endogenous opioids (Terenius 1984). Release of endorphins to the cerebrospinal fluid during acupuncture and its analgesic effects explained the Chinese finding that acupuncture releases a pain-inhibiting substance that is present in the cerebrospinal fluid. If cerebrospinal fluid from one rabbit that had received acupuncture was transferred to another non-treated rabbit the recipient animal showed a similar change in pain sensitivity to that in the acupunctured animal.

It is now well established that acupuncture is a valuable therapeutic modality in the treatment of pain. The mechanisms of pain relief can be described and partly explained in scientific terms, which has allowed acupuncture to be integrated with conventional medicine as a pain-relieving method. Although the philosophy of TCM with regard to its energetic diagnosis belongs to the history of medicine, other aspects resting on empirical findings may be important in the further development and clinical praxis of acupuncture. One example is the existence of anatomically defined acupoints; at least some of these are located close to nerves or in regions with dense innervation, which facilitates generation of nerve impulses in response to mechanical or electrical stimulation producing a subjective sensation (called in Chinese Deqi). This sensation is undoubtedly evoked by activity in thin myelinated and possibly unmyelinated afferent nerve fibres (see Receptors below). It should be noted, however, that needle sensation is found in many locations other than the traditional acupoints; thus, the specificity of the acupoints should be questioned. Interestingly, many of the traditionally selected points used in the treatment of a certain condition are located in somatic tissue innervated from the same spinal segments as the visceral organ assumed to cause the disease. In subsequent research of acupuncture effects it is important to investigate to what extent the empirically selected points have specific effects.

The meridians (channels) have no morphological counterpart in the peripheral structures but they may have a functional basis in referred and projected sensations that are elicited by stimulation of afferent nerve fibres. The concept of channels may still be useful as anatomical coordinates. The nomenclature with meridian numbers is commonly used and internationally accepted. The identification of an anatomical location by its meridian number simplifies the comparison between and the evaluation of studies in which acupuncture has been used. The paradigm of acupuncture according to TCM explains the totality of diseases, their cause and treatment. This explanation is in strong conflict with the concepts of modern biological medicine. The studies of mechanisms in the modern medicine have focused on single mechanisms such as the chemical transmitters involved or the neuronal circuits in the spinal cord but a paradigm that would explain the energetic mechanism has not been proposed. If different aspects of acupuncture could be understood as parts of a general principle both understanding of

the effects and the research should be greatly facilitated.

Recent studies have shown that acupuncture and some other forms of sensory stimulation elicit effects similar in humans and other mammals. This suggests that the generated afferent nerve impulses activate mechanisms of fundamental importance in daily life, such as the control of the cardiovascular and respiratory systems, the neuroimmunological axis and the pain inhibitory systems. These systems need modification of their activity level in stress situations and are involved in homeostasis of individual cells, individual organs and organ systems as well as the body as a whole. In this chapter a hypothesis will be presented and discussed that acupuncture in some situations produces similar effects on certain organ functions to those occurring during long-lasting muscle exercise, such as jogging. Common to exercise and acupuncture, particularly electroacupuncture at low stimulation frequency, are muscle contractions that give rhythmic discharges in nerve fibres. A number of functions are modified similarly in both conditions and with a similar time course. In other respects there are clear differences, such as in metabolic changes and central commands.

Biological background to acupuncture effects

In recent years a large number of publications have appeared dealing with the effects of acupuncture. The underlying mechanisms (e.g. pain relief) are often described and discussed in relation to TCM. Surprisingly, no penetrating discussions have dealt with the physiological background. The paradigm of TCM with balancing of energy may in its way explain any disease or disturbance but it is philosophical rather than biological. The knowledge of biological phenomena was for a long period insufficient to allow an understanding of the endogenous systems that could transform sensory inputs to modification of functions. The scientific understanding of disease processes has since broadened but this has not illuminated the ideas of TCM; instead it provided the possibility of explaining the effects of needle manipulation in Western biological terms. Still, few if any attempts have been made to explain the totality of acupuncture. It should be recognized that any effect of acupuncture must rest on physiological or psychological mechanisms, or both, that have biological significance during evolution. Needle manipulation or the stimulation of cutaneous or subcutaneous tissue should have its effect through artificial activation of systems that have biological effects in functional situations giving similar sensory input.

The use of acupuncture as a pain-relieving method is based on a large number of clinical trials, and no doubt acupuncture has a powerful and sustained effect in the treatment of musculoskeletal pain. The method has also been accepted for pain relief in most countries and is commonly used in general practice and pain clinics as a complement to conventional treatment. Acceptance of the pain relief effect of acupuncture was facilitated by the discovery of endogenous opioids. This gave a logical explanation in Western terms to the effect on the pain sensitivity. In addition to relieving pain, acupuncture is commonly used in TCM to treat a variety of diseases. In recent years this has evoked increasing interest in Western countries, but nevertheless conventional medicine rejects the energetic principle and the metaphysical language of TCM. Still, basic scientific and clinical studies have given evidence that acupuncture may have physiological and therapeutic effects. In fact, acupuncture may have effects related to functional modulation of many different functions. A full understanding of such effects requires a considerable amount of further research. In order to encourage such work it seems important that acupuncture is redefined according to its possible physiological background.

Receptors

In acupuncture many different mechanisms may be involved and similar results may be achieved with other types of mechanical, electrical and thermal stimulation such as transcutaneous electrical nerve stimulation (TENS) massage and physical exercise. The stimuli excite receptors or nerve fibres in the stimulated tissue. According to TCM the needle stimulation should give rise to a specific needle sensation, Deqi or 'attaining the Qi', which is experienced as numbness, heaviness and radiating paraesthesia, a sensation close to deep muscle pain when muscle points are stimulated. The sensation is a sign of activation of thin myelinated nerve fibres, presumably A-delta and possibly also C fibres. Low frequency electrical stimulation of sufficient intensity gives muscle contractions that activate mechanoreceptors with low and high thresholds in muscles and other tissues. Particular significance has been given to a group of receptors in the skeletal muscles that have a high threshold for mechanical stimulation and are innervated by A-delta fibres and possibly C fibres. These receptors are physiologically activated by strong muscle contractions (Kaufman et al 1983, 1984, Kniffki, Mense & Schmidt 1981) and have been denoted ergoreceptors. Functionally these receptors will be excited during muscle contractions. It can be argued that acupuncture, particularly electroacupuncture, and physical exercise with repetitive muscle contractions similarly activate these receptors and afferent nerve fibres. Functional modulation as well as therapeutic effects that have been attributed to acupuncture can also be noted during muscle exercise. Examples of these include decreased pain sensitivity, changes in mood, and changes in blood flow and blood pressure in experimental animals with high blood pressure and in patients with essential hypertension.

Endorphins

Both acupuncture and muscle exercise release endogenous opioids that seem to be essential in the induction of functional changes of different organ systems. Endorphins exert effects by binding to opioid receptors and several types of endogenous opioids have been identified and found to have different affinities to different opioid receptors. Particular interest has been given to β-endorphin. This substance has a high affinity to the μ-receptor and is important in pain control as well as in regulation of blood pressure and body temperature (Basbaum and Fields 1984, Ganten et al 1981, Holaday 1983). It is released via two different systems (Fig. 2.1). One system includes the

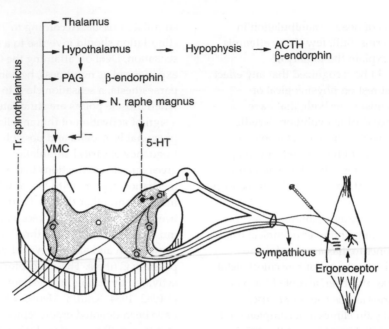

Fig. 2.1 *Schematic outline of some possible physiological principles in the modulation of pain sensitivity and autonomic functions. Stretch receptors (ergoreceptors) in muscles are functionally excited by muscle contraction. The receptors or their afferents (A-delta fibres) may be excited also by electrical or manual needle stimulation in muscle points. The afferents induce different central actions: excitation of the vasomotor centre, release of endogenous opioids via hypothalamic–brainstem pathways and release of β-endorphin and ACTH into the blood from the pituitary. The principle includes both negative and positive feedback; consequently the effects may differ according to the prevailing functional state, with the ultimate goal of preserving homeostasis in different organ systems. (ACTH = adrenocorticotrophic hormone; PAG = periaqueductal gray; VMC = vasomotor centre.) (After Thorén et al 1990. Endorphins and Exercise: Physiological Mechanisms and Clinical Implications. Medicine and Science in Sports and Exercise 22: 417–428. With permission from Williams and Wilkins.)*

hypothalamus and a neuronal network that projects to midbrain and brainstem nuclei; via this route it may influence pain sensitivity as well as autonomic functions (Akil et al 1984, Bloom 1983, Cuello 1983, Smyth 1983). There is evidence that hypothalamic nuclei, particularly the nucleus arcuatus, have a central role in mediating effects of acupuncture. Lesions in this nucleus eliminate the analgesic effects of low frequency but not high frequency electroacupuncture (Wang, Mao & Han 1990). Low frequency electrical stimulation of the deep peroneal nerve induces circulatory changes – effects that are eliminated after hypothalamic lesions.

An increase in the β-endorphin level has been observed in brain tissue of animals after acupuncture and muscle exercise. This substance is probably released at nerve terminals in a β-endorphinergic system projecting from the hypothalamus to the periaqueductal gray (PAG) in the brain stem. In addition to pain relief the increased production of endorphins may give the sensation of joy associated with jogging behaviour. Present data suggest that the pain control systems become more active in long-lasting muscle exercise. The relation between muscle activity and decreased pain sensitivity may partly explain the finding that immobilized and inactive patients suffer more from pain than active patients. In painful conditions it is important to keep the patient mentally and physically active; rehabilitation of pain patients should include a muscle training programme.

Although the details are still unknown, experimental and clinical evidence suggest that acupuncture can also reset the sympathetic system via mechanisms at hypothalamic and brainstem levels. Figure 2.1 suggests that the hypothalamic β-endorphinergic system has inhibitory effects on the vasomotor centre (VMC). This effect elicits a decreased sympathetic tone with vasodilatation and a decreased drive on the heart following the initial excitation of VMC during exercise or nerve stimulation.

Via another system, β-endorphin is released to the blood. Pro-opiomelanocortin in the hypophysis produces equimolar amounts of β-endorphin and adrenocorticotrophic hormone (ACTH) (Crine, Gianoulakis & Seidah 1978) following muscle exercise and, most likely, also after acupuncture. These substances reach different target organs. The two β-endorphinergic systems probably operate independently but both can be stimulated by afferent nerve activity. It has been shown that stress also may give increased levels of β-endorphin and ACTH in the blood (Guillemin et al 1977) independently of the increase of β-endorphin in the brain (Rossier et al 1977). Since the blood–brain barrier is relatively impermeable to circulating peptides the β-endorphin level in the plasma may not have any relevance to the opioid receptors in the brain.

The central effects of endorphins are of importance to understand the effect of acupuncture and muscle exercise; in both situations endorphins are released and they may induce similar changes. This has also been suggested by administration of an agonist to β-endorphin (morphine) or an antagonist (naloxone). As examples can be mentioned the finding that administration of opiates in certain conditions can induce bradycardia and decrease blood pressure via change in the balance between the parasympathetic and the sympathetic systems (Holaday 1983). Sympathetic reflexes induced by pressure or depressor stimuli can be diminished by morphine and potentiated by naloxone (Montrastruc, Montrastruc & Marales-Olivas 1981, Petty and Reid 1981). The cardiovascular system in normal subjects (animals or human) does not change significantly after administration of opioid receptor agonists or antagonists; the effect is evident only when the normal homeostasis is disturbed, for example at blood pressures outside the normal range (Rubin 1984, Yao, Andersson & Thorén 1982). Only small changes in blood pressure or heart rate have been observed with administration of large amounts of naloxone in normotensive animals but the substance can increase blood pressure in hypotension, an effect which is probably mediated via opioid receptors

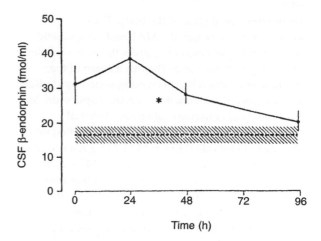

Fig. 2.2 *Time course of CSF immunoreactive β-endorphin elevation after voluntary exercise for 5–6 weeks. Note that the level is still increased 24 and 48 h after termination of exercise. (*P < 0.05.) (From Hoffmann, Terenius & Thorén 1990 with kind permission from Elsevier Science – NL, Sara Burgerhartstraat 25, 1055 KV Amsterdam, The Netherlands)*

(Blake, Stein & Vomachka 1984). Long-lasting but not short-lasting (Metzger and Stein 1984) muscle exercise increases the level of β-endorphin in the brain and cerebrospinal fluid (CSF) for several days after the termination of exercise in rats (Hoffmann, Terenius & Thorén 1990) (Fig. 2.2).

Cardiovascular and nervous system effects

In clinical practice acupuncture is used to treat low blood pressure or circulatory shock. The pressor effect of acupuncture in the hypotensive state has been confirmed in several laboratories. In one study, conscious rats in haemorrhagic shock with a mean arterial pressure (MAP) at 60% of control level before haemorrhage were given acupuncture-like stimulation of the sciatic nerve. The MAP increased to 80% of the control level and was accompanied by a marked increase of sympathetic activity. The pressor effect in hypotensive animals was not antagonized by naloxone but was significantly diminished by intravenous injection of scopolamine, suggesting that the effect is mediated by a cholinergic mechanism (Sun, Yu & Yao 1983).

Experimental and clinical observations indicate that acupuncture and acupuncture-like somatic stimulation exert bidirectional effects on the cardiovascular and sympathetic systems depending on the functional state of the body. Thus, acupuncture decreases the MAP and sympathetic activity in hypertension but gives the opposite effects in the hypotensive state. The mechanism of the regulatory function has been enlightened by studies of the baroreceptor function. Electroacupuncture to the hindleg of conscious rabbits or electrical stimulation of the deep peroneal nerve elicited no change in heart rate (HR) or MAP but gave rise to a significant increase in the slope of the MAP-HR regression line, indicating an increased baroreceptor reflex sensitivity (Wang & Yao 1986). These findings indicate that acupuncture and acupuncture-like somatic stimulation can modulate or reset the function of the baroreceptor reflex. The characteristics of this resetting indicate that the gain of the reflex is increased. In functional terms this means that the ability of the baroreceptor reflex to maintain cardiovascular homeostasis is increased.

It should be realized that changes occurring in the body during muscle exercise are very complex. In addition to changes due to the release of endorphin there is interaction, for example, between central commands and impulses from peripheral receptors, release of other neurotransmitters and hormonal and metabolic changes.

In order to study the effect of afferent nerve impulses on the cardiovascular system, normotensive and spontaneously hypertensive rats (SHR) have been studied in various situations. In awake rats electrical stimulation of the sciatic nerve at an intensity that activates A-delta fibres gives a naloxone-reversible increase of the pain threshold and the threshold elevation remains about 60 min after discontinuation of the stimulation (Hoffmann et al 1990b). Yao, Andersson & Thorén et al (1982a, b) observed that sciatic nerve stimulation at low frequency (2 Hz) induced a poststimulatory and long-lasting (> 10 h) decrease in blood pressure in parallel with the pain threshold increase. Such stimulation in normotensive rats similarly decreased the pain sensitivity but gave only a small decrease in blood pressure (Fig. 2.3). In another type of experiments, stimulation of the sciatic nerve was replaced by direct electrical stimulation of the gastrocnemius muscle. Muscle contractions were induced at a low frequency (3 Hz) and with sufficient intensity to excite A-delta fibres. This

resulted in a similar and even more long-lasting poststimulatory blood pressure decrease. The pain threshold increased similarly following direct muscle stimulation as with sciatic nerve stimulation and the effect was more long lasting. The involvement of endogenous opioids was suggested by the reversal of both pain threshold increase and blood pressure effects after administration of naloxone; the pain threshold increase was reversed by small doses (1 mg/kg), while a large amount (10 mg/kg) was

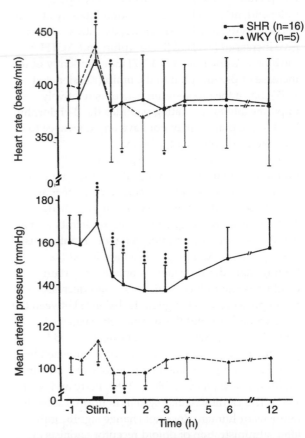

Fig. 2.3 *Blood pressure and heart rate changes induced by electrical stimulation (20 min) of the sciatic nerve in spontaneously hypertensive rats (SHR) and normotensive rats (WKY). The increases in blood pressure and heart rate during stimulation were followed by a long-lasting decrease of blood pressure in SHR but only a small and short-lasting decrease in WKY. Note that the heart rate did not increase during the period of decreased blood pressure. (*P < 0.05, ** P < 0.01, *** P < 0.001.) (From Yao et al 1982 with kind permission from Elsevier Science – NL, Sara Burgerhartstraat 25, 1055 KV Amsterdam, The Netherlands)*

required to reverse the blood pressure effects. The experiments with direct muscle stimulation suggest that muscle afferents contribute significantly both to the autonomic and to the analgesic effects of peripheral afferent stimulation. Furthermore, the reversibility by naloxone suggests that endorphinergic mechanisms are involved.

The sympathetic effects of muscle exercise as well as afferent nerve stimulation can be separated into two phases: excitation and depression. In the first phase there is excitation with increased heart rate, increased cardiac output and regional vasoconstriction together with increased blood pressure. These changes result in a more effective perfusion of the muscles. On the other hand, the blood flow in visceral organs and in the skin may decrease. These actions are adequate to give optimal adaptation to heavy load on the muscles. Provided that the stimulation continues for a sufficient period of time (e.g. due to long-lasting muscle exercise or artificial afferent nerve stimulation) endogenous opioids are released, which produces central inhibition of the autonomic outflow (Reid and Rubin

1987). This sympathetic inhibition is not evident during the ongoing activation owing to excitatory input via certain afferent somatic fibres (flexion reflex afferents) and metabolic effects on chemoreceptors (Rowell 1986). The inhibition via opioid mechanisms appears after termination of exercise or stimulation.

Poststimulatory sympathetic inhibition has been demonstrated in both animals and humans. An example is shown in Figure 2.4 with recordings from visceral sympathetic fibres in spontaneously hypertensive rats. Initially the blood pressure and sympathetic activity increase. After a period of stimulation of the sciatic nerve at low frequency (2 Hz) the blood pressure decrease correlates to a marked decrease in the sympathetic activity. The sympathetic inhibition reaches a maximum after some hours and has a total duration of more than 12 hours. Indirect evidence of the decreased sympathetic activity is the unchanged heart rate during the period of decreased blood pressure (Fig. 2.3). Part of the effect of the acupuncture on circulation may be related to changed sensitivity of the baroreceptors.

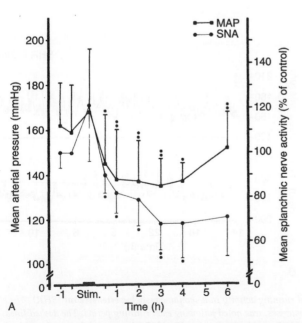

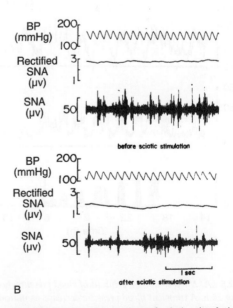

Fig. 2.4 *(A) Changes in mean arterial pressure (MAP) and splanchnic nerve activity (SNA) induced by prolonged sciatic stimulation in five spontaneously hypertensive rats. (B) Recording of splanchnic nerve discharge before and after the sciatic stimulation. (From Yao et al 1982 with kind permission from Elsevier Science – NL, Sara Burgerhartstraat 25, 1055 KV Amsterdam, The Netherlands)*

Moriyama (1987) used a microneurographic technique in humans to analyse the sympathetic activity in the nerve to soleus muscle. During prolonged acupuncture, the sympathetic activity increased initially; in the poststimulatory period the sympathetic activity decreased and recovered only gradually. The sympathetic inhibition could be elicited in several acupuncture points, suggesting that acupuncture elicits a general sympathetic poststimulatory inhibition. Similar results have been reported by Cao, Xu & Lu (1983). They used a finger plethysmographic technique and changes in skin temperature and resistance to investigate correlations between the analgesic effect of acupuncture and changes in galvanic skin response, skin temperature and blood flow. They found a high correlation between increased temperature in the palm of the hand, blood flow and analgesia. The galvanic skin response elicited in the skin by sound or light stimuli decreased markedly following acupuncture. However, this change did not correlate with the degree of acupuncture analgesia.

Hypothetically, acupuncture activates the same types of afferent nerve fibres as do muscle contractions during exercise. Consequently it is of interest to compare effects after muscle exercise and acupuncture in humans. A characteristic feature of both muscle exercise and acupuncture (electrical nerve stimulation at 2 Hz) is increased blood pressure during the initial phase but a decreasing blood pressure with prolonged exercise and particularly after it has finished (Bennett, Wilcox & Mcdonald 1984). As with nerve stimulation, long-lasting regular exercise can give a sustained blood pressure decrease (Jennings et al 1984, Nelson et al 1986). This decrease is more pronounced in hypertensive than in normotensive patients (Bennett, Wilcox & Mcdonald 1984). The decrease is usually short lasting but may last for several hours after a period of muscle exercise (Fitzgerald 1981, Gaal & Freebairn 1979). Physical activity is reported to lower blood pressure in humans with borderline hypertension. Running for 45 min decreased the systolic blood pressure in seven out of nine persons with a mean blood pressure of 13 mmHg (Floras et al 1989). Microneurographic recording from sympathetic fibres in the peroneal nerve 1 h after the exercise showed decreased activity in all patients with decreased blood pressure. In a control situation without muscle exercise no change in either

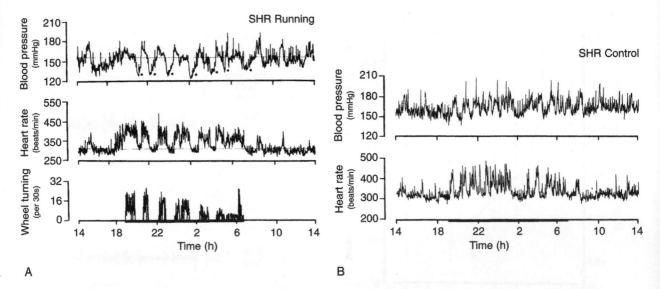

A   B

Fig. 2.5 *(A) Microcomputer printout of blood pressure, heart rate and running activity in a spontaneously hypertensive rat (SHR) during 24 h. A transient blood pressure decrease, as indicated by the asterisks, was noted following each running period. The dashed lines represents the mean reference values (mean arterial pressure, MAP = 155.7 mmHg, heart rate, HR = 317.2 beats/min) during the period 7 a.m. to 7 p.m. in this SHR. The black bar in the time scale indicates the dark period, the night. (B) Similar recordings as in (A) from a hypertensive rat without access to wheel for running.*

sympathetic activity or blood pressure was observed. Administration of nitroprusside giving a similar decrease of the systolic blood pressure increased the sympathetic activity.

Similar observations have been made in the rat. In normotensive and spontaneously hypertensive rats the blood pressure was studied during running in wheels (Fig. 2.5A). The rats used the wheels during the night and after a few weeks the mean running distance per night was equivalent to about 5 km. Typically the rats were running in periods separated by periods of rest. During the resting periods the mean arterial blood pressure decreased markedly (30–40 mmHg) compared with the average mean arterial blood pressure. The blood pressure increased immediately the animals started to run again. SHR without access to wheels showed non-systematic activity during the night and the blood pressure varied with the type of activity but without periods of sustained depression (Fig. 2.5B). Normotensive rats similarly running in the wheel showed no fall in blood pressure during periods of rest.

It would be expected that the marked blood pressure fall in SHR during rest periods should give an increased heart rate but in fact this did not occur. The heart rate does not increase during the blood pressure fall after electrical stimulation of the sciatic nerve or after exercise activity, suggesting a lack of a compensatory increase in sympathetic activity.

Summary and conclusions

Experimental and clinical studies suggest that activity in somatic nerve fibres has a significant effect on, for instance, pain sensitivity and autonomic functions. Hypothetically, the effect has its physiological counterpart in physical exercise and the effect can be reproduced artificially via various types of electrical or mechanical stimulation of certain receptors and nerve fibres. According to Chinese tradition little or no effect of acupuncture should be seen on normal functions; acupuncture has effect only in dysfunction of the "balancing mechanism". The described findings with regard to the cardiovascular system support the idea that acupuncture is most effective when the function is disturbed. When the organism enters a stressful situation, homeostatic modifying mechanisms are

activated in order to maintain optimal function. Physical exercise or artificial activation are such situations; the effects are related to the prevailing condition rather than to the sites of stimulation.

Mechanisms in pain relief by acupuncture

The modulation of biological systems induced by somatic sensory stimulation has been analysed mainly in relation to the analgesic effect. These studies have produced evidence suggesting that changes of pain sensitivity occur in parallel with effects on other systems such as the cardiovascular system. The following section centres on some of the mechanisms that explain at least some of acupuncture is modulatory effects on pain.

Dorsal horn mechanisms

In the entry zone of the spinal cord A-delta and C fibres branch and pass caudally and rostrally over one segment or several forming the tract of Lissauer. Eventually, the fibres terminate in the upper part of the dorsal horn in the substantia gelatinosa (lamina I and II) where cells excited by nociceptive stimuli have been identified. One such group of cells has small receptive fields and responds only to noxious stimuli (nociceptive specific cells, or NS cells). The nociceptive input also reaches other cells in superficial and deeper layers in the dorsal horn. One group of cells receives input from both low threshold and nociceptive afferents and is called multiconvergent or wide dynamic range (WDR) cells. These may be activated by noxious stimuli in a large peripheral area and by, for example, tactile stimuli in part of that area. The cells with multiconvergence seem to be found in conditions with disturbed inhibitory modulation, a condition associated with the appreciation of non-noxious stimuli as painful. Experiments on animals have shown that the receptive field may vary in size and the input modalities can change owing to the condition of the animal, indicating that the efficacy of synaptic transmission is influenced by inhibitory and excitatory input.

The region of termination of the A-delta and C fibres in the dorsal horn corresponds to the distribution of substance P, suggesting that this substance is a transmitter in the pain pathway; however, nociception is mediated also by other transmitters. In this area, opiate-binding sites have also been demonstrated. These binding sites are localized in short axon neurons that inhibit the transmission from the nociceptive afferents to the pain pathway as well as to local motor neurons and the sympathetic system. The inhibition is increased by acupuncture and by other methods exciting non-pain afferent fibres.

The opiate receptor-containing cells in the spinal cord can be activated pharmacologically by administration of morphine to the latter. The morphine diffuses from the CSF into the nervous structures and binds to the opiate receptors giving excitation to inhibitory cells or mimicking their inhibition on the nociceptive pathway. It is likely that, by this type of administration, morphine activates inhibitory cells that are physiologically important in the modulation of nociceptive input at the segmental level in response to stimulation of somatic afferents.

Segmental inhibition of the nociception is empirically well known and described as the gate control theory by Melzack & Wall (1965). Large diameter afferents from low threshold mechanoreceptors ascending in the dorsal column give off collaterals at the segmental level (Fig. 2.6). Terminals from these collaterals excite short axon opiate receptor-containing interneurons, which inhibit the transmission of impulses in nociceptive afferents and produce pain relief. The analgesic effect is strictly topographically arranged and effective pain relief can be obtained by stimulation of low threshold receptors, mainly within the area of pain. The effectiveness of this inhibition can be demonstrated by rubbing the skin or by massage of the painful area. The transmission through pain pathways and motor and sympathetic reflexes is counteracted by inhibitory interneurons that are excited by non-noxious afferent input. Consequently the balance between the inhibitory and excitatory inputs will determine the degree of activity in the pain pathway as well as in local reflexes.

Transcutaneous electrical nerve stimulation (TENS) and acupuncture interact with the segmental transmission from nociceptive efferents. It has been demonstrated that the best pain relief is related to acupuncture stimulation in the region of pain. There seem to be several mechanisms giving the local effect. TENS with high frequency may relieve chronic pain but does not increase the pain threshold. Possibly TENS gives a selective inhibition of the input from C fibres. Low frequency TENS and electroacupuncture give pain relief and also an

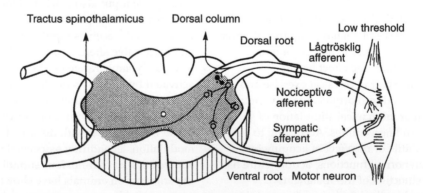

Fig. 2.6 *Schematic drawing of neuronal connections in the pain pathway at the segmental level. An inhibitory interneuron is indicated by the solid circles. The nociceptive afferents excite interneurons with connections to the spinothalamic pain pathway, to motor neurons and to sympathetic neurons. Collaterals of low threshold afferent fibres ascending in the dorsal column excite inhibitory interneurons. Sustained activity from nociceptors may give rise to positive feedforward loops including tonic muscle contraction, sympathetic excitation and pain. On the other hand non-noxious input from the painful region inhibits pain and local nociceptive reflexes.*

increase in the pain threshold, suggesting that the input also from A-delta fibres is inhibited. Acupuncture given manually or as electrostimulation is considered effective when the needle sensation is induced. This suggests that in addition to the inhibitory connection from low threshold afferents as illustrated in Figure 2.6 there are other inhibitory segmental mechanisms related to thin afferent fibres.

It seems likely that different types of afferent fibres may influence the balance between excitation and inhibition in the dorsal horn. Skin afferents as well as certain afferents from joints, ligaments and connective tissue and also some muscle afferents are denoted flexion reflex afferents, since they easily excite the flexion reflex. This is a meaningful action and can be considered as part in the tissue-protecting mechanism of pain. Other afferents from superficial and deep structures have the opposite effect and inhibit the transmission in the pain pathway and the nociceptive reflexes. This dual effect must be taken into account in acupuncture treatment.

Descending inhibitory control

Interest has been given to investigation of systems in the brain controlling the transmission of nociceptive impulses. Experiments on rats showed that electrical stimulation in certain brainstem sites could elicit a complete analgesia without any change in the response to low threshold stimulation. Further experiments showed that several control systems descend from the brainstem to the spinal cord and control the transmission of nerve impulses from the nociceptive afferents to reflexes and ascending paths. Most interest has been focused on the endorphinergic system. Microinjection of morphine or electrical stimulation of the PAG in the midbrain suppresses behavioural nociceptive reactions in animals and gives a profound inhibition in the spinal cord of neuronal responses to noxious stimuli. Nerve fibres from the PAG descend to the nucleus raphe magnus (Fig. 2.1), which is one of the midline nuclei in the medulla oblongata. The cells in the nucleus raphe magnus send their axons via the dorsolateral funiculus of the spinal cord to the spinal segmental level. The fibres terminate in the substantia gelatinosa of the dorsal horn. One group of descending fibres is serotoninergic and seems to activate enkephalinergic interneurons in the spinal cord, inhibiting the transmission from the nociceptors. The endorphinergic nature of this descending system is demonstrated by the reversal of its effect by administration of naloxone. This drug may reverse the descending inhibition from PAG as well as acting directly on spinal interneurons. The link between serotoninergic descending fibres and endorphinergic interneurons suggests that serotonin reuptake inhibitors should potentiate the effect of acupuncture.

Morphine exerts parts of its action on opiate receptors in the brainstem. This effect can be demonstrated by local application of small amounts of the drug in the PAG. The effective pain relief obtained by intrathecal morphine injection shows that activation of spinal opiate receptors also plays an important role in morphine analgesia. Morphine analgesia is easily reversed by naloxone and it would be expected that acupuncture analgesia should also be influenced similarly by naloxone. Such effects have been reported; however, other studies have given divergent results. The analgesic effect of acupuncture in pain patients appears to be reversed by naloxone. Experiments on healthy volunteers show that acupuncture increases the pain threshold but naloxone gives only partial reversal. This finding suggests that there are several systems controlling the input to the pain pathways. Furthermore the control systems may differ between the healthy state and in pain.

Acupuncture and treatment of diseases

In TCM acupuncture has been used to treat many different symptoms and diseases. The method is used in many countries and is probably one of the most popular in the developing countries. Several conferences have dealt with indications for the use of acupuncture. In 1979 a WHO inter-regional seminar drew up a provisional list of diseases that lend themselves to acupuncture treatment. The list was based on clinical experience and not necessarily on controlled clinical research. Furthermore, the inclusion of specific diseases was not meant to indicate the extent of acupuncture efficacy in treating the listed conditions. The list contains a large number of diseases; in summary, the conditions can be divided into the following groups:

- pain
- dysfunction of autonomic nervous system
- infections and inflammation
- diseases of the peripheral and central nervous system.

A large number of clinical reports deal with effects of acupuncture in various diseases. Many of the publications are in Chinese and are sometimes available for Western readers as abstracts. Some general problems with the clinical reports on acupuncture effects are the small number of patients included, the absence of placebo-controlled studies and the large amount of variation in acupuncture technique. It is difficult to find reliable scientific proof of specific effect on any condition. The experimental evidence from animals and humans sometimes gives supporting evidence. In the following text some diseases are discussed on the basis of clinical reports as well as mechanisms that possibly can explain the effect. Further evidence of clinical effects is given elsewhere in this volume.

Cardiovascular conditions

The cardiovascular effects should be separated into generalized and local effects. Changes in sympathetic tone give general effects such as changes in blood pressure and heart rate. A decrease in blood pressure has been reported in acupuncture-treated patients with essential hypertension (Rutkowsky 1980, Smith 1992, Tam and Yiu 1975). In most patients the decrease in systolic and diastolic pressure is small (5–10 mmHg). The effect seems to be related to the cause of hypertension; blood pressure decrease has been observed in essential hypertension, and such an effect occurs also in an animal equivalent, SHR rats with high sympathetic activity. In these rats cardiovascular depression is observed after low frequency (2 Hz) nerve stimulation and exercise. Hypertension due to ligation of the renal artery is not, however, decreased by electrical stimulation of sciatic nerve (Hoffmann and Thorén 1986). The

importance of the involvement of the sympathetic system in the depressive effect of acupuncture is at least partly mediated via the pressure sensitivity of the carotid sinus baroreceptor reflex (Wang and Yao 1986). Acupuncture seems to modulate the receptor sensitivity via the sympathetic innervation.

The sympathetic inhibition results in vasodilatation in the skin with increased skin temperature. Kaada (1982, 1985) reported increased skin temperature and decreased pain in patients with Raynaud's disease as a result of transcutaneous electrical stimulation of the hands. The temperature increase was 7–10°C in the affected extremities but the changes were small in regions at normal temperature (0.5–2°C). Chronic ischaemia with ulceration of the legs was also affected by the low frequency hand stimulation and the ulcers healed after treatment in 3–9 weeks.

In several studies ischaemic heart diseases have been treated with transcutaneous nerve stimulation or acupuncture. Richter, Herliz & Hjalmarsson (1991) compared the effect of acupuncture and placebo in 21 patients with severe and stable angina pectoris. Acupuncture was given three times per week for 4 weeks. During this treatment the number of pain attacks decreased significantly compared with placebo, the working capacity increased and the pain at maximal load during ergometer bicycling decreased significantly ($P < 0.01$). At corresponding load the ST-segment* was reduced from 1.3 to 0.7 mm following acupuncture. The patients reported a significant increase in the quality of life. Similar results were obtained by Ballegaard et al (1986, Ballegaard 1990). They investigated groups of patients with stable angina pectoris and could also observe significant changes in working capacity, decreased number of anginal pain attacks and a decrease in ECG pathology. The consumption of nitroglycerine also decreased significantly. Mannheimer et al (1985, 1989) investigated the effect of TENS in patients with severe angina pectoris. Electrical stimulation (70 Hz) in skin areas of referred cardiac pain increased the tolerance for pacing, decreased the lactate metabolism and reduced the ST-segment decrease at maximal workload.

---

* The ST-segment represents the electrical potential between the deviations named S and T in the electrocardiogram.

The mechanisms of the reported effects on the heart are speculative. The central control of the sympathetic system seems to be important. In experiments on rabbits, cardiac ischaemia was induced by ligation of the left ventricle coronary artery over 10 min. The ECG recovery was compared with and without acupuncture. In the acupuncture group the recovery was significantly faster than in the control group as measured by the ECG recordings. After hypothalamic lesions (nucleus arcuatus) the faster recovery following acupuncture was eliminated and there was no significant difference in the recovery between the groups receiving acupuncture or not. Possibly the segmental reflex elicited by the nociceptive afferent activity in the ischaemic heart to the sympathetic output to the heart is modified. Needling in somatic tissue innervated from the same spinal segments as the heart (T1–4) may inhibit the sympathetic activity, as suggested from Figure 2.6. Descending systems from hypothalamic/brainstem levels may further modify the sympathetic output to the heart. It is interesting that at least some of the traditionally selected acupoints in treatment of heart diseases are usually localized in relevant spinal segments.

The reported results above should be interpreted with caution, as the contribution of unspecific effects (placebo) is generally not properly controlled. The pills used by Richter, Herliz & Hjalmarsson 1991 have much less placebo effects than needling. Ballegaard (1986, 1990) compared the effects of deep needling with superficially inserted needles. Both treatments gave a significant improvement compared with the situation before acupuncture, but there was no significant difference between the two treatments. The question is therefore open whether the effect is due to placebo or whether deep and superficial needling are both equally effective in the treatment of angina pectoris.

A significant improvement of the peripheral circulation can be achieved by electrical stimulation of nerves innervating an ischaemic area. This effect is most probably related to local mechanisms with release of vasodilating substances from peripheral terminals of afferent nerve fibres owing to antidromic activation. Possibly inhibition of the sympathetic system also plays a role. The increased circulation following stimulation of the nervous supply has been demonstrated in surgical flaps. In reconstructive surgery using tissue flaps ischaemia and necrosis easily ruin the result. In experimental studies on rats the effect of different modes of sensory stimulation was evaluated (Di Marzo, Tippins & Morris 1989, Jansen et al 1989, Kjartansson & Lundeberg 1990). The results suggest that sensory stimulation has effects similar to the increased blood flow obtained by injection of the neurotransmittors substance P (SP) or calcitonin gene-related peptide (CGRP) into the flaps. The results in animal experiments suggest that sensory stimulation in order to increase the blood flux in ischaemic tissue could be of clinical value in reconstructive surgery. This has been supported by a study using TENS to reverse ischaemia in patients undergoing reconstructive surgery for mammary carcinoma. In 12 out of 14 patients in the treatment group, repeated TENS restored capillary filling to normal and reduced oedema and stasis; only two out of 10 in the control group given placebo TENS for 7 days showed any improvement with capillary filling returning to normal.

Another long-standing ischaemic condition is ischaemic leg ulcers. These are a common complication in diabetes mellitus and some other diseases. Studies on the effect of sensory stimulation in ischaemic ulcers indicate that it may induce enhanced healing. In a controlled study of the effect of TENS in combination with standard treatment for healing of chronic diabetic ulcers the TENS group showed a significant improvement in ulcer area and healed ulcers compared with the control group after 12 weeks of treatment (Lundeberg, Eriksson & Malm 1992, Lundeberg 1993). The results of this study further indicate that electrical stimulation for 40 minutes a day is sufficient.

Asthma bronchiale

The effect of acupuncture on asthma bronchiale has been investigated in a large number of studies. Most authors report that acupuncture decreases the airway resistance significantly. The problem is, however, that many studies do not have adequate placebo controls and the number of patients included is small. According to the Chinese tradition acupuncture should be given repeatedly to asthmatic patients if the condition is to be improved. This has not been taken into account and in some studies only one or a few treatments have been given. Berger and Nolte (1977) used plethysmographic measurements in 12 patients. Acupuncture in thoracic points gave a significant decrease in the airway resistance compared with placebo in nine of the patients. The measurements were made 1 or 2 h after the treatment. Virsik et al (1980) studied 20 patients who received acupuncture in thoracic segments and placebo stimulation in the gluteal region. Compared with placebo, acupuncture gave significant increases in peak respiratory flow rate and vital capacity. In several studies the effect on pulmonary function was compared after acupuncture and inhalation of sympathomimetic or anticholinergic drugs. The drugs gave a more pronounced effect than acupuncture. When the drugs were given after acupuncture the respiration could be further improved, indicating that acupuncture did not fully counteract the bronchoconstriction. Tashkin et al (1977) compared acupuncture in thoracic points with placebo acupuncture in methacholine-induced asthma. In this condition also acupuncture gave significant improvement of the respiration compared with placebo, but isoprenaline was more effective in decreasing the airway resistance.

The effect of acupuncture seems to relate to the origin of the asthmatic problems. Takishima et al (1982) reported that a requirement for improved respiration following acupuncture is that the patients should react with decreased airway resistance following inhalation sympathomimetics. Tandon & Philip (1989) compared acupuncture and placebo acupuncture in histamine-induced asthma; neither acupuncture nor placebo produced any significant effect on respiratory functions.

In some studies a series of acupuncture treatments were given. In a Danish study patients received acupuncture treatment twice weekly over 5 weeks and were compared with a group given placebo acupuncture (Christensen et al 1986). Both groups were improved and in the treatment group the improvement was significant during the treatment period compared with the placebo group. The effect persisted for 2 weeks after the end of treatment. A similar finding was made by Jobst, Chen & McPherson (1986) in patients with disabling

breathlessness. The effects of acupuncture and placebo were compared, using the walking distance over 6 min, the subjective experience and the respiratory tests. Acupuncture or placebo treatment 13 times during 3 weeks increased the walking distance in the acupuncture group with 48% compared with 17% in the control group. The subjective improvement was also significant in the acupuncture group but the respiratory values were unchanged in both groups.

The difference between placebo and real acupuncture reported in most studies suggests that acupuncture decreases the airway resistance in asthmatic patients. Most studies have shown an immediate short-lasting effect following acupuncture but there is also some evidence that a more long-lasting effect is possible. There is, however, a need of more studies particularly those concerning long term effects on asthma.

The cause of the improvement of airway resistance by acupuncture is not settled. It seems from the placebo-controlled studies that stimulation in thoracic segments is needed to obtain an improvement. The autonomic control of airways is presumably partly related to the segmental innervation of thoracic respiratory muscles. It seems reasonable that stimulation of somatic afferents in these segments may influence output to the sympathetic chain and further to the lungs. On the other hand, it cannot be excluded that the effect of acupuncture on the respiration is unspecific with regard to the stimulated area. Stimulation in the paravertebral muscles has been combined with stimulation of other muscle points. As discussed previously, muscle points are effective in inducing endorphin release and possibly also release of other neurotransmitters. Placebo stimulation has usually been given in non-muscle points or superficially in the skin and this technique is less effective in releasing such substances. Although there is no evidence that endorphins influence airway resistance directly such an effect may occur via other routes. The changes in central sympathetic control of the cardiovascular system could be paralleled by changes in the autonomic output to the airways. The facilitation of respiration following a period of exercise – the "second breath" – is well known among sports enthusiasts. If the hypothesis is correct that acupuncture induces similar functional changes to those of muscle exercise then a decrease in airway resistance should be expected.

Another cause of the effect could be release of ACTH, which is produced from pro-opiomelanocortin in the hypophysis in equal amounts with β-endorphin. ACTH stimulates the release of cortisol with a secondary effect on inflammatory reactions. Still another cause of decreased inflammatory reactions in the airways could be the production of calcitonin gene-related peptide (CGRP) from the region of acupuncture stimulation (Lundeberg 1993). Changes in the immune system have also been reported after acupuncture, which could influence the asthmatic disease.

Psychological factors may contribute to the severity of asthmatic attacks. Important components in acupuncture treatment are decreased stress and increased relaxation, experienced by many patients independent of the reason for the acupuncture treatment (Widerström 1993). The anxiety and stress felt by many asthmatic patients may be positively influenced by acupuncture.

Immunological reactions

According to TCM infectious diseases can be treated with acupuncture. It has been reported that acupuncture is as effective as antibiotics in the treatment of gastrointestinal infections (Rogers & Bossy 1981). Most information is anecdotal, however, and few controlled studies have been performed. There are reports that the immune defence system may be strengthened from muscle exercise. Many joggers, for instance, believe that they will get infections if they discontinue running regularly. Some scientific reports support this idea. Edwards et al (1984) reported changes in the population of lymphoid cells in human peripheral blood following physical exercise. The number of lymphocytes increased as did activity associated to natural killer cells. Enhancement of human natural killer cell activity related to enkephalins has been observed in in vitro experiments (Faith et al 1984). Neil, Allen & Morley (1984) reported a significant increase in natural killer cell activity from lymphocytes incubated with β-endorphin; morphine had no such effect. In experiments on spontaneously hypertensive

rats the natural killer cell activity increased significantly ($P < 0.005$) in rats running in a wheel compared with sedentary controls (Jonsdottir, personal communication 1995). If the preliminary results on the effect on the immune system can be verified they may have important clinical applications in modulation of specific immune-mediated diseases.

Tinnitus

In TCM acupuncture is used for relief of tinnitus. Scientific documentation indicating that acupuncture may have specific effects on tinnitus is lacking, however. It could also be noted that the WHO list of 1979 does not include tinnitus as a condition suitable for acupuncture treatment. During the last decades, several studies have been carried out in Western countries. Hansen, Hansen & Bentzen (1982) compared the effect of acupuncture and placebo on tinnitus. They found a small reduction of the condition after both placebo and real acupuncture but the effect was not significant. Marks et al (1984) gave traditional acupuncture in a placebo-controlled trial. No significant difference was found between the groups. In both these studies some patients reported improvement but this was considered unspecific. Thomas, Laurell & Lundeberg (1988) reported that 40% of their patients experienced reduced tinnitus during the acupuncture treatment period, but within 3 months the tinnitus had returned to the original level. A similar effect was reported by Nilsson, Axelson & Gu (1992). In their study, patients ($n = 46$) with severe tinnitus were given 10 treatments. Only three patients reported improvement, which lasted at least 10 days after the treatment. One-third of the patients reported a transient reduction lasting from hours to days. Statistical analyses of the whole group did not show any significant treatment effects. In a study by Lindholm et al (1991) acupuncture treatment was given twice weekly over 2 months, a total of 15 treatments for each patient ($n = 57$). They reported significant effects on tinnitus in 56% of the patients, in which the tinnitus was reduced or disappeared completely for an undefined period of time.

It should be noted that the studies of Thomas, Laurell & Lundeberg (1988), Lindholm et al (1991) and Nilsson, Axelson & Gu (1992) did not include control groups or placebo, which may explain at least partly both the difference in results and the positive outcome reported by Lindholm et al (1991). In a placebo-controlled study of noise-induced tinnitus (Axelson et al 1994) a similar acupuncture technique was used to that in the investigation by Lindholm et al 1991. The positive results of the former were not reproduced. Some patients in both the acupuncture and the placebo groups experienced a small reduction in tinnitus, but without any significant difference between the groups. The effect lasted only for hours or a few days except for one patient who reported a marked and long-lasting improvement already after the first acupuncture treatment.

It is concluded that the specific effect of acupuncture on tinnitus is small or absent. Many patients, however, experienced positive concomitant effects such as improved sleep, better acceptance of the disturbing noise and better quality of life. Therefore, acupuncture may have some beneficial effects, which could be valuable for some patients owing to general stress reduction and relaxation. In this respect acupuncture may be preferable to other treatment modalities that also are without specific effects on tinnitus but may have adverse instead of positive side-effects.

Drug abuse and obesity

Acupuncture treatment of opiate dependent persons was initiated in Hong Kong in 1973. The method has gained increasing popularity as a complement to other methods in different types of drug abuse. Needles are placed in the vagus-innervated part of the ear and stimulated manually or electrically at high frequency for periods of 10–30 min. The treatment has decreased the abstinence symptoms and facilitated treatment with other methods. Several publications support the value of acupuncture in treatment of opiate abstinence (Wen 1977, Wen & Chung 1978, Wen et al 1979). The main effect of acupuncture seems to be a marked reduction of the abstinence symptoms. The levels of plasma ACTH and cortisol, which are elevated during abstinence, decrease following acupuncture but not with methadone treatment. A fast narcotic detoxification

in opiate-addicted patients has been used (Kroening and Olessen 1985, Wen 1977). Electroacupuncture in the ear was combined with repeated small doses of naloxone (0.04 mg). This method was reported to give detoxification during 1 or 2 days with an almost total absence of adverse abstinence symptoms.

Acupuncture has also been used to treat alcohol abuse. Smith et al (1988) reported that a combination of body and ear acupuncture gave valuable results. Acupuncture treatment was given daily and according to the report 50% of those who continued the treatment were free from the drug at least 6 months after the end of the treatment. The most convincing results have been reported by Bullock, Culliton & Olander (1989). This study included 80 persons with severe alcoholism, divided into one group with real acupuncture and one group with placebo stimulation. Treatment was given for 8 weeks with increasing intervals between the treatments. In the acupuncture group 21 out of 40 patients completed the programme but only one patient completed it in the placebo group.

There is a common belief that acupuncture, in particular ear acupuncture, is a useful method for stopping smoking or decreasing body weight. However, only a few controlled studies have been performed to elucidate this possibility. Gillams et al (1984) divided people who wanted to stop smoking into three groups. One group was treated with ear acupuncture, another group received placebo acupuncture at the same points and the third group participated in group therapy. The result showed no significant difference between the three groups with regard to number of persons who stopped smoking. Clavel (1985) compared the stop-smoking effect in smokers who were randomized to acupuncture and nicotine gum. Both treatments reduced the smoking during the months of treatment in comparison to an untreated control group but did not differ with regard to tendency to resume smoking later.

Similar results were obtained by Lamontagne et al (1980). Heavy smokers ($n = 75$) were randomly divided into three groups. One group received ear acupuncture for 20 minutes twice weekly. The second group received acupuncture in other points assumed to give relaxation. The patients in the third group were asked to try to stop smoking. They met a therapist twice a week during 20 minutes to report about their smoking habits. The result of the study showed that the groups who received acupuncture had a significantly less cigarette consumption than the third group 14 days after the end of the treatment. The difference was, however, not significant 1, 3 and 6 months after the treatment.

As a method of stopping smoking, acupuncture appears to have a value similar to that of other methods. It appears to have some effect on the abstinence and it may be of value to combine acupuncture and other methods (Jiang and Cui 1994).

A few studies report acupuncture treatment of obesity. Mok (1976) compared the effect of acupuncture in a group of 24 persons weighing 5–33% over the ideal weight. Their weight was followed over three periods. During the first period acupuncture was given in points in one ear, during the second period the same points were stimulated in both ears, and during the third period the needles were placed in different points supposed not to influence the body weight. The result showed no significant effect on the weight in any of the treatment periods. Shafshak (1995) confirmed that ear acupuncture itself did not reduce the weight. On the other hand overweight patients who were set on a low calorie diet were able to stay on this diet if they were simultaneously given acupuncture.

In conclusion, acupuncture seems to be of some value in the treatment of opiate and alcohol addiction owing to its ability to reduce adverse abstinence symptoms. The long term effect is, however, uncertain and the reports emphasize the importance of the psychosocial care following detoxification. Acupuncture is a complement in the treatment but does not by itself give sustained result in the treatment of overweight persons or smokers.

Treatment of mood and behaviour

After acupuncture many patients experience changes in mood such as feelings of sedation and well-being and improved sleep. Regular muscle exercise often gives decreased psychological tension, and euphoria or joy. Exercise (Wood 1977) and acupuncture (Greist et al 1979, Hechun, Yunkui & Zhan 1985) appear to be almost as effective as antidepressive drugs in the treatment of some patients with anxiety and depression. Behavioural effects are seen in animals

after both electrical nerve stimulation and long-lasting muscle exercise.

In a series of experiments the motor activity of spontaneously hypertensive rats was followed over a period of several weeks (Hoffmann, Thorén & Ely 1987). The test group but not the controls had access to a wheel in their home cage. The runners showed significantly less spontaneous locomotor activity than did the controls. Parallel with the decrease in exploratory activity, the aggressive behaviour decreased in runners as did the aggression towards an intruder compared with the controls. The locomotor activity was significantly less in the runners during a period of 45 days when these animals had access to a wheel. In a further experiment the wheels were locked to prevent running; after a few days the previous runners became significantly ($P < 0.01$) more aggressive than the controls probably as a side-effect of abstinence.

Discussion

Acupuncture is a method of utilizing endogenous mechanisms to influence a variety of functions. Its effects are unreliable since our present knowledge of the control mechanisms are limited and the practice of the method rests on tradition and intuition rather than on scientific research. Judged from our understanding of the biological principles it seems as if the use of sensory stimulation may be developed to offer a valuable complement to conventional methods.

Most practitioners using acupuncture rely on the traditional Chinese view of its influence on various functions in the body. It is understandable that healers who belong to the school of alternative medicine have limited knowledge and understanding of the biological mechanisms on which medical science rests and easily accept ideas that do not conform to this paradigm. In all fields of Western medicine a rapid development of methods has occurred during the last century; in contrast, the practice of acupuncture is essentially unchanged. It is surprising, therefore that a fair number of medical practitioners with an education in biological medicine accept the traditional view.

In this chapter the physiological background to the clinical effects of acupuncture has been described and discussed. Acupuncture is a method of stimulating certain types of afferent nerve fibres. The result of this stimulation is related not only to the site and type of stimulation but even more to the condition of the subject who is stimulated. In normal conditions no or only small effects are seen. The natural counterpart to acupuncture is long-lasting physical exercise, which is a stressful situation requiring adjustment in the body to keep the correct homeostasis. To survive in a changing and stressful environment adjustment via inherent control systems must be necessary. These systems are local and associated with segmental reflexes and central modifying functions of general importance such as the cardiovascular and hormonal systems. Although our knowledge of how the homeostatic systems operate and are influenced by internal and external stimuli is limited, it seems very important to utilize present knowledge to improve the practice of acupuncture.

This will increase the efficacy in treatment and encourage research in the field. The traditional view creates suspicion from the great majority of medical health professionals and creates a barrier to research. Most of the research today is carried out by enthusiastic practitioners lacking proper training in research. The result is low quality of many of the published articles.

Changes in biological parameters occur as a result of somatic afferent stimulation whether this is from normal physical exercise, electrical stimulation of afferent nerve fibres or mechanic or electrical stimulation via acupuncture needles. The direction of changes seems to be towards an optimal performance of different functions. The details in the underlying mechanisms are largely unknown but there is good evidence that autonomic nervous system and hormonal controls are involved. In further research the physiological mechanisms in physical exercise should be helpful in understanding acupuncture mechanisms.

Our biological system has developed over a very long period of time and is adapted for a life as hunters and collectors where persistence in physical activity is of fundamental importance for survival. In modern society psychosocial stress is high but the motor activity minimal. The emotional tension that is the result of unresolved stress cannot often be transformed into physical exercise in accordance with the inherited biological needs. Instead the stress-induced changes remain and give long-lasting functional disturbances, for example in muscle tone and the autonomic nervous system. A contributing factor to disturbance in health is therefore probably too-limited physical exercise with an insufficient afferent input for an optimal performance. The physical fitness obtained as a result of training is often pointed out but the fact that sufficient afferent input is essential for other functions also is easily forgotten.

An important conclusion must be that regular physical exercise should be encouraged to strengthen physical and mental fitness and to prevent functional disturbances. Some people with diseases have practical problems in performing certain types of physical exercise. Acupuncture, TENS and other methods for afferent stimulation may be a complement or an alternative to physical training for such patients. It is evident that sensory stimulation can only to a certain extent replace physical activity, which has many other positive components.

In treatment of pain and diseases with any method the engagement of the patient is important. The psychological factor becomes particularly important in methods that rely on endogenous modulation of various functions in which psychological factors (often referred to as placebo) are integrated. No doubt, all types of somatic sensory stimulation and particularly acupuncture have very strong placebo effects. Acupuncture is possibly an uniquely effective method in activation of positive placebo effects. It must be realized that placebo is as physiological as any other mechanism. Mental activity, conscious or unconscious, may modulate somatic mechanisms as effectively as any peripheral stimulus. The somatic and psychological factors must act in harmony to utilize endogenous mechanisms most effectively.

References

Akil H, Watson S J, Young E, Lewis M E, Khachaturian H, Walker J M 1984. Endogenous opioids: biology and function. Annual Review of Neurosciences 7: 223–255

PHYSIOLOGICAL MECHANISMS IN ACUPUNCTURE 37

Axelson A, Andersson S, Gu Li-De 1994 Acupuncture in management of tinnitus: a placebo controlled study. Audiology 33: 351–360

Ballegaard S 1990 Effects of acupuncture in moderate stable angina pectoris: control study. Journal of Internal Medicine 227: 25–30

Ballegaard S, Jansen G, Pedersen K, Nissen W H 1986 Acupuncture in severe stable angina pectoris: a randomized trial. Acta Medica Scandinavica 220: 307–313

Basbaum A I, Fields H L 1984 Endogenous pain control systems: brain-stem spinal pathways and endorphin circuitry. Annual Review of Neurosciences 7: 309–338

Bennett T, Wilcox R G, Mcdonald I A 1984 Post-exercise reduction of blood pressure in hypertensive men is not due to acute impairment of baroreflex function. Clinical Science 67: 97–103

Berger D, Nolte D 1977 Acupuncture in bronchial asthma: bodyplethysmographic measurements of acute broncholytic effects. Comparative Medicine East and West 5: 265–270

Blake M J, Stein E A, Vomachka A 1984 Effects of exercise training on brain opioid peptides and serum LM in female rats. Peptides 5: 953–958

Bloom F E 1983 The endorphins. A growing family of pharmacologically pertinent peptides. Annual Review of Pharmacology and Toxicology 23: 151–170

Bullock M L, Culliton P D, Olander R T 1989 Controlled trial of acupuncture for severe recidivist alcoholism. Lancet 8652: 1435–1439

Cao X-D, S-F Xu, W-X Lu 1983 Inhibition of sympathetic nervous system by acupuncture. Acupuncture and Electrotherapy Research 8: 25–35

Christensen P A, Laursen L C, Taudorf E, Sörensen S C, Weeke B 1986 Akupunktur til asthmapatienter. Ugeskr laeger 27: 241–243

Clavel F 1985 Helping people to stop smoking: randomised comparison of groups being treated with acupuncture and nicotine gum with control group. British Medical Journal 291: 1538–1539

Crine P, Gianoulakis C, Seidah N G 1978 Biosynthesis of beta-endorphin from beta-lipotropin and a larger molecular weight precursor in rat pars intermedia. Proceedings of the National Academy of Sciences USA 75: 4719–4723

Cuello A C 1983 Central distribution of opioid peptides. British Medical Bulletin 39: 11–16

Di Marzo V, Tippins J R, Morris H R 1989 Neuropeptides and inflammatory mediators: bidirectional modulatory mechanisms. TIPS 10: 91–92

Edwards A J, Bacon T H, Elms C A, Verardi R, Felder M, Knight S C 1984 Changes in the populations of lymphoid cells in human peripheral blood following physical exercise. Clinical and Experimental Immunology 58: 420–427

Faith R E, Liang H J, Murgo A J, Plotnikoff N P 1984 Neuroimmunomodulation with enkephalins: enhancement of human natural killer (NK) cell activity in vitro. Clinical Immunology and Immunopathology 31: 412–418

Fitzgerald W 1981 Labile hypertension and jogging: new diagnostic tool or spurious discovery. British Medical Journal 282: 542–544

Floras J S, Sinkey C A, Ayleard P E, Seals D R, Thorén P N, Mark A L 1989 Post-exercise hypotension and sympathoinhibition in borderline hypertensive men. Hypertension 14: 28–35

Gaal C M, Freebairn C 1979 Ear acupuncture relaxation therapy in alcoholics. Medical Journal of Australia 2: 179–180

Ganten D, Unger Th, Schilkens B, Rascher W, Speck G, Stock G 1981 Role of neuropeptides in regulation of blood pressure. Disturbances in neurogenic control of the circulation. American Physiological Society pp 139–151

Gillams J et al 1984 Acupuncture and group therapy in stopping smoking. The Practitioner 228: 341–344

Greist J H, Klein M H, Eischens R R, Faris J, Gurman S A, Morgan W P 1979 Running as treatment for depression. Comparative Psychiatry 20: 41–53

Guillemin R, Vargo T, Rossier J 1977 Beta-endorphin and adrenocorticotropin are secreted concomitantly by the pituitary gland. Science 197: 1367–1369

Hansen P E, Hansen J H, Bentzen O 1982 Acupuncture treatment of chronic unilateral tinnitus: a double blind crossover trial. Clinical Otolaryngology 7: 325–329

Hechun L, Yunkui J, Zhan L 1985 Electro-acupuncture vs. amitriptyline in the treatment of depressive states. Journal of Traditional Chinese Medicine 5(1): 3–8

Hoffmann P, Friberg P, Ely D, Thorén P 1987 Effect of spontaneous running on blood pressure, heart rate and cardiac dimensions in developing and established spontaneous hypertension in rats. Acta Physiologica Scandinavica 129: 535–542

Hoffmann P, Skarphedinsson J O, Delle M, Thorén P 1990 Electrical stimulation of the gastrocnemius muscle in the spontaneously hypertensive rat increases the pain threshold: role of different serotonergic receptors. Acta Physiologica Scandinavica 138: 125–131

Hoffmann P, Terenius L, Thorén P 1990 Cerebrospinal fluid beta-endorphin concentration is increased by long-lasting voluntary exercise ink the spontaneously hypertensive rat. Regulatory Peptides 28: 233–239

Hoffmann P, Thorén P 1986 Long-lasting cardiovascular depression induced by acupuncture-like stimulation of the sciatic nerve in unanesthetized rats. Effects of arousal and type of hypertension. Acta Physiologica Scandinavica 127: 119–126

Hoffmann P, Thorén P, Ely D 1987 Effect of voluntary exercise on open-field behavior and on aggression in the spontaneously hypertensive rat (SHR). Behavioral and neural biology 47: 346–355

Holaday J W 1983 Cardiovascular effects of endogenous opiate systems. Annual Review of Pharmacology and Toxicology 23: 541–594

Jansen G, Lundeberg T, Samuelsson U B, Thomas M 1989 Increased survival of ischemic musculocutaneous flaps after acupuncture in rats. Acta Physiologica Scandinavica 135: 555–558

Jennings G L, Nelson L, Esler M D, Leonard P, Korner P I 1984 Effects of changes in physical activity on blood pressure and sympathetic tone. Journal of Hypertension 2 (suppl 3): 139–141

Jiang H, Cui M 1994 Analysis of the therapeutic effect of acupuncture in abstinence. Journal of Traditional Chinese Medicine 14: 56–63

Jobst K, Chen J H, McPherson K 1986 Controlled trial of acupuncture for disabling breathlessness. Lancet 20/27: 416–418

Kaada B 1982 Vasodilatation induced by transcutaneous nerve stimulation in peripheral ischemia (Raynaud's phenomenon and diabetic polyneuropathy). European Heart Journal 3: 303–314

Kaada B 1985 Behandlung chronischer Ulzera und peripherer Ischämie mit transkutaner Nervenstimulation (TNS). In: Bischko J (ed) Handbuch der Akupunktur und Aurikulotherapie, Haug Verlag, Heidelberg, pp 16–35

Kartjansson J, Lundeberg T 1990 Effects of electrical nerve stimulation (ENS) in ischemic tissue. Scandinavian Journal of Plastic Reconstructive Surgery 24: 129–134

Kaufman M P, Longhurst J C, Rybycki K J, Wallach J H, Mitchell J H 1983 Effects of static muscular contraction on impulse activity of groups III and IV afferents in cats. Journal of Applied Physiology: Respiration and Environmental Exercise Physiology 55(1): 105–112

Kaufman M P, Waldrop T G, Rybycki K J, Ordway G A, Mitchell J H 1984 Effects of static and rhythmic twitch contractions on the discharge of group III and IV muscle afferents. Cardiovascular Research 18: 663–668

Kniffki K-D, Mense S, Schmidt R F 1981 Muscle receptors with fine afferent fibers which may evoke circulatory reflexes. Circulation Research 48: (suppl I) I25–I31

Kroening R J, Olessen T D 1985 Rapid narcotic detoxification in chronic pain patients treated with auricular electroacupuncture and naloxone. International Journal of the Addictions 20: 1347–1360

Lamontagne Y, Annable L, Gagmon C-M 1980 Acupuncture for smokers: lack of long-term therapeutic effect in a controlled study. CMA Journal 122: 787–790

Lindholm S, Berg S, Larsson B, Hybbinette J-H 1991 Öronkliniken, Länssjukhuset i Kalmar. Akupunkturbehandling mot tinnitus. Läkartidningen 10: 847–849

Lundeberg T 1993 Peripheral effects of sensory nerve stimulation (acupuncture) on inflammation and ischemia. Scandinavian Journal of Rehabilitation Medicine (suppl) 29: 6186

Lundeberg T, Eriksson S V, Malm M 1992 Electrical nerve stimulation improves healing of venous ulcers. Annals of Plastic Surgery 29: 328–331

Mannheimer C, Emanuelsson H, Waagstein F, Wilhelmsson C 1989 Influence of naloxone on the effects of high frequency transcutaneous electrical nerve stimulation in angina pectoris induced by atrial pacing. British Heart Journal 62: 36–42

Mannheimer C, Karlsson C A, Emanuelsson H, Vedin A, Waagstein F, Wilhelmsson C 1985 The effect of transcutaneous electrical nerve stimulation in patients with severe angina pectoris. Circulation 71: 308–312

Marks N J, Emery P, Onisphoron C 1984 A controlled trial of acupuncture in tinnitus. Journal of Laryngology and Otology 98: 1103–1109

Melzack R, Wall P D 1965 Pain mechanism: a new theory. Science 150: 971–979

Metzger J M, Stein E A 1984 B-endorphin and sprint training. Life Sciences 34: 1541–1547

Mok M S 1976 Treatment of obesity by acupuncture. American Journal of Clinical Nutrition 29: 832–835

Montrastruc J L, Montrastruc P, Marales-Olivas F 1981 Potentiation by naloxone of pressor reflexes. British Journal of Pharmacology 74: 105–109

Moriyama T 1987 Microneurographic analysis of the effects of acupuncture stimulation on sympathetic muscle nerve activity in humans: excitation followed by inhibition. Nippon Seirigaku Zasshi 49: 711–721

Neil K, Allen J, E Morley J E 1984 Endorphins stimulate normal, human peripheral blood lymphocyte natural killer activity. Life Sciences 35: 53–59

Nelson L, Esler M D, Jennings G L, Korner P I 1986 Effect of changing levels of physical activity on blood-pressure and haemo-dynamics in essential hypertension. Lancet ii: 473–476

Nilsson S, Axelson A, Gu Li De 1992 Acupuncture as a method in tinnitus management. I Tinnitus 91: 535–540

Petty M, Reid J L 1981 The effect of opiates on arterial baroreceptor reflex function in the rabbit. Naunyn Schmiedebergs Archives of Pharmacology 319: 206–211

Reid J L, Rubin P C 1987 Peptides and central neural regulation of the circulation. Physiological Review 67: 725–749

Richter A, Herliz J, Hjalmarsson Å 1991 Effect of acupuncture in patients with angina pectoris. European Heart Journal 12: 175–178

Rogers F, Bossy J 1981 Activation of the defence system of the body of animals and men by acupuncture and moxibustion. Acupuncture Research Quarterly 5: 47–54

Rossier J, French E D, Rivier C, Ling N, Guillemin R, Bloom F E 1977 Foot-shock induced stress increases beta-endorphin levels in blood but not brain. Nature 270: 618–620

Rowell L B 1986 Human Circulation. Oxford University Press, Oxford

Rubin P C 1984 Opioid peptides in blood pressure regulation in man. Clinical Science 66: 625–630

Rutkowski B 1980 Electrical stimulation and essential hypertension. Acupuncture and Electrotherapy Research 5: 287–295

Shafshak T S 1995 Electroacupuncture and exercise in body weight reduction and their application in rehabilitating patients with knee osteoarthritis. American Journal of Chinese Medicine 23: 15–25

Smith F W Jr 1992 Acupuncture for cardiovascular diseases. Problems in Veterinary Medicine 4: 125–131

Smith M O, Khan I 1988 An acupuncture programme for the treatment of drug-addicted persons. Bulletin of Narcotics 40: 53–41

Smyth D G 1983 Beta-endorphin and related peptides in pituitary, brain, pancreas, and antrum. British Medical Bulletin 39: 25–30

Sun X-Y, Yu J, Yao T 1983 Pressor effect produced by stimulation of somatic nerve on hemorrhagic hypotension in conscious rats. Acta Physiologica Sinica 35: 264–270

Takishima T, Mue S, Tamura G, Ishihara T, Watanabe K 1982 The bronchodilating effect of acupuncture in patients with acute asthma. Annals of Allergy 48: 44–49

Tam K-C, Yiu H-H 1975 The effect of acupuncture on essential hypertension. American Journal of Chinese Medicine 3: 369–375

Tandon M, Philip F T 1989 Comparison of real and placebo acupuncture in histamine-induced asthma. A double-blind crossover study. Chest 96: 102–105

Tashkin D P, Kroening R J, Bresler D E, Simmons M, Coulson A H, Kerschner K 1977 Comparison of real and simulated acupuncture and isoproterenol in methacholine-induced asthma. Annals of Allergy 39: 376–387

Terenius L 1984 The endogeneous opioids and other central peptides. In: Wall P D, Melzack R (eds) Textbook of pain Churchill Livingstone, Edinburgh

Thomas M, Laurell G, Lundeberg T 1988 Acupuncture for the alleviation of tinnitus. Laryngoscope 98: 664–667

Thorén P, Floras J S, Hoffmann P, Seals D R 1990 Endorphins and exercise: physiological mechanisms and clinical implications. Medicine and Science in Sports and Exercise 22: 417–428

Virsik K, Kristufek P, Bangha O, Urban S 1980 The effect of acupuncture on pulmonary function in bronchial asthma. Progress in Respiration Research 14: 271–275

Wang Q, Mao L, Han J 1990 Great nucleus of hypothalamus mediates low but not high frequency electroacupuncture analgesia in rats. Brain Research 9: 60–66

Wang Wei, Yao Tai 1986 Role of the cervical sympathetic nerve in the resetting of carotid sinus baroreceptor reflex during somatic nerve stimulation in the rabbit. Chinese Journal of Physiological Science 2: 319–326

Wen H L 1977 Fast detoxification of heroin addicts by acupuncture and electrical stimulation (AES) in combination with naloxone. Comparative Medicine East and West 5: 257–263

Wen H L, Chung S Y C 1978 Reduction of adrenocorticotropic hormone (ACTH) and cortisol in drug addicts treated by acupuncture and electrical stimulation (AES). Comparative Medicine East and West 6: 61–66

Wen H L, Ho W K K, Wong H K, Mehal Z D, Ng Y H, Ma I 1979 Changes in adrenocorticotropic hormone (ACTH) and cortisol levels in drug addicts treated by a new and rapid detoxification procedure using acupuncture and naloxone. Comparative Medicine East and West 6: 241–245

Widerström-Noga E 1993 Analgesic effects of afferent stimulation – a psychobiological perspective. Doctoral thesis, University of Göteborg

Wood D T 1977 The relationship between state anxiety and acute physical activity. American Corrective Therapy Journal 67–69

Yao T, Andersson S, Thorén P 1982a Long-lasting cardiovascular depression induced by acupuncture-like stimulation of the sciatic nerve in unanesthetized spontaneously hypertensive rats. Brain Research 240: 77–85

Yao T, Andersson S, Thorén P 1982b Long-lasting cardiovascular depressor response following sciatic stimulation in SHR. Evidence for the involvement of central endorphin and serotonin systems. Brain Research 244: 295–303

3

Basic points for pain relief acupuncture

Val Hopwood

This chapter contains tables of the major acupuncture points together with composite illustrations showing the rough location of the points. Precise anatomical detail is to be found in the tables. The Chinese proportional measure, the Cun, is referred to occasionally. One Cun is roughly equal to 2.5 cm or 1 inch and is taken as the width of the first distal interphalangeal joint of the patient, or sometimes the distance between the first and second joints of the index finger of the patient. This gives a very rough guide to the relative positioning of the acupuncture points and will obviously be of greater importance when considering the location of points on abnormally tall or short people or, indeed, on children. Figure 3.1, shows the general proportions of the body and will enable the student to apply

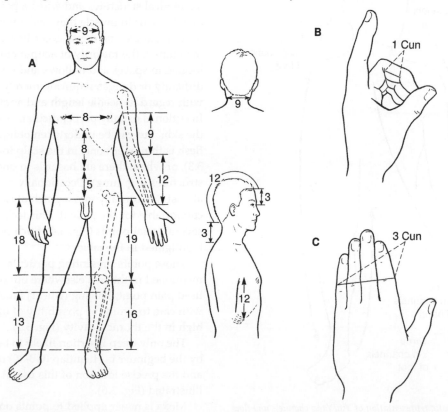

Fig. 3.1 *Proportional (Cun) measurements: (A) Applied to the entire body. (B) Across one finger. (C) Across four fingers.*

these measurements when point locations are given only in terms of Cun in other texts.

The points are grouped logically according to their primary situation and the Yin/Yang designation of the channels (see Tables 3.1–3.3). It is a useful rule of thumb when trying to locate channels and the points on them to remember that the Yang channels mostly lie where the sun supposedly shines, mainly on the outside of the limbs and the back (which is exposed to the sun when working), while the Yin channels are situated on the inner side of the limbs and the front of the trunk (Fig. 3.2).

Selecting points for a particular painful condition is essentially a subjective exercise. Every

acupuncturist is likely to include certain points but, equally, each therapist will have their own favourites according to their analysis of the symptoms.

The list of points included in this book is not exhaustive. It is assumed that the practitioner will select local and distal points according to the guidelines printed elsewhere. The points selected in the course of the channels are those most commonly used for painful conditions; where points are frequently used as distal points this is mentioned. The more effective acupressure points are also noted.

Most of the points thus selected also have other actions and these have been mentioned where interesting or relevant. True traditional Chinese acupuncture is a complex and demanding discipline and the information given here only scratches the surface of basic therapy.

Specific needling details have generally not been included. It is assumed that all physical therapists have a basic knowledge of, and familiarity with, anatomical structures and when a point is directly over bone or in muscle they will adjust their needling angle and depth accordingly. As previously mentioned, the majority of acupuncture points are located in spaces and hollows and present little difficulty or danger, requiring merely common sense with regard to needle length and angle of insertion. Insertion is usually perpendicular, at right angles to the skin, but can be undertaken obliquely where the flesh is thin over bone, in the scalp for instance (Fig. 3.3), or where there are hazards to underlying structures (e.g. lung). Occasionally an insertion almost horizontally into a pinch of skin will be most comfortable for the patient. This technique is used on several facial points (Fig. 3.4). Such points have been highlighted in the table.

Those points presenting particular problems are mentioned in the text elsewhere but one commonly used pain point, Jianjing (GB-21) must be needled with care to avoid the possibility of lung tissue lying high in the thoracic cavity (Fig. 3.5).

The only deep insertion likely to be encountered by the beginner is Huantiao (GB-30) on the thigh, and the precise location of this useful point is also illustrated (Fig. 3.6).

Moxa is never applied to points on the Lung channel since this can be harmed by heat, but

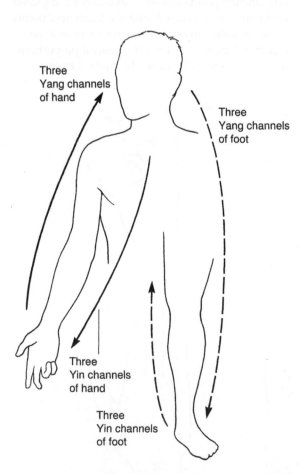

Fig. 3.2 *Schematic representation of Yin/Yang channels and flow of Qi.*

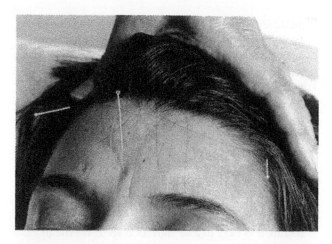

Fig. 3.3 *Oblique insertions. ST-8 Touwei, bilaterally, EX-3 Yintang.*

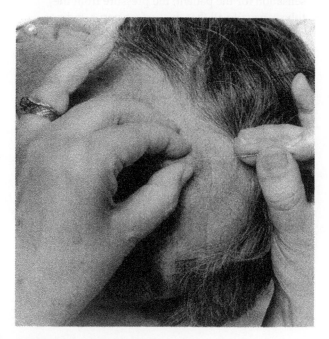

Fig. 3.4 *Pinch insertion, GB-14 Yangbai.*

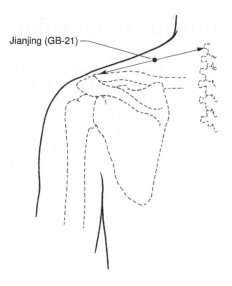

Fig. 3.5 *Needling GB-21 Jianjing.*

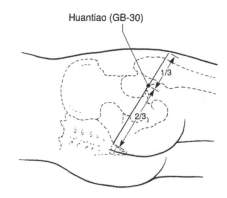

Fig. 3.6 *Location of GB-30 Huantiao.*

reference should be made to Chapter 8 for the use of this heating technique on other points. Cupping (see p. 105) is applicable on any point where the thickness of the flesh will accommodate the sucking action without causing pain to the patient. Cupping over bony protruberances is impractical; similarly, a sufficient vacuum will not be achieved in hirsute areas.

Treatment combinations

Some examples of treatment combinations include abdominal points (Fig. 3.7), points on the hand (Fig. 3.8) and points on the foot (Fig. 3.9).

It is rare that one point is used alone, in isolation. This is said to be the mark of an expert acupuncturist, but it takes considerable skill and a lengthy training to be certain that the effect will be exactly what is required. However, 'less is more' in acupuncture, as well as in homeopathy, and too many points are a sign of poor practice. The beginner should aim for 4–5 needles when working unilaterally.

Having decided which points will be appropriate, it will be necessary to position the patient carefully and make sure they are well-supported with plenty of pillows. Most treatments will last for at least 20 minutes. It has been suggested that an extra 10 minutes will do no harm and will probably allow a full placebo effect to develop. This is a powerful additional effect and better used than ignored.

Where a choice of points has included a selection on different aspects of the body, a choice needs to be made with regard to treatment time. It is perfectly acceptable to treat for 10 minutes on one aspect, and 10 minutes on the other. The other alternative would be to treat the two aspects at separate sessions, alternating the groups of points used. This depends on being able to see the patient within a week from the previous treatment.

As a rule, needles should be inserted in a definite order, distal to proximal, and removed proximal to distal. This has the advantage of making it difficult to forget a lone needle and have the patient indicate it accusingly! Take special care when using GV 20, Baihui, it is easy to lose sight of a short needle in grey hair!

Guidance tubes do reduce the initial needling sensation for the patient; the pressure from the tube is usually all that the surface nerve endings detect. However more care is needed as the tube is slipped off. The needle will not be very deeply embedded in the skin, and if it is a long one, will cause some skin pain if it is allowed to lean over, and drag on the skin, before being inserted to the correct depth.

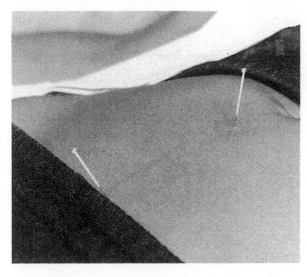

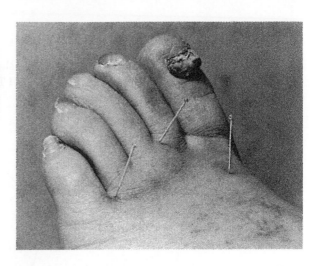

Fig. 3.9 *Example of treatment combination; GB-43 Xiaxi, ST-44 Neiting and LI-3 Taichong. All needles 25 mm.*

Fig. 3.7 *Abdominal points. 25 mm needles, CV-3 Zhongji and CV-6 Qihai.*

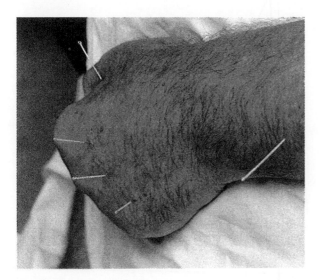

Fig. 3.8 *Example of treatment combination; Baxie points with TE-5 Waiguan. All needles 25 mm.*

Arm channels

Major points on the Yin channels of the inner arm are shown in Figure 3.10 and Table 3.1. Points on the Yang channels of the outer arm are shown in Figure 3.11 and Table 3.2.

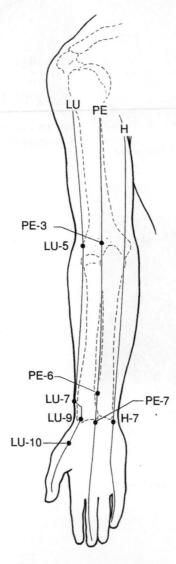

Fig. 3.10 *Yin channels of the arm.*

Table 3.1 *Points on the Yin channels of the arm*

Number	Name	Location	Additional actions
Heart 7 (H-7)	Shenmen	Transverse crease of the wrist in depression at radial side of FCU posterior to the pisiform bone	Luo point Sedating and calming effect Insomnia
Pericardium 3 (PE-3)	Quze	The middle of the transverse cubital crease on the ulnar side of the tendon of biceps brachii	Dispels Heat
Pericardium 6 (PE-6)	Neiguan	2 Cun proximal to the transverse wrist crease between palmaris longus and flexor carpi radialis	Luo point linking with TB-4 Yangchi Key point of Yin Wei Mai Particularly useful for nausea and vomiting Acupressure point
Pericardium 7 (PE-7)	Daling	On the transverse wrist crease between palmaris longus and flexor carpi radialis	Point of choice for carpal tunnel syndrome Insomnia
Lung 5 (LU-5)	Chize	On the lateral aspect of the anterior elbow crease, lateral to the biceps tendon	Sedation point. Useful in sore throat and respiratory disorders involving the pathogen Heat
Lung 7 (LU-7)	Lieque	Radial side of the forearm, in a hollow 1.5 Cun proximal to the transverse wrist crease (oblique insertion)	Luo linking point to LI-4 Hegu Major point for lung conditions and key point for Ren channel
Lung 9 (LU-9)	Taiyuan	Depression on radial side of the radial artery on the anterior wrist crease	Influential point for pulse and circulation
Lung 10 (LU-10)	Yuji	Halfway along the shaft of the first metacarpal bone where the red and white skin meet	Point of choice for osteoarthritis pain in the thumb

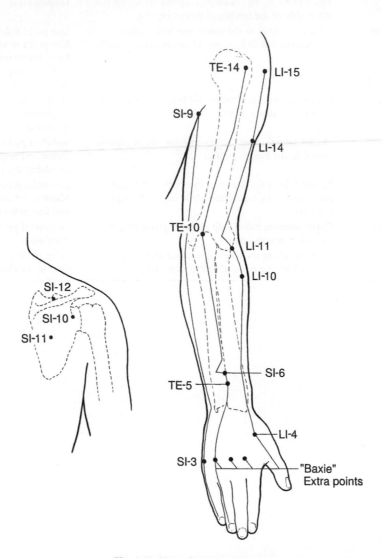

Fig. 3.11 *Yang channels of the arm.*

Table 3.2 *Points on the Yang channels of the arm*

Number	Name	Location	Additional actions
Large Intestine 4 (LI-4)	Hegu	On the dorsum of the hand between the 1st and 2nd metacarpal bones and on the radial side of the midpoint of the 2nd metacarpal bone	Major anaesthetic point for the whole body. Used for toothache and headache. Commonly used bilaterally in combination with Taichong LIV-3 to calm patients Acupressure point
Large Intestine 10 (LI-10)	Shousanli	On the radial side of the dorsal surface of the forearm and on the line connecting LI-5 and LI-11, 2 Cun below the cubital crease	Motor point for the forearm
Large Intestine 11 (LI-11)	Quchi	At the lateral end of the cubital crease with the elbow flexed	Important homeostatic and immune enhancing point. He Sea point
Large Int. 14 (LI-14)	Binao	At the insertion of the deltoid muscle, on the line connecting LI-11 and LI-15, 7 Cun above LI-11	Local pain point only
Large Int. 15 (LI-15)	Jianyu	In the depression anterior and inferior to the acromion when the arm is abducted	Anterior "eye" of the shoulder Used in paralysis of the arm
Triple Energiser 5 (TE-5)	Waiguan	On the dorsal side of the forearm, 2 Cun proximal to the dorsal wrist crease, between the radius and the ulna	Torticollis, temporal headache, common cold and fever Luo connection to PE-7 Daling
Triple Energiser 10 (TE-10)	Tianjing	On the lateral side of the upper arm, in the depression 1 Cun proximal to the tip of the olecranon when the elbow is flexed	Local point for elbow pain
Triple Energiser 14 (TE-14)	Jianliao	Posterior to Jianyu, in the depression posterior and inferior to the acromion when the arm is abducted	Posterior "eye" of the shoulder
Triple Energiser 21 (TE-21)	Ermen	On the face, anterior to the supratragic notch, in depression behind the posterior border of the condyloid process (see Fig. 3.18)	Used for deafness, tinnitus and dizziness
Small Intestine 3 (SI-3)	Houxi	Junction of red and white skin at the ulnar end of the distal palmar crease	Torticollis, all neck pain, tinnitus, deafness and headache Opens Governor channel
Small Intestine 6 (SI-6)	Yanglao	Ulnar side of posterior surface of the forearm, depression proximal to and on the radial side of the head of ulna	Acute pain along the channel
Small Intestine 9 (SI-9)	Jianzhen	1 Cun above end of the posterior axillary crease with arm adducted	Periarthritis of the shoulder
Small Intestine 10 (SI-10)	Naoshu	On the shoulder above the posterior end of the axillary crease in the depression below the lower border of the scapular spine	Local point for shoulder pain
Small Intestine 11 (SI-11)	Tianzong	On the scapula, in the depression of the centre of the subscapular fossa, at the 4th vertebral level	Scapular pain
Small Intestine 12 (SI-12)	Bingfeng	On the scapula at the centre of the suprascapular fossa, directly above SI-11 Tianzong	As Above
Small Intestine 18 (SI-18)	Quanliao	On the face directly below the outer canthus, in the depression below the zygomatic bone (see Fig. 3.18)	Trigeminal neuralgia, use on opposite side Toothache, facial paralysis
Small Intestine 19 (SI-19)	Tinggong	On the face, anterior to the tragus and posterior to the condyloid process, in the depression found when the mouth is opened	Local point for tinnitus and deafness

Leg channels

Points on the Yin channel of the inner leg are shown in Figure 3.12 and Table 3.3.

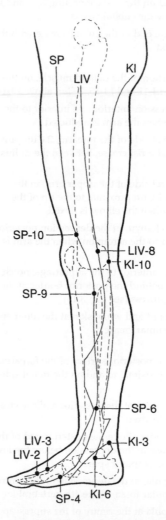

Fig. 3.12 *Yin channels of the leg.*

Table 3.3 *Points on the Yin channels of the leg*

Number	Name	Location	Additional actions
Spleen 4 (SP-4)	Gongsun	On the medial border of the foot, anterior and inferior to the proximal end of the 1st metatarsal bone	Luo point for Stomach channel, diarrhoea and constipation
Spleen 6 (SP-6)	Sanyinjiao	On the medial side of the leg, 3 Cun above the tip of the medial malleolus, posterior to the medial border of the tibia	Meeting point of three Yin channels Important general tonification point for any metabolic deficiency Acupressure point
Spleen 9 (SP-9)	Yinlingquan	On the medial side of the leg, depression posterior and inferior to the medial condyle of the tibia	Oedema of the lower limb
Spleen 10 (SP-10)	Xuehai	Highest point of vastus medialis, 2 Cun proximal to the upper border of the patella	Important immune-enhancing point Used for skin disorders, allergies, etc.
Kidney 3 (KI-3)	Taixi	Medial side of the foot, posterior to the medial malleolus, depression between the tip of the malleolus and the achilles tendon	Important point in deficiency conditions like osteoporosis, gynaecological problems, dysmenorrhoea, etc.
Kidney 6 (KI-6)	Zhaohai	Medial side of the foot, in the depression below the tip of the medial malleolus	Dysmenorrhoea Not advisable during the first months of pregnancy
Kidney 7 (KI-7)	Fuliu	On the medial side of the leg, 2 Cun above Taixi KI-3, anterior to the achilles tendon	Tonification point. Cystitis Lumbago Night sweats
Kidney 10 (KI-10)	Yingu	Medial side of the popliteal fossa, between the tendons of semitendinosus and semimembranosus, knee flexed	Good local point for medial knee pain Regulates Lower Jiao
Liver 2 (LIV-2)	Xingjian	At the margin of the web between the first and second toes	Dispels heat Soothes the Liver Regulates circulation of Qi
Liver 3 (LIV-3)	Taichong	Between the first and second metatarsal bones, 2 Cun proximal to the margin of the web	Used with Hegu, LI-4 for mental agitation. Lowers blood pressure Eye disorders. Metabolic problems Acupressure point
Liver 8 (LIV-8)	Ququan	At the medial end of the popliteal crease, at the anterior border of semimembranosus and semitendinosus	Good local point for knee problems

Urinary Bladder channel

The Urinary Bladder channel (Table 3.4) includes points on the back of the trunk (Fig. 3.13) and the leg (Fig. 3.14).

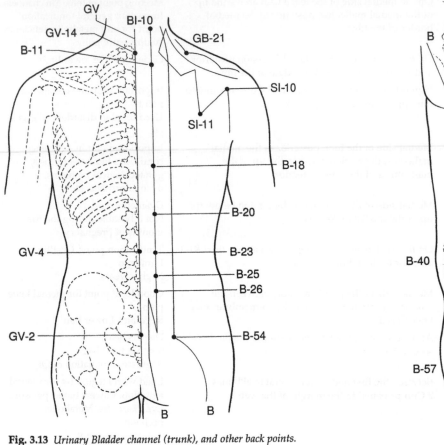

Fig. 3.13 *Urinary Bladder channel (trunk), and other back points.*

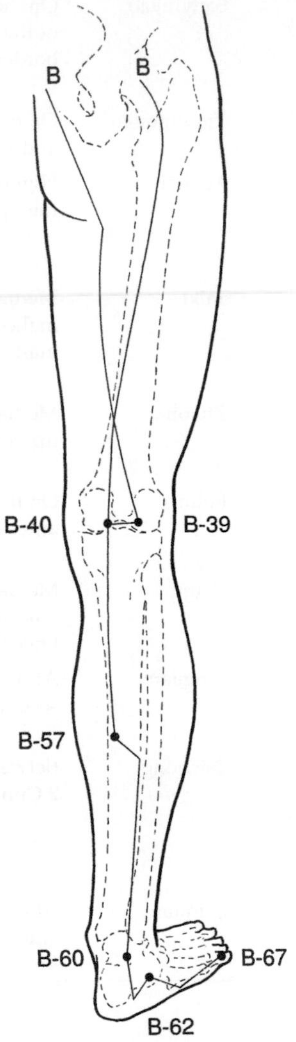

Fig. 3.14 *Urinary Bladder channel (leg).*

Table 3.4 *Urinary bladder channel points*

Number	Name	Location	Additional actions
Bladder 2 (B-2)	Zanzhu	On the face, in the depression at the medial end of the eyebrow, at the supraorbital north (see Fig. 3.18)	Sinusitis and eye disorders
Bladder 10 (B-10)	Tianzhu	On the nape, in the depression of the lateral border of the trapezius muscle and 1.3 Cun lateral to the midpoint of the posterior hairline	Headache Common cold
Bladder 11 (B-11)	Dashu	Below the spinous process of the 1st Thoracic vertebra, 1.5 Cun lateral to the midline	Influential point for bone
Bladder 18 (B-18)	Ganshu	Below the spinous process of the 9th Thoracic vertebra, 1.5 Cun lateral to the midline	Thoracic pain Tonification point for the Liver
Bladder 20 (B-20)	Pishu	Below the spinous process of the 11th Thoracic vertebra, 1.5 Cun lateral to the midline	Tonification point for the Spleen
Bladder 23 (B-23)	Shenshu	Below the spinous process of the 2nd Lumbar vertebra, 1.5 Cun lateral to the midline	Used for bone and joint disorders and any loss of Kidney Qi
Bladder 25 (B-25)	Dachangshu	Below the spinous process of the 4th Lumbar vertebra, 1.5 Cun lateral to the midline	Local point for low back pain
Bladder 26 (B-26)	Guanyuanshu	Below the spinous process of the 5th Lumbar vertebra, 1.5 Cun lateral to the midline	As above
Bladder 39 (B-39)	Weiyang	At the lateral end of the popliteal crease, medial to the tendon of biceps femoris	Useful when treated with moxa for knee pain
Bladder 40 (B-40)	Weizhong	Midpoint of the popliteal crease, between tendons of biceps femoris and semitendinosus muscle	Skin conditions Removes heat from blood Distal point for lumbar pain
Bladder 54 (B-54)	Zhibian	On the buttock, level with the 4th sacral foramen, 3 Cun lateral to the median sacral crest	Local low back pain point
Bladder 57 (B-57)	Chengshan	On the midline of the calf, in the pointed depression formed below gastrocnemius belly when the heel is lifted	Haemorrhoids Muscle cramp
Bladder 60 (B-60)	Kunlun	Posterior to the lateral malleolus, between the tip and the achilles tendon	Important distal point to the channel Particularly used in neck pain
Bladder 62 (B-62)	Shenmai	On the lateral side of the foot in the depression directly below the external malleolus	Used in combination with Houxi SI-3 for autoimmune disorders, e.g. rheumatoid arthritis
Bladder 67 (B-67)	Zhiyin	On the lateral side of the distal phalanx of the little toe, 0.1 Cun from the corner of the toenail	Used with moxa to turn a breech baby

Gall Bladder channel

Important points on the Gall Bladder channel are listed in Table 3.5. Leg points on this channel are shown in Figure 3.15 (see also Figs 3.13, 3.18).

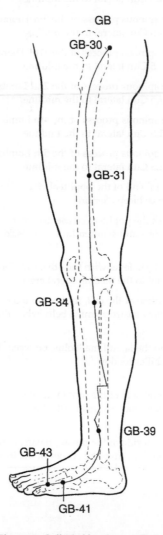

Fig. 3.15 *Gall Bladder channel (leg).*

Table 3.5 *Gall Bladder channel points*

Number	Name	Location	Additional actions
Gall Bladder 2 (GB-2)	Tinghui	On the face, anterior to the intertragic notch, in depression posterior to the condyloid process with the mouth open (see Fig. 3.18)	Deafness, tinnitus
Gall Bladder 14 (GB-14)	Yangbai	On the forehead, 1 Cun above the centre of the eyebrow Pinch insertion, down towards eye (see Fig. 3.18)	Headache, migraine, sinusitis, and trigeminal neuralgia
Gall Bladder 20 (GB-20)	Fengchi	On the nape, below the occipittal bone, in the depression between the upper ends of Sternocleidomastoid and Trapezius (see Fig. 3.18)	Torticollis, cervical spondylosis, dizziness, hypertension Headache
Gall Bladder 21 (GB-21)	Jianjing	On the shoulder directly above the nipple on the midpoint of the line connecting Dazhui (AV-14) and the acromion. Care!	Periarthritis of the shoulder Neck problems
Gall Bladder 30 (GB-30)	Huantiao	On the lateral side of the thigh, at the junction of the middle third and lateral third of the line connecting the greater trochanter and the sacral hiatus, hip slightly flexed	Sciatica, low back pain, paralysis of the leg
Gall Bladder 31 (GB-31)	Fengshi	Lateral midline of the thigh, 7 Cun above the popliteal crease	Motor point for paralysis of the leg
Gall Bladder 34 (GB-34)	Yanglingquan	On the lateral side of the leg, in the depression anterior and inferior to the head of the fibula	Influential point for muscles and tendons. Acupressure point
Gall Bladder 39 (GB-39)	Xuanzhong	On the lateral side of the leg, 3 Cun above the tip of the lateral malleolus, on the anterior border of the fibula	Influential point for marrow Distal point for torticollis
Gall Bladder 41 (GB-41)	Foot Linqi	Posterior to the 4th metatarsophalangeal joint, in the depression lateral to the extensor muscle of the little toe	Deafness, mastitis, dysmenorrhoea
Gall Bladder 43 (GB-43)	Xiaxi	Proximal to the margin of the web between the 4th and 5th toes	Important distal point for knee pain

Stomach channel

Important points on the Stomach channel are listed in Table 3.6. Leg points on this channel are shown in Figure 3.16 (see also Figs 3.17, 3.18).

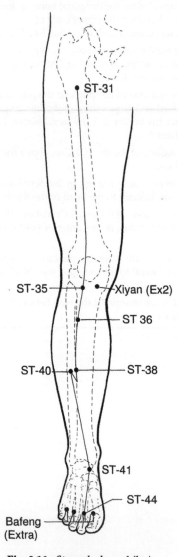

Fig. 3.16 *Stomach channel (leg).*

Table 3.6 *Stomach channel points*

Number	Name	Location	Additional actions
Stomach 7 (ST-7)	Xiaguan	On the face, anterior to the ear, in the depression between the zygomatic arch and mandibular notch (see Fig. 3.18)	Facial palsy
Stomach 8 (ST-8)	Touwei	On the lateral side of the head, 0.5 Cun above the anterior hairline at the corner of the forehead, 4.5 Cun lateral to the midline. Oblique insertion (see Fig. 3.18)	Migraine, frontal and parietal headache. Excessive lacrimation
Stomach 25 (ST-25)	Tianshu	On the middle abdomen, 2 Cun lateral to the centre of the umbilicus (see Fig. 3.17)	Acute and chronic gastric problems including diarrhoea and constipation
Stomach 31 (ST-31)	Biguan	On the anterior side of the thigh and on the line connecting the anteriosuperior iliac spine	Local for anterior hip pain Paralysis of lower limb
Stomach 35 (ST-35)	Dubi	With the knee flexed, on the knee, in the depression lateral to the patella and its ligament	Lateral "eye" of the knee
Stomach 36 (ST-36)	Zusanli	On the anterolateral side of the leg, 3 Cun below Dubi (ST-35), one finger breadth from the anterior crest of the tibia	Major general tonification point Acupressure point
Stomach 38 (ST-38)	Tiaokou	On the anterolateral side of the leg, 8 Cun below Dubi (ST-35), one finger breadth from the anterior crest of the tibia	Used in shoulder pain
Stomach 40 (ST-40)	Fenglong	As Tiaokou, but two fingerbreadths from the anterior crest of the tibia	Bronchitis, hay fever
Stomach 41 (ST-41)	Jiexi	Central depression between tendons of extensor hallucis longus and extensor digiti longus on the ankle crease	Local point for ankle pain
Stomach 44 (ST-44)	Neiting	Proximal to the margin of the web between 2nd and 3rd toes	Important distal point. Toothache, headache. General anaesthesia

Head points

Many channels cross the head. Some important points are shown in Figure 3.17.

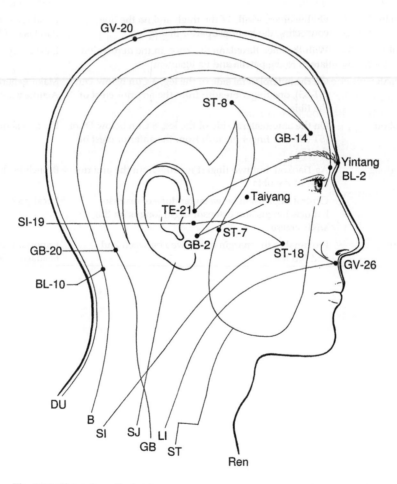

Fig. 3.17 *Channels on the head.*

Trunk channel points

The Conception Vessel runs down the front of the trunk. Some important points are listed in Table 3.7. Other points include those in Figure 3.18. The back of the trunk includes points on the Governor Vessel (Table 3.8). Other back channels are shown in Figure 3.13.

Extra points

Extra points not on meridians are listed in Table 3.6. Points on the back are shown in Figure 3.19.

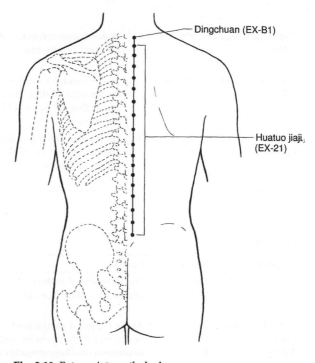

Fig. 3.19 *Extra points on the back.*

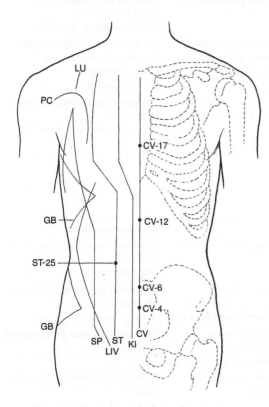

Fig. 3.18 *Channels on the front of the trunk.*

Table 3.7 *Conception vessel points*

Number	Name	Location	Additional actions
Conception Vessel 4 (CV-4)	Guanyuan	On the lower abdomen, on the midline, 3 Cun below the centre of the umbilicus	Dysmenorrhoea Good moxibustion point Acupressure point
Conception Vessel 6 (CV-6)	Qihai	On the lower abdomen, on the midline, 1.5 Cun below the centre of the umbilicus	General tonification point Acupressure point
Conception Vessel 12 (CV-12)	Zhongwan	On the lower abdomen, on the midline, 4 Cun above the centre of the umbilicus	Gastritis Nausea and vomiting
Conception Vessel 17 (CV-17)	Shanzhong	On the chest, on the midline, at the level of the 4th intercostal space, on the xiphisternum. Oblique insertion	Bronchial asthma, tight chest

Table 3.8 *Governor vessel points*

Number	Name	Location	Additional actions
Governor Vessel 2 (GV-2)	Yaoshu	On the sacrum, on the midline at the sacral hiatus	Useful point for central low back pain
Governor Vessel 4 (GV-4)	Mingmen	In the depression below the spinous process of the 2nd lumbar vertebra	Lumbago and sciatica Important point for treating depleted body energy. Suitable for Moxibustion
Governor Vessel 14 (GV-14)	Dazhui	In the depression below the spinous process of the 7th cervical vertebra	Occipital headache. Fever Depression Immune-enhancing effect
Governor Vessel 20 (GV-20)	Baihui	On the head, 5 Cun directly above the midpoint of the anterior hairline at the midpoint of the line connecting the apices of both ears. Oblique insertion	Psychologically effective point Sedation, harmonization Used in prolapse No stimulation
Governor Vessel 26 (GV-26)	Renzhong or Shuigou	On the face at the junction of the upper third and middle third of the philtrum. (Pinch insertion, up towards nose)	Emergency stimulation, in shock, or collapse Used to mobilize stiff lumbar spine

Table 3.9 *Extra points*

Number	Name	Location	Additional actions
Extra, Head and Neck (EX-2)	Yintang	On the forehead at the midpoint between the eyebrows Oblique insertion (see Fig. 3.18)	Rhinitis, frontal headache, frontal sinusitis Mood lightener
Extra, Head and Neck (EX-5)	Taiyang	At the temporal part of the head, between the lateral end of the eyebrow and the outer canthus, in the depression one fingerbreadth behind them (see Fig. 3.18)	Headache, migraine, toothache, trigeminal neuralgia
Extra, Upper Extremity (EX-30)	Baxie	Four points on the dorsum of each hand, proximal to the edge of the webs between the fingers. Hegu (LI-4) is often used as one of the Baxie points (see Fig. 3.11)	Particularly useful in arthritis of the hand
Extra, Lower Extremity (EX-45)	Bafeng	Four points on each foot, proximal to the margins of the webs between the toes (see Fig. 3.16)	Arthritis and parasthesia of the toes
Extra, Lower Extremity (EX-2)	Xiyan or Neixiyan	In the depression medial to the patellar ligament when the knee is flexed (see Fig. 3.16)	Medial "eye" of the knee Knee pain
Extra points of the Back (EX-1)	Huatuojiaji	On the back and low back, 17 points on each side, below the spinous processes from the 1st Thoracic to the 5th Lumbar vertebrae, 0.5 Cun lateral to the posterior midline	Pain along the spine, segmental radiation
	Dingchuan	On the back, below the spinous process of the 7th verterbrae, 0.5 cun lateral to the midline (sometimes known as EX-B1)	Asthma

4

Safe practice, needle techniques and types of needle

Val Hopwood

This chapter will consider some of the practicalities associated with acupuncture treatment and some of the problems that physiotherapists are likely to encounter when starting to practice.

It must be borne in mind that acupuncture is a very emotive topic; it is probably the ultimate in invasive techniques available to a physiotherapist and the idea of penetrating the skin is one that a lot of health professionals are not very comfortable with. The concept alone is enough to produce a quick negative reaction from many physiotherapy managers and certainly from those higher or lower management personnel without a clear picture of what is involved.

That said, there are many sensible ways of minimizing the risk and the trauma both to the therapist and the patient. The newspapers are full of stories about AIDS, and the association with infections caused by sharing needles for whatever reason strike a chill into most hearts. Physiotherapists who undertake a training in acupuncture have a responsibility to themselves and their patients to be sure from the outset of their practice that the principles of safe, hygienic insertion and needle disposal will be adhered to.

Needles and hygiene

It cannot be stated strongly enough that those physiotherapists who cannot guarantee complete sterilization of used needles should not be practising. Presterilized, disposable needles are the obvious choice and are strongly recommended for use in those countries with a health service able to afford them.

Disposal of these needles is then crucial and the needles and any associated dressing material or used cotton wool must be incinerated as close to the site of use as is possible. Sharps are usually disposed of by high temperature incineration at special plants; they must never be discarded at the local rubbish tip!

It is recognized, however, that one-use disposable needles are an expensive item in what is likely to be an already stretched physiotherapy budget in most countries. Autoclaving of used needles is quite safe, provided the temperature is high enough and the holding times after sterilization are carefully followed. Care must be taken to keep the needles in sterile, lidded containers afterwards. If disposable needles are too expensive then autoclaving is the best way to guarantee sterility.

Table 4.1 shows the minimum acceptable holding time for each temperature, when autoclaving needles.

Glass bead sterilizers are sometimes used for acupuncture needles but not enough is known about their effect on the needles and research on the optimal width, depth and temperature of the units and the length of time for the sterilization of the needles is inconclusive (Morrison 1989). They are not recommended at present.

Table 4.1 *Minimum holding times for needles in an autoclave*

Temperature (°C)	Minimum holding time (min) after temperature is achieved
121	15
126	10
134	3

Where needles are being reused and sterilized any risk is to the therapist rather than to the patient as long as the autoclaving procedures are followed. The therapist should never handle the shaft of the needle and great care should be taken on withdrawing the needle from the patient that the patient's body fluids, either blood or plasma, do not come into contact with those of the operator. This means essentially that any open wounds or breaks in the skin on the hands must be covered by a plaster before treatment commences. All patients should be assumed to be HIV positive when being given acupuncture treatment, so that it is not necessary to ask the question. The therapist should always keep a sharps box or lidded container beside the patient.

The AIDS virus is in fact rather less viable than the hepatitis virus (A, B and C forms) so equally great care must be taken to eliminate all risk of passing the latter on. The hepatitis virus is easy to catch, has long term health consequences and is more difficult to destroy by disinfection or sterilization. The same rules apply as with HIV precautions: all patients must be assumed to be infected, the needles must either be safely disposed of by burning or correctly autoclaved and any open areas on the operator's skin must be covered. The part of the needle which has been in contact with the body fluids of the patient must not be handled by the therapist. There is always a danger of a needlestick injury when handling any kind of needle. All health authorities will have a procedure for dealing with this and the physiotherapist must be familiar with it for his or her own protection.

Since large numbers of patients with AIDS have now turned to alternative therapies, including acupuncture, this means of transmission may become increasingly important, not only to thousands of patients, but also to the acupuncturists themselves, through needlestick accidents.

Swabs

Basic needling technique usually involves the use of some sort of skin-cleansing agent before insertion of the needle. It is debatable whether a quick wipe with an alcohol swab truly serves to disinfect the skin

surface. Certain groups of regular needle users, such as diabetics, use the same needle again and do not routinely swab the skin prior to injection. Yet these people do not get infections at their injection sites and dentists have been injecting local anaesthetics without skin preparation for years (Korista & Felig 1992).

The host will usually have acquired resistance to their own bacteria and new bacteria must be injected through the skin in some concentration in order for an infection to occur. The amount varies with the type of organism. Wiping the skin with an alcohol swab has been shown to remove a large proportion of the resident bacteria but will not sterilize the skin (Dan 1967). Washing the skin with soap and water also reduces the number of organisms present so it is most important that the practitioner removes excess bacteria from their own hands before commencing treatment. It is also true that a hollow needle has a greater potential for conveying organisms into the body than a thinner, solid acupuncture needle. Hence for normal patients all that is required for safe penetration of the skin is to ensure that the skin is clean and the practitioner has washed their hands thoroughly. It is not necessary to wear gloves.

It is of course possible to treat immunodeficient patients; these are a group that will often benefit greatly from acupuncture. T Cells, B Cells and phagocytes complement one another and work in the body combining natural and adaptive immunity mechanisms to provide a versatile and durable defence system against microbial invaders. Thus in those patients who are immunologically challenged a defect of a trivial nature may show in chronic or recurrent infections, or incomplete recovery or unsatisfactory responses to treatment.

Immunodeficiency may be primary, due to genetic defects, or secondary, due to malignancy, autoimmune disease, protein-losing states or chronic infections. Immunodeficiency may also be caused by some drugs and radiotherapy.

Patients who may be at increased risk from infections and who would benefit from having the sites of acupuncture sterilized include those with some of the following:

- lymphoproliferative diseases e.g. Hodgkin's lymphoma

- leukaemia
- malignancies
- autoimmune diseases
- organ transplants e.g. kidney
- AIDS
- organ damage e.g. heart valves.

To achieve skin sterilization in as short a time as 2 min, a 1–2% solution of iodine in 70% alcohol can be used. This can be obtained as a preprepared skin wipe. Alternatively 2% chlorhexidine can be used.

Since information on the sorts of conditions above may not always be available it is wise to ask the patient the following questions:

- Do you have any current medical problems for which you are receiving treatment?
- Are you on any medication, and do you know if it is an immune-suppressing drug?
- Are you given antibiotic cover when dental work is done?

If answers to any of the above lead you to suspect a compromised immune system then sterilize the skin prior to treatment. This is a simple procedure. First, locate the acupuncture points, wipe the skin with an iodine swab and while waiting the required 2 min wash your own hands.

Needling techniques

It is difficult to be dogmatic about needling techniques, as most practitioners evolve their own over the years and there seems to be a wide variation. Two main things emerge, however: it is essential that the process is relatively painless for the patient, and it seems to be necessary that "Deqi" or needling sensation is achieved most of the time. (Professor Andersson has gone into the physiological reasoning behind this in more detail in Chapter 2, so it will not be repeated here.)

Chinese literature is full of details of precise needling techniques claiming to have different needling effects. The most important of these are those for sedating and those for tonifying an acupoint. If the practitioner is from the Five Element school of practice this is a very important distinction.

When a needle is inserted to a certain depth, the patient may feel soreness, numbness or distension around the point. The operator may also feel some tenseness around the needle. This is known as the "arrival of Qi" or Deqi. If it does not manifest itself then the needle may be lifted and rotated quickly a couple of times to encourage it. Scraping the wound part of the handle with the fingernail gives a gentle vibration which can sometimes be effective in producing the Qi sensation. Gentle flicking to the needle is also sometimes used.

According to what is perceived as the clinical situation, either Excess or Deficiency of Qi, the needle can then be further manipulated. To reinforce or tonify the Qi the needle is lifted gently and slowly and then thrust down again rapidly. To sedate or reduce, the reverse action is performed. It is difficult to state precisely what is achieved by either technique, however, and some practitioners use only an even method, trusting to the homeostatic inclination of the body to obtain appropriate stimulation.

If patients are treated with acupuncture they will generally require at least three treatments before the therapist can be certain that there is a reaction. Strong reactors will show changes immediately after the first treatment, and may even grow slightly worse, but the majority of patients experience a gradual change in symptoms. TCM holds that 10 treatments form a course of treatment and often patients can be given as many as three courses. However, economic medicine, as it is frequently practised in the countries where physical therapists use acupuncture, demands results much more quickly. Most patients do not receive more than seven or eight treatments in total and still achieve good results. Where the problem is chronic then patients should be encouraged to return every 6 months or so for "top-up" treatments to keep the symptoms under control, bearing in mind that they will need only one or two.

Types of needle

The most commonly used needles are made of stainless steel with a solid shaft. The classic needle has a layer of fine coiled wire as a handle, but some have a light plastic handle with varying colours to indicate the gauge of the needle shaft. Thicker needles are easier to use when a deep insertion is required, especially for a beginner, since it is easy to buckle a long, fine needle. Some practitioners use thicker needles in order to gain more stimulation at the acupoint and there is no doubt that a very fine needle produces less sensation.

In order to use the thinner variety, a guide tube is necessary. Some practitioners prefer to use these at all times since the sensation of pressure on the skin where the tube is pressing detracts from the initial pin prick. Others find that the important feedback to the operator is missing and it is more difficult to achieve instant Deqi.

It is necessary to use all-metal needles when using moxabustion but otherwise selection is guided by the preference of the therapist. Needles come in varying lengths from 10 mm to 125 mm.

Intradermal needles

These are like tiny thumb tacks and can be used under a piece of sticking plaster to maintain a constant stimulation at an acupoint. They are not recommended for use on body points and should be used for ear acupuncture, but only with care since infection is always possible when a foreign body is left in the tissues for any length of time. Their use is no longer advocated by physiotherapists in the UK and non-invasive seeds under plaster are thought preferable.

Seven Star or Plum Blossom needles

These comprise several smaller needles inlaid into a small round plate attached vertically to a flexible handle 12–15 cm long. These are still used in some parts of the world but not generally recommended since the prevalence of AIDS as some light bleeding may occur and the needles themselves are difficult to sterilize.

Short wedge-shaped needles

These have a cutting edge and are specifically designed to cause a drop of blood to be produced, particularly in conditions where there is excess heat.

However, they must be used with great care and they are no longer recommended for the same reasons as the others mentioned previously.

How the needle is inserted and what type of manipulation is given to it subsequently would seem to be a relatively straightforward topic. However, many books have been written on the subject and there are many variations on the simple insertion technique, all claiming to have a different effect on the body. Since this information is presented essentially to persuade those who know little or nothing of acupuncture to seek out a formal training and begin to practise themselves, it is better not to confuse the issue with complicated theories that have little scientific validation.

Simple needling technique consists of the following steps:

1. Wash hands.
2. Locate the acupuncture point.
3. Swab the skin over the point.
4. Select a needle of the correct length.
5. Hold at the far end or handle; do not handle the shaft. (This will not apply initially if using an insertion tube.)
6. Push the needle quickly into the skin in order to minimize the skin pain. The other hand can be used to exert gentle distracting pressure or stretch the surrounding skin.
7. Slowly and gently advance the needle to the required depth. A degree of rotation is optional but it should be equally in clockwise and anticlockwise directions in order to prevent muscle tissue being caught up painfully.
8. When the needle has been retained for the desired period of time it should be gently withdrawn, using finger pressure from the other hand to help release it.
9. As a general rule a cotton wool ball should be applied immediately to the hole to prevent a minor bleed and possible bruise.
10. Both needle and cotton wool should then be disposed of carefully as explained previously.

It is immediately clear that the preceding description leaves a lot out. There are many techniques for needle insertion; some practitioners enter the skin very slowly with a degree of rotation, others favour a short, sharp entry and advance rapidly to the required depth. Some use a single-handed technique only; others use guidance tubes or stabilize the base of a longer needle with a small piece of sterile cotton wool (Figs 4.1, 4.2, 4.3).

The most important thing about acupuncture needling is that it must be painless for the patient, or they will not return, and the needling sensation should be obtained at nearly every point. This

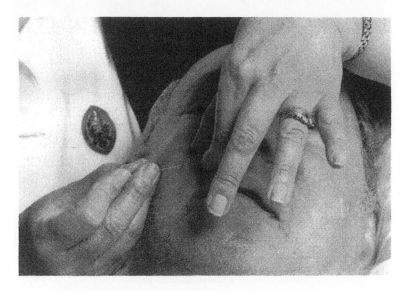

Fig. 4.1 *Beginning of insertion into a pinch of skin (25 mm needle LI-20 Yingxiang).*

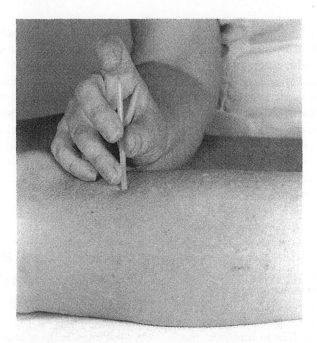

Fig. 4.2 *Simple one-handed insertion using guide tube (40 mm needle GB-34 Yanglingquan).*

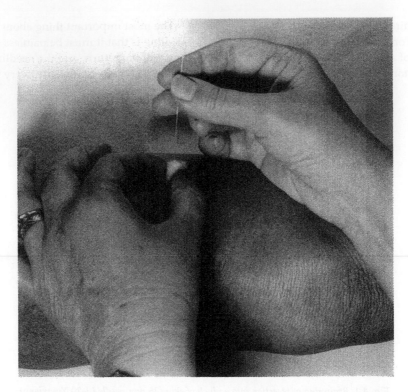

Fig. 4.3 *Simple insertion, left fingers stretching skin (40 mm needle ST-40 Fenglong).*

needling sensation or "Deqi" is almost unique to acupuncture and is difficult to describe precisely. Most people describe it as either a numbness, a spreading sensation, a feeling of fullness, warmth or, occasionally, like an electric shock. It can sometimes be felt along the course of the meridian and skilled . practitioners are able to direct the energy up or down according to the effect they want.

It is said to be possible to control the type of stimulus and hence the treatment given by the way the needle is subsequently manipulated. A sedating technique can be used for pain relief, but the point may also be tonified and more energy supplied to the area where a deficiency is suspected. Sedation requires that the needle be inserted and left with no further manipulation for up to 20 min. The more complicated Chinese techniques need considerable needling experience to accomplish.

When using acupuncture for pain relief, the simplest form of treatment will be to "unblock" the channel concerned. Points should be selected at or near the painful site on channels that pass over or near the area. Points proximal and distal to the site of pain are usually added, together with local trigger points or "Ah Shi" points. Many acupuncture textbooks have been published giving groups of recommended points for the treatment of common painful conditions and these formulae may help in the selection for an individual patient. However, ultimately the above guide is likely to be the most effective for a simple painful problem and this is all that a novice should attempt to tackle without further training.

Precautions and contraindications with acupuncture treatment

A good knowledge of anatomy is essential in order to be able to insert acupuncture needles safely and intelligently. There are obviously some areas of the body that pose a greater risk than others. When using the simple selection of points commonly used for pain relief given elsewhere in this book the possible hazards are highlighted with each point, but as a general guide the following areas should be avoided at all times:

- the scalp area of infants before the fontanelles have closed
- nipples and breast tissue
- the umbilicus
- external genitalia.

The following guidelines have been taken from the 1995 revision of the Acupuncture Association of Chartered Physiotherapists in the UK.

General precautions

Painful treatment The needle may be painful on insertion but the pain should not persist after the initial stimulation is achieved. If pain persists the needle should be removed.

Broken needle If the needle breaks in situ, the point of entry should be marked and immediate medical help sought. Using a needle of the correct length at each point will minimize this risk.

Uncontrolled movements Patients with uncontrolled movements who are unable to remain still for any length of time are not suitable for treatment.

Drowsiness Some patients may feel very relaxed and even sleepy after treatment. They should be advised not to drive until they have fully recovered (Brattberg 1986).

Infection The skin should always be carefully examined for infection prior to treatment, if there is any indication of possible infection then medical advice should be sought. Very thin and fragile skin should not be needled.

Needlestick injury Those physiotherapists working in the NHS should follow their health authority needlestick policy. Those in private practice should consult their own doctor or seek advice from the nearest casualty department.

Allergy Some patients are allergic to specific metals and any known allergy of this nature should be ascertained prior to treatment with needles.

Special precautions

Special care should be taken when needling the groups of patients in the following sections.

Pregnant patients There is a danger of miscarriage when treating patients in the first trimester of pregnancy and of premature labour in the last 2 months if the wrong points are used. It is essential that practitioners are aware of these. Extra care must be taken with the selection of points at all times during a pregnancy. As a general rule the following points should not be used:

- LI-4 Hegu
- SP-6 Sanyinjiao
- B-67 Zhiyin
- B-60 Kunlun
- KI-3 Taixi
- GB-21 Jianjing.

Diabetics Care should be taken when needling diabetic patients because of the danger of poor peripheral circulation and the effect of some points on blood sugar levels.

Hazardous acupoints Certain points are located in potentially dangerous areas of the body. The practitioner must be aware of the hazard and needle with appropriate care.

Some points are useful, but need special care and are not for beginners. The most commonly used point in this category is GB-21, Jianjing. Since it is situated right over the apex of the lung, an injudicious needle here has been known to cause pneumothorax. However it would be evident to any physical therapist that the lung is close by. The technique for needling this point safely is to raise the tissue on the edge of trapezius into a pinch and needle horizontally into this, from back to front. GB-21 is a very useful point for both neck and shoulder pain (possessing other actions that make it also useful in TCM) and should not be left out of the prescription but just needled very carefully. Care should also be taken when needling CV-17 Shanzhong, as it is occasionally possible to penetrate the thoracic cavity here, but if care is taken always to needle obliquely there is no danger. These two aside, there are no other particularly hazardous points in the tables of suggested points in this book.

Frail patients Patients with a weak constitution after prolonged chronic illness will tolerate acupuncture poorly. Minimal treatment must be given. Extra care should be taken with those with known low blood pressure. Do not use a combination of Hegu (LI-4) and Quchi (LI-11) bilaterally since this combination is known to lower blood pressure.

Pacemakers Patients with pacemakers should not be given electroacupuncture.

Confused patients Great care must be taken with patients who are unable to understand the procedure. Those unable to cooperate must not be treated.

Acknowledgements

Thanks to PAPMA, the New Zealand group members of IAAPT, for permission to use material from the PAPMA training course in this chapter. Thanks also to AACP for permission to reprint part of their Guidelines for good practice.

References

Acupuncture Association of Chartered Physiotherapists 1995 Guidelines for safe practice. AACP

Brattberg G 1986 Acupuncture treatment: a traffic hazard? American Journal of Acupuncture 14(3): 265–267

Dan T C 1967 Routine skin preparation before injection. Lancet July 12: 96–98

Korista V A, Felig P 1992 Is skin preparation necessary before insulin injections? Lancet May 20: 1072–1073

Morrison S C 1989 Sterilization of acupuncture needles. Physiotherapy Canada 41(6): 31–32

5

Assessment procedures

Maureen Lovesey

Health is defined by the World Health Organization as physical, mental and emotional well-being of the person providing the ability to maintain a balance in life and participate in a fully active life to achieve a full potential as a human being. This follows the triangle of health put forward by TCM and other traditional philosophies (Fig. 5.1). In ancient China traditional doctors were paid to keep their patients well; patients paid regularly to maintain health – their aim being to prevent illness, not to cure it. In fact the doctor would be responsible for paying for medicines and treatment if their "service" failed to keep the patient healthy. In contrast, Western medicine is largely concerned with managing illness and relieving symptoms; however, development of health care in Western industrial societies is moving towards a more preventative approach.

Physiotherapy is usually recommended when a physical loss of function or ability is found. The reasons that the public seek out acupuncture may be for much vaguer reasons such as "restoring energy", overcoming exhaustion and stress – problems not usually referred to a physiotherapist in the first instance, unless they are specialists working in mental illness teams. However, there are problems for which a person would seek either a physiotherapist or an acupuncturist. There are also many conditions met in physiotherapy practice in which acupuncture can be added as an adjunct to treatment. Examples of the first instance include musculoskeletal disorders and pain or discomfort. Further training in a more comprehensive approach is required in order to treat a wider range of conditions such as neurological, respiratory, urogenital, skin disorders or addictions, to mention a few conditions which are seen by physiotherapists.

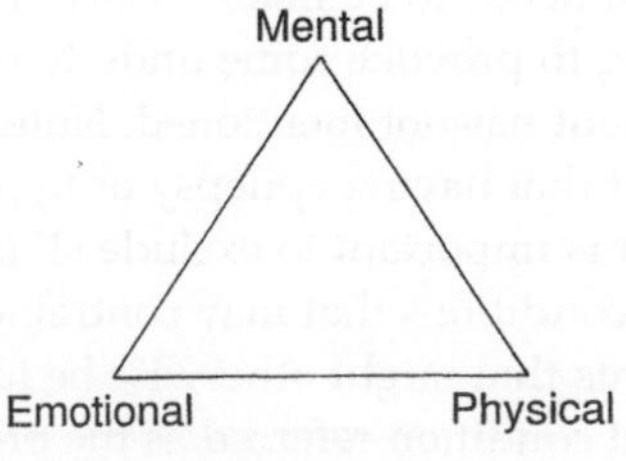

Recording

The physiotherapist must make a full assessment of the patient's condition on first consultation and all appropriate findings must be recorded and kept up to date within 24 hours of seeing the patient.

Note: Do not forget that this is a legal record.

Accurate assessment is an essential tool in formulating an effective programme. A clear assessment and recording of practice using a standardized system means that clinical practice can be monitored and evaluated, which can be used as a research tool. It also facilitates treatment changeovers where treatment has to be carried out by different practitioners.

Fig. 5.1 *The WHO "triangle of health" of traditional medicine.*

Assessment procedures

There are many methods of assessment. Whichever method is used, however, it should follow a logical sequence but not be so rigid as to fail to allow for personal preference on the part of the person being assessed or the assessor. It is essential that the patient's reasons for seeking assistance are fully understood by the assessor and that these are taken into account when planning a treatment programme as the assessor's views on the situation may differ from those of the patient.

As this book is primarily concerned with an introduction to acupuncture for the treatment of pain involving mainly musculoskeletal or superficial/external problems, it is beyond the scope of this book to deal with more deep-seated or internal problems, except possibly for the relief of pain in terminally ill patients. Two possible assessment procedures are put forward that are suitable for the above cases; it is possible to use a mixture of the two.

The first is a Western-type approach, which is particularly suited to musculoskeletal problems and follows both subjective and objective routes (Cyriax 1975). The second is an introduction to TCM assessment. It can be seen that there is much common ground between the two and they may be used in conjunction. Other methods include a Western approach of measuring and balancing electrical potential at different points.

In making a request for help some people feel nervous or apprehensive at being in surroundings that are perhaps new to them, being asked numerous questions and then being offered a treatment that may seem completely alien to them. Every effort should be made to put the person being assessed at ease and to establish some empathy with him/her and to treat them as a whole and not just an interesting case. The assessment should of course start with the individual's details which should include, name, address, telephone number, occupation, hobbies, method of referral, general practitioner and/or consultant.

Information will be particular to the set of problems but questions about feelings, thoughts and attitudes to illness are important. Recent research on the placebo effect indicates that the patient's expectations of outcome and beliefs influence the treatment. What is often called the placebo effect is the very important variable of motivation and patient belief that what he or she does will influence his or her health. Lack of participation with treatment indicates that the full resources that are available have not been engaged. To make the treatment most effective, patient participation with the treatment programme is a *sine qua non* (which directly translated means 'without which nothing').

Method one

Subjective

It is helpful to start with questions about the areas and behaviour of the pain. The pain should be mapped in on a chart (Fig. 5.2) with different areas of pain marked and numbered in order of severity and the type of pain, for example, ache, boring, tension, sharp, shooting, tingling, burning, throbbing, marked, and frequency (i.e. constant, periodic, occasional).

Details should be taken of the problem and how long it has been present, whether it came on suddenly or gradually, whether it has changed and whether it is getting worse, better or remaining the same. The patient should be asked if he or she knows what may have caused the problem and a list should be made of what aggravates it and what helps, including time of day and sleeping patterns. When the pain is aggravated it is important to find out how long it takes to ease or to settle down again to its previous level as this can be used as a benchmark for assessing progress. A condition that takes more than a few minutes to settle down from a higher level is known as irritable. Medication, general health, X-rays and past history should be noted.

When first seeing the patient, a thorough investigation needs to be made to ensure that you are not going to provoke some underlying condition that the patient has not mentioned. Note the effects on treatment that having epilepsy or hypertension may have. It is important to exclude all known underlying conditions that may contraindicate any of the treatments that might otherwise be ideal for the specific local condition referred as the presenting problem. Assessment in Chinese medicine includes a

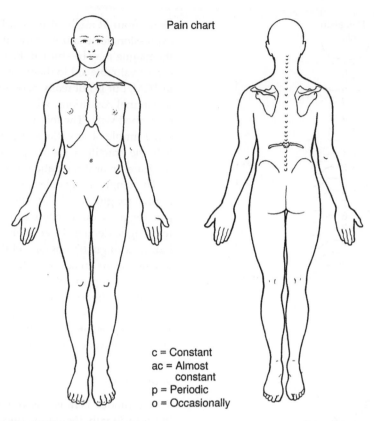

Pain chart

c = Constant
ac = Almost
     constant
p = Periodic
o = Occasionally

Fig. 5.2 *Outline for pain chart.*

systematic questioning on all the body systems – cardiovascular, neurological, respiratory, ear, nose and throat, skin, digestion, sensation, blood pressure scores, menstrual history and any symptoms, including past medical history as well as medication. Before proceeding to treatment if there is any doubt about the patient's condition further discussion should take place with the patient's physician with a view to possible further medical screening.

Objective

Gait should be observed and noted; a note should also be made of general posture and any deformities. Passive and active movements and muscular testing should be carried out that are relevant to the problem and measurements noted. If appropriate a neurological check should be carried out. The area should then be palpated for temperature, accessory

movements, stiffness, tenderness, trigger spots, etc. The findings must be accurately recorded; diagrams can be helpful particularly for spinal problems (Fig. 5.3).

Note: The above testing is not described in detail as it assumes that the assessor is familiar with normal joint range and muscle strength and testing from previous training.

Method two

This is based on a simple form of TCM assessment that comprises:

- listening
- looking
- smelling
- palpation.

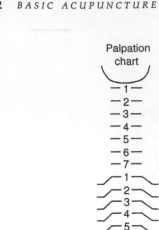

Fig. 5.3 *Spine chart.*

It will be seen from the above headings that there is much similarity between the two approaches.

1. Listening

A careful history of the problem should be taken, including what aggravates and what eases it as in method one, and a pain chart made out. Additional questions might include whether the problem is affected by the weather. Patients with arthritis often mention they are worse when the weather is damp or cold; cold would indicate that the use of moxa or heat would be appropriate, whilst the use of spleen points can be useful in patients affected by the damp (see Chapter 1).

2. Looking

This would again include observation and noting of gait, posture and deformities, etc., and also general demeanour. It might also include facial colour and expression, for example dark circles under eyes; also the tongue may be studied. Examining the tongue is a very valuable aid to diagnosis of internal problems in TCM, but is not really necessary for the treatment of external conditions, which this book is most concerned with. The following gives a description of some simple observations of the tongue that may help the practitioner when planning the treatment programme or if the patient is not improving.

The tongue body colour is very important; a normal tongue should be a healthy pink colour. A pale tongue would denote a lack of Qi or energy. A red tongue denotes Heat. A blue/purple tongue indicates stagnation of Qi and Blood. A swollen tongue means an accumulation of fluid in the body. A thick coating usually denotes something like catarrh or a digestive upset. A white coating indicates Cold and a yellow one indicates Heat (see Chapter 1). It is important to note, however, that the colour etc. of the tongue can be distorted by medication.

3. Smelling

This technique is rarely used in Western medicine, but occasionally there is a noticeable smell to the skin or the patient remarks that he has an unpleasant taste in his mouth.

4. Palpation

The area is palpated for hot or cold, swelling and sore or trigger spots. The state of the internal organs can be gauged from taking the pulse. Pulse diagnosis is highly skilled in TCM, and this is beyond the scope of the present book. For external conditions it is not really necessary to take the pulse as the pulse should not be much changed. Generally, in internal conditions a slow pulse denotes Cold, a fast pulse denotes Heat and a wiry pulse denotes tension.

As mentioned earlier it may well be a good idea to use a combination of the above methods.

Treatment plan

After examination the problem should be discussed with the patient and a treatment plan put forward.

The pros and cons and aims of such a programme and alternatives should also be discussed so that the patient is aware of the choices available and can agree a treatment plan with the therapist. This is of paramount importance as any treatment or testing undertaken without the patient's consent, however innocuous, could constitute assault. If the patient is reluctant or refuses treatment the therapist may be able to persuade them to go ahead with treatment, but it must be born in mind that there is a fine line between persuasion and coercion. If the patient refuses treatment or testing this should be recorded in the notes. Consent is often implied by the patient positioning him/herself for testing or therapy, but a simple explanation such as "I am going to bend your knee to test your range of movement" is a better option and leaves no room for ambiguity.

If acupuncture is a treatment that the therapist feels would be of particular benefit to the patient, it must be remembered that to some people this will seem very alien. A careful explanation of the method will often overcome fears. Some people of course have an aversion to needles. If needling seems to be the best method of giving acupuncture then needle phobia may sometimes be overcome by talking through the situation and showing how fine the needles are and even inserting one. If the patient is not willing to go ahead with needle acupuncture they may be very happy with non-invasive methods (acupressure, etc.).

Treatment effects

When using acupuncture, patients should be advised that they need to 'take it easy' for an hour or so after treatment and rest if possible as they may feel slightly tired, light headed or both. It is often a good idea to use a smaller number of points than usual in the first treatment, particularly if the patient is not particularly robust, so that the effects of acupuncture on that patient can be observed. The patient should also be advised that the effects of acupuncture can vary considerably, from someone who gets off the bed and feels better, through someone who feels better some time after treatment (often the next day), to a slight worsening of the condition. (This is normally temporary and usually means the treatment will be successful.) A few people do not

respond to acupuncture, but it is worth trying six to eight treatments particularly in chronic conditions, which are often slow to respond.

Choosing points

When choosing acupuncture for a musculoskeletal problem such as a sprain or osteoarthritis of a joint, consideration should be given to which channels, nerve roots or dermatomes pass through the problem area; trigger or "Ah Shi" points should also be identified. Both local and distal points should be chosen. Ear points can also be used.

For more generalized conditions such as rheumatoid arthritis, general points to help the immune system and swelling such as ST-36 and SP-4 or SP-6 may be used as well as local points. For generalized pain or cancer pain, potent points such as LI-4 can be very helpful. Internal problems are more complex and are beyond the scope of this book, but for conditions such as asthma the points would include lung points and/or bladder points on the upper dorsal spine.

Monitoring treatment outcomes

Whichever method of treatment is used it is most important to identify some benchmark tests for monitoring and reassessment purposes. These might include range of movement tests from the objective findings, and from the subjective assessment the length of time that a patient can do an activity such as sitting before the pain comes on or gets worse. It is best to choose one treatment only at first so that the effects of this treatment can be taken into account before additional treatment (excluding advice) is included. Patients can be poor historians and do not always remember how bad they were. Subtle improvements such as the ability to do more before the onset of pain or taking less analgesics are often not noticed unless carefully questioned and recorded at subsequent visits. It is often useful to get the patient to keep a record of pain. This can be done as a graph or by using a simple chart such as the example in Figure 5.4. In this the pain is often noted on a scale of 0–10, (where 0 = no pain; 10 = very severe pain). The chart can be further enhanced by including T = treatment, M = medication, * = extra activity etc., with further details entered under 'comments' (e.g. 'walked 2 miles'). If appropriate, notes on sleeping can also be included.

The above method is very easy to see at a glance, provides a good way of monitoring patients with predominantly painful conditions and is generally liked by patients who find it easy to use. Criticism is sometimes levied that keeping a pain chart encourages the patient to dwell on his/her "pain". However, the author of this chapter has been using the above method for many years and has found the reverse to be true; patients can be encouraged to think about their pain only four times a day instead of constantly dwelling on it as some do. Both patient and therapist can soon see from the record whether the treatment is having some effect; this is particularly important for patients with chronic pain who may have tried many other methods and for whom even a small percentage decrease in their pain can improve their mood and quality of life.

Other recording methods, including visual analogue scales, pain questionnaires, etc., may be used if desired but these are often more complicated and sometimes difficult to interpret.

Day	am	noon	pm	evening	comments
Mon					
Tues					
Wed					
Thurs					
Fri					
Sat					
Sun					

Pain to be noted on a scale of 0 -10 (10 =Very severe).
The chart can be further enhanced by including T or M (T=treatment, M =medication).
*marked by time of day to indicate extra activity, etc. and described under comments, e.g. walked 2 miles. If appropriate, notes on sleeping can also be included.

Fig. 5.4 *Pain record.*

Summary

- **Subjective assessment** Includes:
  referring problem
  past medical History
  lifestyle observations
  X-ray evidence
  pain profiles.
- **Objective assessment** Findings on examination
- **Treatment plan** Selection of acupuncture points
- **Goals.**

CASE STUDY 5.1

Mrs K   Age: 60   Occupation: housewife/supply teacher
Hobbies: golf, travel

Reason for referral Acute pain in neck and shoulder (see Fig. 5.5).

Assessment findings Mrs K presented as an emergency on New Year's Eve 1994. She had had pain in her neck and shoulder for about a month and this had become much worse in the last 2 days. The problem had come on suddenly and started in her neck and scapula; she had had a similar problem about 12 years previously, which had gradually cleared up and was helped by massage. She had continued to have massage once a week for 5–6 years as she found this was beneficial. She had started to have massage again about a month before and just after this her neck

became painful; this of course may have had nothing to do with her problem recurring. The only other thing that she thought may have attributed to causing her neck ache was that she started golf not long before. The problem had become more acute after lifting heavy boxes. Her problem was aggravated by driving, dressing herself and doing her hair. She was very bad at night, being kept awake for most of the night and also waking when she dozed. Medication included arthrotec, hormone replacement therapy, oil of evening primrose and occasionally paracetamol. She had not had an X-ray.

When I saw her she was in acute pain so I was not able to examine her fully. She had a lot of problem undressing, which increased her pain. Her neck movements were quite good but all her shoulder movements were grossly limited. Other findings were as follows:

Elevation: (R) 170; ↑   (L) 30 (active),   80 (passive).
Hand behind back: (R) D 4–5; ↑   (L) ↑ midsacrum.
Tenderness: Subacromion +; anterior shoulder +++;
posterior shoulder +; sore left cervical 5.

Treatment plans and goals I concluded that this was
an acute capsulitus with some degeneration in the
cervical spine. The first aim was to ease the acute pain
and mobilize her shoulder to help her with daily living
tasks and then advise her on lifestyle.

The points chosen included left LI-15, 14 and 4; G-21;
TE-14, 5; S-38; jianneiling (extra). These were chosen
as they are all points around the shoulder (local points)
or on channels passing through the affected area (distal
points); S-38 is an empirical point for shoulder problems.
As the pain was severe electroacupuncture was used
between LI-15 and janeiling, also from TE-14 to TE-5
and a lamp was used over the shoulder.

Outcomes Mrs K was seen again the next day; she
had gone out for a New Year's Eve dinner and the
shoulder had become very painful during the evening
and she had had a bad night but since the morning she
had felt easier. The acupuncture treatment was
repeated.

At the next treatment on 3/1/95 she reported that she
felt much better; on 4/1/95 elevation had improved to
100 and hand behind back to L3; on the next treatment
6/1/95 elevation had increased to 140 but she still had a
low grade constant ache.

She reported on 11/1/95 that she was pain free
after the last treatment but still having some intermittent
pain. She was given a few more treatments including
manual therapy to loosen up left C5 and supplied with
a support pillow. By the third week in January she had
full movement and was getting occasional discomfort
only.

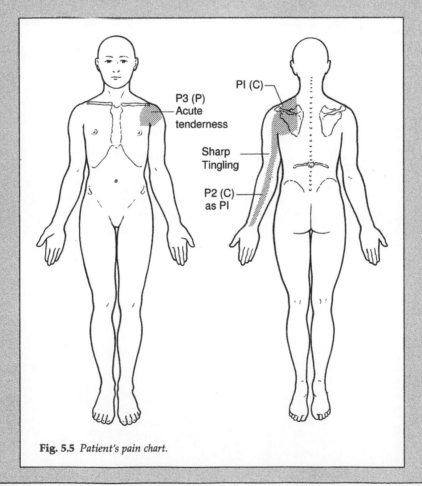

Fig. 5.5 *Patient's pain chart.*

References

Cyriax J 1975 Textbook of orthopaedic medicine. Balliére Tindall, London

Further reading

Ellis N 1994 Acupuncture in clinical practice. Chapman & Hall, London
Lewith G T, Lewith N R 1983 Modern Chinese acupuncture. Thorsons, London
Maciocia G 1987 Tongue diagnosis in Chinese medicine. Eastland Press
Stux G, Pomeranz B 1991 Basics of acupuncture, 2nd edn. Springer Verlag
Zhen Li Shi 1985 Pulse diagnosis. Paradigm

Some specialized techniques

6

Introduction to acupressure

Sara Mokone and Val Hopwood

Introduction

Acupressure is a healing art that uses the fingers of the therapist to press key acupuncture points on the surface of the skin to stimulate the self-curative ability of the body. It is a safe technique with no serious side-effects and requires minimal equipment – only a pair of trained, sensitive hands.

History

Acupressure has been used in healing for over 5000 years. It has many guises, with a variety of techniques and theories, but it is firmly linked to TCM and the points used are those on the acupuncture meridians. A description of these meridians is found elsewhere in this book (see Chapter 3). It is useful for the physical therapist to investigate both traditional and modern aspects of this art in order to arrive at a personal technique. Physical therapists, osteopaths and chiropractors are particularly suited to the use of acupressure because they have a "hands on" approach to treatment and understand most of the anatomical and physiological complexities of the human body. In addition, massage is a "core skill" of physical therapy.

The knowledge that massage and touch not only give relief from pain, but also invigorate and improve the condition of the tissues, dates from the earliest times. Early texts describing touch as a healing modality are those in the "Huang ti nei ching" (The Yellow Emperor's manual of corporeal medicine), where acupressure is described together with needle acupuncture, herbs, diet and moxabustion. The Yellow Emperor's book gives a detailed account of the relationship of the elements with the human body, citing time, seasons and weather as influences on general well-being, and includes acupressure massage as a treatment modality for imbalances in the flow of Qi.

Traditional approaches documented from ancient India and Japan and other parts of the Orient have many links with the traditional Chinese school of medicine and also include acupressure-like techniques, the most well-known of which is probably Japanese shiatsu. More recently connective tissue massage, applied kinesiology and craniosacral therapy have evolved from analysis of theories explaining the techniques.

Techniques and methods

Table 6.1 and Figure 6.1 describe some of the acupressure massage techniques and the areas of the body they are commonly used on. All the massage techniques can be freely adapted according to the condition under treatment and the constitution of the patient. The actual touch employed can be defined as either light or deep (An Fa, or firm pressure). Options include light or deep touch on a point, gentle or stimulating massage on a point, or light or stimulating massage along a meridian or on an area. Combinations of local or distal points on the same meridian, parallel points on different meridians and meridian massage can all be used.

Table 6.1 *Acupressure massage techniques*

Name of technique	Method	Particular application
Slow motion kneading (Jou Fa)	Use thumbs and fingers to squeeze	All large areas of muscle
Push-rub method	Circular frictions, deep or light	Stimulates blood and lymph, use in areas of stagnation
Wiping or quick tapping	Self-explanatory	Use mainly on tender areas of the face
Rolling	(See Fig. 6.1)	Used on shoulders, back, waist and buttocks
Press-rotate (Mo Fa)	Use palm and fingers to press points with a slight circular motion, or use elbow on back	Generally for use on the abdomen
Grasping method (Na Fa)	(See Fig. 6.1)	Shoulders, neck, underarm and extremities
Dig, press or "finger needle" technique	(a) Single finger: use thumb, middle finger, braced between thumb and index finger (b) Bent finger or knuckle: use bent index or middle finger, brace with thumb, use proximal interphalangeal joint to exert pressure (c) Elbow: brace elbow using the other arm, hand placed on the forearm	Useful when treating fairly thick muscle tissue. Particular use on GB-20, LI-4, PE-6 and ST-36

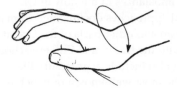

Kneading method

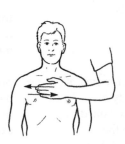

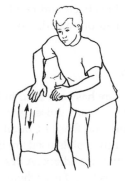

Push-rub method

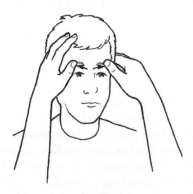

Wiping method (Mo-Fa)

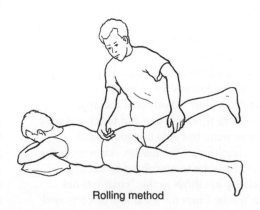

Rolling method

Fig. 6.1 *Acupressure massage techniques.*

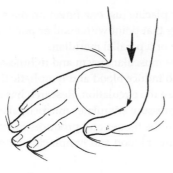

Press-rotate (Mo-Fa) method

Grasping method

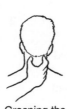

Grasping the
Fengchi point

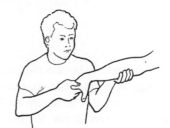

Grasping the Hegu point

Pressing method (An-Fa)

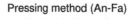

Pressing with knuckle
of index finger

Press with ball
of thumb

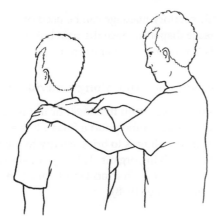

Grasping the shoulders

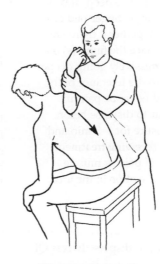

Elbow-pressing-on-the
-back technique

Fig. 6.1 *Acupressure massage techniques.*

Light touch

Technique

Light touch can be defined as the placing of the finger on the acupressure point without any pressure at all. The forefinger or the middle finger are those usually employed. No other part of the hand should be in contact with the patient. The more acute the pain, the more gentle or subtle the touch.

Uses

Light touch is thought to be effective on recognized powerful energy or acupoints, to transfer Qi to another point or area. It is generally used on distant points to treat acute conditions. No pressure is applied since the theory behind this form of treatment is that the Excess Qi (heat and inflammation) will be drained away from the area.

Light touch can also be used to balance Qi between two points on the same meridian or a proximal point and a distal point on different meridians.

Deep touch

Technique

This technique involves prolonged finger pressure on the acupuncture point; this should be deep, steady and penetrating. Use either a single finger pad or the index, middle and ring finger together if there are adjacent points to be treated. Place the finger(s) on the points gently at first, progressively going deeper into the tissues and working to the tolerance of the patient. This technique should never be painful; allow any pain that does occur to disperse before continuing. Maintain the pressure for 1–3 min and up to 5 min while the person receiving treatment continues to experience relief of pain or muscle spasm, or until there is total relaxation in the area.

Effects and uses

1. In local inflammatory areas, to disperse Excess Qi

either by placing just one finger on the area, or by balancing that point with another point, either on the same or a parallel meridian.
2. To release muscular spasm and tightness in the tissues, to induce blood and lymphatic flow and harmonize the circulation. Research has shown that acupressure stimulates microcirculatory activity in the tissues and produces more efficient movement of blood and lymph circulation (Coseo 1991).

Gentle massage

A gentle rotatory massage can be used over the point to increase dispersal, once the pain has lessened, and there is less heat and inflammation.

Stimulating massage along a meridian

This is performed with the finger or thumb pad or the inner border of the middle finger. It is essentially used in chronic illness to bring energy to the area and the underlying organs. This type of stimulation is known to have both a local mechanical effect and a reflex effect (Ebner 1978).

Uses

This acupressure technique clears stagnation of Qi, which results from a build-up of fatty deposits, scar tissue or cellulitis. Massage in the direction of energy flow has been shown to have optimal results in clinical practice. An example of this technique would be thumb pad massage along the course of the Large Intestine meridian together with the Lung and Small Intestine meridians in the treatment of chronic catarrh. Two examples of these techniques for emphysema and for pain in pregnancy are given in Case Studies 6.1 and 6.2.

CASE STUDY 6.1

Mr P is a retired caretaker/gardener aged 66, who suffers with chronic obstructive airways disease. Chest X-ray shows long-standing collapse of left lower lobe. He has compensatory emphysema of the left lung upper lobe and inflammatory changes in left middle and lower zones.

Other tests: blood gases: PO_2 44 mmHg
PCO_2 44 mmHg
Medication: O_2 via nasal canuli continuous 24 h, 2 l/min
nebulized bronchodilators
inhaled corticosteroid

CASE STUDY 6.1 *cont'd*

diuretic
cyclical antibiotics

Between 1988 and 1992 Mr P completed an 8 month pulmonary rehabilitation programme in which he undertook an individually tailored exercise programme and inspiratory muscle training using a resistive device; relaxation techniques, advice on managing dyspnoea and various sputum clearance techniques were also taught. By 1992 admissions to hospital became frequent; he was unable to walk outside the house. The increase in dyspnoea reduced mobility and caused anxiety. He was experiencing general pain in shoulders, neck and chest wall due to the increased effort and work of breathing. Carpopedal tetany and leg muscle cramps caused further discomfort.

At this stage he was again referred for physiotherapy, which was carried out in the patient's own home on a weekly basis.

Treatment goals To reduce pain and anxiety by increasing air entry, using gentle acupressure and meridian massage, in an attempt to maintain maximum mobility and quality of life.

Treatment Clothes do not have to be removed for acupressure treatment and this can be advantageous with dyspnoeic patients who find the activity of undressing extremely distressing.

In sitting and leaning forward with forehead supported:

acupressure was given down the neck and across the shoulder, paying particular attention to the Gall Bladder, Bladder and Small Intestine meridians. Light pressure, during expiration, on the upper Shu points – mainly for the lungs, pericardium and heart (T2, 3, 4 and 5 – 1.5 cm from spinous processes) were all effective in reducing muscle tension and soreness, which facilitated more upper limb assisted-active movement.

In sitting: working along the Yin meridians of the arms was perceived to be very comforting and reduced anxiety readily. Direction was from proximal to distal, gently tapping and stroking.

Sidelying: meridians Massage along the Gall Bladder meridian on the leg dramatically improved muscle tremors, pain and cramps for a duration of 4 days. The Yin meridians on the leg were easily treated in this position which allowed work on Spleen and Kidney points SP-9 and KI-6, which can assist in relieving pedal oedema, together with LU-7 and CV-9. The Back Shu points were treated with light pressure and some deep pressure. Moxa and heat packs were used, as appropriate.

The overall effect of the acupressure and light touch was to reduce anxiety and perceived dyspnoea. The feelings of well-being lasted for several days after the treatment session, which, in turn, enabled the patient to perform with confidence a few simple activities of daily living.

CASE STUDY 6.2

Reason for referral Ms S, a 24-year-old Afro-Caribbean woman, was referred for a home visit. She had acute back pain 34 weeks into her second pregnancy, and was unable to attend an outpatient department for treatment as pain was too acute. She had missed two antenatal classes, and the midwife was concerned.

Findings on first visit Ms S lived in a maisonette, two bedrooms upstairs, and lounge and kitchen downstairs. This was relevant to the pressures on her, as she had an 18-month-old son, who expected to be carried up and downstairs. She was having difficulty standing up, and no position, lying or sitting, was providing any relief from pain, which had been continuous for 2 weeks. She was worried about her pending delivery, as she had had a very long and painful delivery on the first occasion.

Examination was difficult to perform, because of the acute pain. I started treatment straight away by asking her to kneel over a large number of pillows, with her weight on knees and bent arms – forward semi-kneeling. My theory was that the position of the baby was causing pressure on LI-2, and congestion internally.

In this position, through her clothing, I used light pressure on B-23 and GB-30, while listening to her fears and worries, and talking through various strategies for being able to cope with her quite demanding 18-month-old son.

General meridian massage and two-point pressure above and below the painful spot were used. She was able to lie in side-lying immediately after this initial treatment.

On the following visit, the acute pain had disappeared and she was able to attend the following antenatal session.

Applications of acupressure in clinical practice

1. First Aid. Useful in emergency situations such as fainting or acute back pain, or earache in a small child at 3 a.m. in the morning!
2. To be applied as self-treatment by patients between clinical appointments (Mittiskus 1991).
3. To use as an adjunct to other physical therapy modalities, including acupuncture.
4. A specific use for acupressure in pregnancy is autopressure on PE-6 Neiguan in order to reduce symptoms of nausea (Belluomini et al 1994).
5. Acupressure is a useful technique to teach unskilled care assistants or relatives in order to implement care plans in a community setting both with children and with adults.
6. Some adults have needle phobia or cannot cooperate with the acupuncture process. Acupressure makes it possible to treat this group and is also an ideal modality for use with young children and babies.

Helpful hints

- the middle finger is the longest and strongest finger and has the sensitivity best suited to acupressure
- the thumb is stronger but lacks sensitivity
- choose a comfortable, relaxed atmosphere and the most comfortable position for the patient; this is important because relaxation is needed for a successful treatment session
- the calves, the face and the genital areas are sensitive; the back, buttocks and shoulders need firmer pressure
- for sustained pressure, utilizing body weight will reduce fatigue

Precautions

Acupressure is very safe. It is found in clinical practice that if, by chance, pressure is applied to the wrong points, the energy will rebalance itself within a few days with no ill-effects. However, do not apply pressure to open wounds or directly to an area of inflammation or oedema. Avoid areas of scar tissue, boils, blisters, rashes or varicose veins. Treat the corresponding point on the opposite side of the body if possible. For example, for varicose veins on the inner side of the left leg, treat SP-6 Sanyinjiao on the right leg.

Note: It is wise to avoid LI-4 and SP-6 during pregnancy, as they are traditionally forbidden for expectant mothers (Catherine Bauer 1987).

As acupressure is a gentle form of treatment, negative emotional and physical reactions to treatment are rare. In general: "If the Qi is strengthened and moves suddenly after a long period of stagnation, it can move accumulated toxins with it. The body will try to rid itself of these toxins and this will cause a range of physical symptoms such as headaches or skin rashes" (Jarmey & Tindall 1991). There may be emotional reactions and mood changes but these will be short lived as treatment continues. A general warning about this should be given to the patient.

Major acupressure points

Table 6.2 shows the major acupressure points. They are frequently used for the treatment of pain and offer considerable therapeutic benefit. Other uses are mentioned that have been found empirically and recommended for uses mentioned in traditional texts. They are easily accessed by patients for self-treatment between appointments and the technique is simple to learn.

Description of the locations can be found in Chapter 3.

Examples of conditions treated with acupressure

Distal point acupressure

Conjunctivitis

Use the Tsing or end points on the Bladder and

Table 6.2 *Major acupressure points*

Point	Uses
LI-4 Hegu	Headaches, toothaches, sinusitis, cold and pain in the upper body. Not used in pregnancy
TB-5 Waiguan	Pain in posterior aspect of the shoulder, upper arm and ulnar border of the forearm
SI-3 Houxi	Pain in the posterior aspect of the shoulder
PE-6 Neiguan	Relieves anxiety, nausea and travel sickness
HE-7 Shenmen	Insomnia, calming point
GB-20 Fengchi	Neck pain and headache and to dispel Cold
CV-17 Tianzhong	For opening the chest, in respiratory problems; 'calms the diaphragm'
GB-34 Yanlingquan	Special point for tendons. Calms the Liver
ST-36 Zusanli	Headaches, toothaches, pain in the leg and knee, digestion problems, anxiety and poor circulation
LIV-3 Taichong	Digestive disorders, migraines, period pains, irritability and insomnia
B-62 Shenmai	Pain in the lumbar spine, hip joints and sciatica. Posterior knee pain
KI-6 Zhaohai	Pain in lower abdomen, the adductor region, the medial side of the knee
SP-6 Sanyinjiao	Poor digestion, difficult labour, insomnia, bladder problems. Swollen joints. Not used in pregnancy
SP-4 Gongsun	Pain on the medial aspect of the lower leg and ankle. Swollen joints
KI 1 Yongquan	Back pain and pain in lower legs. Calming point. Entry point of Kidney channel.

Stomach meridians. The technique is to use a light touch for 1 min, followed by slightly stimulating massage if there appears to be no immediate result. Supplement by advising the patient to bathe the eyes or apply a slice of cucumber on the eye.

Toothache

Common distal points for treatment of toothache are LI-4 and ST-44 for the upper and lower jaw respectively. ST-4, 6 and 7 can be used as local or "Ah Shi" points.

Combinations of local and distal points

Headaches

Various point combinations can be used, according to which meridian crosses the precise location of the pain. Self-treatment can occasionally abort a serious headache, particularly with migraine attacks.

- ■ *Points for occipital pain –*
  1. GB-20; SI-3
  2. GB-20; B-60
  3. GB-20; B-65
  4. GV-20; B-67

- ■ *Points for frontal headache –*
  1. EX-HN 3 Yintang; EX-HN 5 Taiyang; LU-7
  2. GB-14; ST-44

- ■ *Points for parietal headache –*
  1. EX-HN 5 Taiyang; LI-4; GB-20
  2. ST-8; GB-38

- ■ *Points for vertex pain –*
  1. GV-20; LIV-3
  2. B-7, bilaterally.

Earache

- ■ *Points used –*
  TE-17 Yifeng; TE-3 Zhongzhu
  Use of these points may provide welcome relief in emergency situations (for example, for a small child in the early hours of the morning), where symptomatic treatment is needed, rather than being able to get at the underlying cause of the problem.

Temperomandibular joint pain

- ■ *Points used –*
  ST-6, 7, 44; LI-4; TB-17; Ah Shi points

Neck strain

- **Points used –**
B-10; LU-7; LI-4, 10; GB-20; GV-14; Ah Shi
points; SI-3
Use a combination of these as local and distal
points in pairs. Technique, as before, is to start
with light pressure on the point, go to deep
and firm pressure, and on to massage along
the meridian if not responding.

Shoulder pain

- *General points used –*
LI-4, 11; GB-34; ST-38; B-57; SI-10

- *Points according to the symptoms –*
Supraspinatus tendinitis: LI-16, 15; SI-12, 14;
combine any of these with LI-4, as a distal
point
Perifocal inflammation of the shoulder joint:
SI-11
Infra-acromial bursitis: TE-14

Elbow pain

Tendon strain or injuries to the joint following

jerking or small, rapid movement: LI-11, 12. Use the
following as distal points: LI-10, TE-5, and LI-4.
Positioning the fingers on LI-12 and LI-10 will
facilitate easy treatment of points above and below
the painful site. A light touch is used at first,
especially with acute inflammation. Progression to a
deep touch may follow. For painful joints in general
GB-34 can be used as a distal point (see influential
points, Chapter 1).

Hand and wrist pain

This is often the result of a jarring injury, after a fall.
The many ligaments and small joints may be
inflamed. Treat with LI-4 and SI-3.

Back pain

When treating back pain the Ah Shi points should be
used primarily. The patient can be taught to do this
for themselves, either in standing or lying, using
either finger pads or the flexed proximal
interphalangeal joint of the middle finger (see
Techniques). The following points can also be used;
pressure is applied in B-22, 23, 25, 32; GV-4.

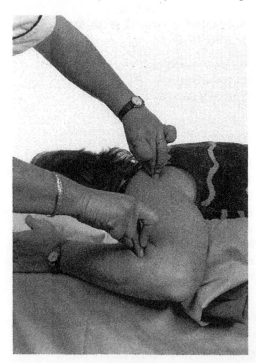

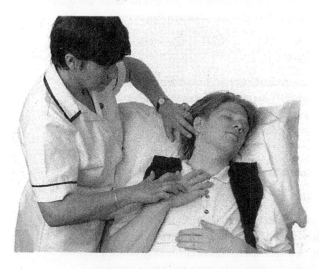

Fig. 6.2 A, B *(A) Acupressure using supported middle finger. Pressure
LI-11 and SI-10, points distal and proximal to the painful elbow joint. (B)
Demonstrating, on a care assistant, the points to use for ear ache: TE-17
and TE-3.*

Sciatica

It is assumed that a correct physical therapy assessment has been made to determine the possible cause of this type of pain. Treat on the affected side or bilaterally, depending on how one-sided the problem seems to be. Use points above and below the pain as in normal acupuncture. Select from the following points: GB-30, 31, 34, 39; B-40, 57, 60.

Knee pain

This is an easy site to teach patients self-treatment. For knee pain on flexion the eyes of the knee are used together with GB-34. For knee pain on extension select SP-9 and ST-36 below the knee and ST-34 and SP-10 above the knee.

Specific meridian point acupressure

The following points have useful and specific actions and have been included for interest. Not all are included in the section in this book on point location so they may need to be checked from the diagrams.

LU-1 Zhongfu Situated on the lateral aspect of the chest, in the interspace between the first and second ribs, 6 Cun lateral to the midline. This can be used as a local point in the treatment of chronic respiratory conditions such as bronchitis, emphysema and bronchiectasis. Use stimulating massage at this point to increase secretions and soothe an irritating cough.

LU-9 Taiyuan Situated on the anterolateral aspect of the wrist crease in the depression at the radial side of the radial artery. This point can be used in conjunction with the previous point and for the same conditions. It is also useful in shoulder pain and as a local wrist pain point.

PE-8 Laogong Laogong is located in the centre of the palm. The exact point is where the tip of the middle finger touches the palm when the fingers are clenched. The two points, one on each palm are known in Chinese massage as the gates for communicating between the body energy and the outside world. They can be held and massaged with the thumb of the other hand for calming. Hands are rubbed together to release tension.

LI-11 Quchi Situated at the anterolateral aspect of the elbow at the extreme end of the elbow crease when the elbow is flexed. This point is often used in combination with LI-4 particularly for painful neck and shoulder.

LI-20 Yingxiang Situated on the nasolabial groove, beside the midpoint of the lateral border of the ala nasi. Can be used for sinusitis, sneezing and catarrh. For acute sinusitis the point should be held and another finger should be placed on the distal point, at either LI-4, LU-7 or LU-9.

GV-26 Renzhong Situated below the nose in the furrow between the upper lip and the nose. Apply firm pressure with the tip of the thumb. This point can be used in emergency situations to revive a person who has fainted. Please note that the usual first aid precautions should be taken first. A special point for relieving acute low back pain.

ST-25 Tianshu Situated 2 Cun lateral and level with the umbilicus. Local point used for gastritis and acute abdominal discomfort. It can be used either bilaterally or unilaterally with ST-36 as a distal point. Light pressure initially. Used with a fairly stimulating massage it can be used for the relief of constipation.

SP-21 Dabao Situated in the midaxillary line in the sixth intercostal space. This ranks as one of the great energy giving points of the body, together with ST-36. Deep and stimulating massage is given in cases of lethargy and tiredness. It can be used during convalescence to revitalize the energy and stimulate the immune system. As with all other acupressure, take care to start with a light touch because this point is nearly always tender to touch. Self-massage or the assistance of a carer is necessary as it should be done regularly, at least four times a day for about 3 min at a time. It has also been used in the treatment of exhausted athletes!

Summary

This chapter has attempted to introduce the physical therapist to the techniques of acupressure used in clinical practice. Some techniques have been described and illustrated but, within the constraint of light and deep touch, the practitioner will evolve their own technique as experience is gained. There are many other combinations of points recommended in the literature and the student is encouraged to read further. There is little clinical research available at present indicating the long term benefits of this modality and it is most often used in conjunction with orthodox acupuncture and for self-treatment between sessions.

Acknowledgements

Grateful thanks for the material that has been contributed to this chapter by: John Cross, MCSP, Editor of AACP Journal 1994–6; Edwin H. Groll, RPT, Public Relations Officer for IAAPT 1991–5; Joseph H. Yao CA RPT, Member of IAAPT.

References

Bauer C 1987 Acupressure for women. Crossing Press, California, USA

Belluomini J et al 1994 Acupressure for nausea and vomiting of pregnancy, a randomised, double blind trial. Obstetrics and Gynaecology 84(2): 245–248

Coseo M 1991 Acupressure homework for faster recovery time. Journal of Chinese Medicine 149 (Sept 1995): 21

Ebner M 1978 Connective tissue massage physiotherapy. 64(7): 208–210

Jarmey C, Tindall J 1991 Acupressure for common ailments. Gaia, London

Mittiskus P 1991 Study of acupressure techniques for back pain. Longmont United Hospital Physical Therapy Department, USA

Further Reading

Bauer C 1987 Acupressure for women. Crossing Press, California, USA

Carballo A 1992 Digitopuntura – Masaje Chino Tui-na. KIER, Buenos Aires, Argentina

Kenyon J 1987 Acupressure techniques – a self-help guide. Thorsons, London

Kenyon K 1974 Do it yourself acupuncture without needles. Arco, New York

State Standard of the People's Republic of China 1990 The location of acupoints. Foreign Language Press, Beijing, China

Wang Zhao-Pu 1991 Acupressure therapy. Point percussion treatment of cerebral birth injury, brain injury and stroke. Churchill Livingstone, New York

Jwing-Ming (2nd Printing 1994) Chinese qigong massage. YMAA, Boston MA

7

Myofascial pain syndromes, trigger point therapy and dry needling acupuncture

Charles Liggins

The myofascial pain syndrome is a very common condition that causes pain, discomfort and other manifestations. It is often not diagnosed in its own right but may mimic many other diagnoses, leading to incorrect medical interventions, both conservative and surgical. Non-response or disappointing response to these measures is often the source of serial referral of patients. The condition does not respond well to many medications, nor to some conventional physiotherapeutic measures, even when they appear to be indicated by the presenting symptoms. Yet its treatment may be relatively simple and in many cases can bring rapid relief to patients suffering from a wide range of incapacitating painful conditions.

Historical perspective

The ancient Chinese physicians formulated a medical system that among many other therapies, included acupuncture, which works on balancing the Qi in the "channels" or meridians. Along many of these channels lie acupuncture points that are sites of access to the channels and are stimulated by various means, including needling, to harmonize (regulate) the flow of Qi. When the normal Qi flow is compromised a pattern of disharmony arises that can result in various clinical manifestations including pain. Under such circumstances, acupuncture points may become spontaneously tender and other tender spots associated with the disordered pattern may arise. These tender spots (many of which are called "trigger points" in the Western literature) have been given the name "Ah Shi" points. As well as needling indicated acupuncture points to harmonize the flow of Qi, it is usual to needle the tender Ah Shi points when treating the associated symptoms.

It is noteworthy that the distribution of tender spots and acupuncture points is similar. An investigation carried out by Liu, Varela & Osutald (1975) showed that there was a high correlation between the two. A more definitive study was made by Melzack, Stillwell & Fox (1977) and the findings showed that for every recorded trigger point there is a corresponding acupuncture point. Furthermore there is a very high correlation of 71% between the two and the pain syndromes with which they are associated.

Through the ages Western physicians became well aware of tender spots and the painful conditions with which they were often associated, and many forms of therapy were devised to deal with them. In the early part of this century the condition that is now called myofascial pain syndrome was given various names that included fibrositis, fibromyositis, myofibrositis and others. Although this diverse terminology gave rise to confusion the feature common to all of them was the presence of tender spots, many of which gave rise to referred pain.

According to Baldry (1989) a major historical landmark in the understanding of myofascial pain and related phenomena was the investigations carried out by Kellgren (1938). In performing experimental work with normal subjects Kellgren found that pain could be artificially induced by injecting hypertonic saline into fascia and muscles. Injection of the fascia gave rise to local pain while injection of muscle could produce diffuse pain in that muscle. In some cases pain was not felt in the injected muscle but in other structures that, depending on the muscle injected, could include joints – for example the knee joint (vastus medialis), shoulder joint (infraspinatus), teeth (masseter) and organs. It is of interest that the pain produced often fell into predictable patterns of referral.

Baldry describes how Kellgren applied his findings from experimental work to the clinical situation, in which he clearly defined the differences between the "exquisitely tender" spots and the referred pain with which they were associated. He also describes how the terminology relating to tender spots and the associated referred pain evolved, and relates that the term "myofascial" is attributable to Steindler (1940), while Kellgren's term "tender spot" changed to the currently used one "trigger point", the latter having been introduced by Travell & Rinzler (1952). Travell is also responsible for the introduction of the terms "myofascial trigger point" and "myofascial pain" into general use and the medical literature.

Definitions

Myofascial syndrome

This syndrome is defined as: "pain and/or autonomic phenomena referred from active trigger points with associated dysfunction".

Examples of autonomic dysfunction include local vasoconstriction, pilomotor activity, perspiration, salivation and lacrimation. There may also be proprioceptive/autonomic dysfunction such as vertigo, tinnitus, imbalance and inability to judge the weight of objects held in the hands. A clinical example of this syndrome is given in Case study 7.1.

Myofascial trigger point

A myofascial trigger point is a: "hyperirritable spot, usually in a taut band of skeletal muscle or in the muscle's fascia, that is painful on compression, and

can give rise to characteristic referred pain, tenderness and autonomic phenomena".

Both of these general definitions are attributable to Travell & Simons (1983) who have also formulated more precise definitions for the different types of trigger points they have identified. For competent examination and successful therapeutic intervention it is important that the practitioner is aware of these differences.

Types of trigger point

These are classified as follows (Travell & Simons 1983).

Active "A focus of hyperirritability in a muscle or its fascia that is symptomatic with respect to pain; it causes a pattern of referred pain at rest and/or on motion that is specific for that muscle. An active trigger point is tender, prevents full lengthening of the muscle, weakens the muscle, usually refers pain on direct compression, mediates a local twitch response of its taut muscle fibres when adequately stimulated, causes tenderness in the pain reference zone, and often produces specific referred autonomic phenomena, generally in its pain reference zone."

Latent "A focus of hyperirritability in a muscle or its fascia that is clinically quiescent with respect to spontaneous pain; it is painful only when palpated. A latent trigger point may have all the other clinical characteristics of an active trigger point, from which it is to be distinguished."

Primary "A hyperirritable focus within a taut band of skeletal muscle. The hyperirritability was activated by acute or chronic overload (mechanical strain) of the muscle in which it occurs, and was not activated as the result of trigger point activity in another muscle of the body. To be distinguished from secondary and satellite trigger points."

Secondary "A hyperirritable spot in a muscle or its fascia that becomes active because its muscle was overloaded as a synergist substituting for, or as an

CASE STUDY 7.1 Myofascial pain syndrome

Reason for referral A single lady of 38 was referred to the Physiotherapy Pain Clinic complaining of facial and temperomandibular joint (TMJ) pain, as well as headaches and a "buzzing" sound in the right ear. On examination she appeared to be in great distress and had to be accompanied to the clinic by a relative. The patient reported that she had initially been prescribed analgesics by her general practitioner but these had no effect on her pain. She was referred to an Ear, Nose and Throat surgeon and an operation was performed 'on one ear' (stapedectomy) but this did not relieve the pain. Subsequently two further operations were performed on the ear with minimal effect on the pain but an "echoing" sound developed in the ear and her hearing acuity diminished to an extent that necessitated the wearing of a hearing aid.

She underwent further surgery to straighten her nasal septum and remove polyps after a diagnosis of sinusitis was made. The TMJ and facial pain persisted, as did the headaches. After further unsuccessful treatment with analgesics she was referred to the Department of Facio-maxillary Surgery and an observant surgeon, who had recently attended a lecture on the myofascial pain syndrome given by the author, referred her on to the Physiotherapy Clinic for opinion.

The distribution of the facial pain was diffusely spread over the cheeks and was concentrated over the right TMJ, while the head pain was situated over the frontal, temporal and occipital regions. She had a "buzzing" sound in the right ear.

She was reluctant to move her neck and tension in both sternocleidomastoid muscles (SM) was evident. Palpation of these muscles resulted in great local tenderness and exacerbation of face and head pain, and the pain in the right ear and TMJ area worsened on palpation of the right SM. A diagnosis of myofascial pain syndrome was made with multiple trigger points in both divisions of the SM.

Treatment Initial treatment consisted of the stretch and spray technique described by Travell & Simons (1983), using ethyl chloride as the cooling agent. This resulted in a willingness to move the neck and to allow ischaemic compression to be performed on several of the trigger points. She was shown how to perform this herself and given advice on neck care, sleeping positions and the application of moist heat over the SM muscles and given an appointment to return 1 week later. At her next appointment she attended on her own and reported that since the treatment commenced she no longer needed to be accompanied by a relative when she went out. On re-examination she said that she still had pain in all the previously recorded areas but that it was considerably diminished. The buzzing sound was still present.

The second treatment consisted of dry needling of the most tender trigger points using disposable 30 mm 0.30 gauge stainless steel needles. This was followed by the spray and stretch routine. She was told to continue her home care routine and attend the clinic the following week.

On her third attendance, she reported that the pain was very much better and that the buzzing sound had gone. It was noted that the patient was now smiling and all her distress had disappeared. Her neck movements were full and there was only slight tenderness on palpation of the SM.

After six treatments, given at weekly intervals, her original symptoms were diminished to the extent that she was considered for discharge, though the patient requested to attend periodically for maintenance treatment. This request was acceded to and she remains reasonably well with no recurrence of her symptoms. However she has received treatment for occasional attacks of sinusitis, which respond well to acupuncture.

Discussion This patient presented with an almost classical case of myofascial pain syndrome due to trigger points in both SM. The cause of the trigger points was obscure though her history of sinusitis and breathing difficulties could have resulted in mechanical overload of the affected muscles. The echoing and subsequent buzzing sounds she experienced could have been due to the original surgery on the right ear and, though it is of interest that the latter sound disappeared with trigger point therapy, it would be speculative to consider that her original symptoms were of myofascial origin and, had she received the appropriate treatment, surgical intervention might not have been required and she would still be able to hear properly.

antagonist countering the forces of, the muscle that contained the primary trigger point. To be distinguished from a satellite trigger point."

Satellite "A focus of hyperirritability in a muscle or its fascia that becomes active because the muscle was located within the zone of reference of another active trigger point. To be distinguished from a secondary trigger point."

Associated "A myofascial trigger point in one muscle that develops in response to compensatory overload, shortened position, or referred phenomena caused by trigger point activity in another muscle. Satellite and secondary trigger points are types of associated trigger points."

Trigger points found in other tissues

Although this chapter pertains particularly to myofascial trigger points, the practitioner should be aware that trigger points can occur in other tissues. Travell & Simons (1983) relate the possible presence of cutaneous, ligamentous, periosteal and scar trigger points. In post-traumatic or operative situations the latter should be suspected as a source of pain that has proved resistant to therapy. An example of pain from failed back surgery is given in Case study 7.2.

Where is the myofascial trigger point situated?

Travell & Simon's (1983) definition indicates that the trigger point is situated in the skeletal muscle or in the muscle's fascia. However a study carried out by Kawakita, Miura & Iwase (1991) suggests that the trigger point may be more related to the fascia than to the muscle. This study related to dry needling, pressure algometry and pulse algometry. The authors stated that when needling a trigger point, a stiffness (readily detected by an experienced acupuncturist) usually occurs at a given depth and postulated that this is where the most hyperalgesic site in the tender

point is located, and the site was likely to be on or near the fascia. In their investigation they located a tender trigger point using pressure algometry, then, using pulse algometry (a monitoring needle) and ultrasonic tomography, they confirmed that the point of maximal tenderness was on or near the fascia. They state that the fascia is one of the most pain-sensitive tissues in the deep structures. In their discussion they considered that the hyperirritability of the trigger point could be due to an inflammatory response taking place at the fascia as a result of mechanical damage by acute overload of contracting muscle.

Features of myofascial pain

Myofascial trigger points can occur in both sexes at any age, though it appears that women are more susceptible. They may also be a source of musculoskeletal pain in children.

Characteristics of trigger point pain

Subjective

Most patients report a history of spontaneous pain, stiffness, tenderness and weakness of muscle, tendency towards fatigue and insomnia.

Objective

Objective examination in the myofascial syndrome usually reveals a palpable, firm (taut) band in muscle, a twitch response, restricted range of movement both in shortening and lengthening of muscle, and weakness without atrophy or neurological deficit; sustained pressure may induce pain in a predictable pattern.

Activation of trigger points

Trigger points may be activated directly or indirectly. Direct activation can be the result of acute overload,

CASE STUDY 7.2 Failed back surgery syndrome

Reason for referral A 55-year-old male was referred to the Acupuncture Section of the Pain Management Clinic with a diagnosis of "failed back surgery syndrome". He complained of persistent pain in the right lower back and buttock with radiation down the back of the thigh and into the posterior leg. The pain had responded minimally to many forms of therapy including medication, physiotherapy, chiropractic adjustment, epidural blocks and surgery. The latter had included laminectomy, spinal fusion and several "revisions". The patient had lost much time from work and was being considered for boarding on medical grounds.

Examination revealed that the pain was of a burning nature and mainly concentrated in the centre of the buttock. The patient confirmed that the pain was identical with that experienced before the first operation. Movements of the lower spine were restricted. Kinesiological testing showed a right pelvic imbalance. Examination of the operation scars with a metal probe revealed several scar trigger points, while deep palpation elicited a very tender area over the sciatic notch, and sustained pressure reproduced the thigh and leg pain. In addition there was a tightening of the soft tissues in the posterolateral aspect of the gluteal region. The piriformis syndrome complicated by the presence of scar trigger points was suspected.

Treatment The aims of the treatment were to correct the pelvic imbalance, to desensitize the scar trigger points and then to deactivate the piriformis trigger points. The first treatment tackled the pelvic imbalance and the scar trigger points. The pelvic imbalance was corrected and the scar trigger points were needled with 7 mm 0.20 gauge stainless steel needles, which were left in situ for 15 min and stimulated manually at 5 min intervals. At his second attendance, a week later, the patient reported that he had experienced a more comfortable week and that the burning component of his pain had lessened. Re-examination of the scar trigger points indicated that they were much less sensitive and the pelvis remained balanced; however, palpation of the piriformis muscle caused discomfort and reproduced pain in the original distribution.

The second treatment consisted of needling the scar trigger points as before; then two 75 mm 0.30 gauge needles were inserted deeply into the tender area over the gluteal notch. Both needles elicited a vigorous twitch response. All needles were left in place for 20 minutes, those in the scar being stimulated at 5 min intervals. The other two needles were not stimulated at this treatment session. After removal of the needles the tender area over the sciatic notch was sprayed with ethyl chloride and the tight area was manually stretched to obtain fascial release. The patient was advised on the application of moist heat over the area and instructed to attend a week later.

On his third attendance he reported that there had been an exacerbation of pain on the evening of treatment and this extended to the next day. However, on the third day he experienced great relief that had been sustained. It was noted that the scar trigger points were no longer sensitive and the tenderness over the sciatic notch very much reduced. He subsequently attended for five more treatments at weekly intervals, after which he was discharged with instructions to report back to the clinic if the pain recurred. Follow-up at 3 months revealed that he remained relatively pain free and had resumed work with no further time off.

Discussion Whenever there has been surgery or trauma to an area in which there is pain, it is always advisable to check the scar for trigger points as they can act as low level antagonists and activate myofascial trigger points. They respond well to dry needling and although they are often very painful a vigorous approach should be pursued.

It is a known fact that myofascial trigger points can cause pain and other phenomena that can mimic an apparently more serious condition. It is the author's contention that many operations have been carried out because patients have presented with "classical" symptoms that suggest that a surgical approach is indicated, but surgery should never be carried out with only pain as the diagnosis. Soft tissue causes of low back are often either overlooked or disregarded; however they are extremely common and if they are of myofascial origin the treatment is usually straightforward. A meticulous assessment of the status of the soft tissues, and their possible contribution to the patient's pain and dysfunction, should be made by orthopaedic surgeons and neurosurgeons before surgery is contemplated.

fatigue due to overwork, direct trauma and that from chilling. Indirect activation can occur as a result of pathology in underlying or adjacent areas, for example visceral disease or arthritic disorders. Emotional distress is another recognized factor.

Perpetuating factors

Perpetuating factors are features which can cause the symptoms of myofascial pain syndrome to persist despite judicious local treatment of the tender trigger points. Thus the elimination of these factors can be regarded as the most important part of the treatment regimen for the condition. Travell & Simons (1983) suggest that the perpetuating factors may also be viewed as predisposing factors to the condition, "since their presence tends to make the muscles more susceptible to the activation of trigger points".

There are many different perpetuating factors associated with the syndrome. These have been conveniently classified by Travell & Simons (1983) as follows:

- **Mechanical stresses** Body asymmetry, for example short leg; muscular stress, such as poor posture, prolonged immobility and unnatural pressure on muscles
- **Nutritional inadequacies** Certain vitamin and trace element deficiencies
- **Metabolic and endocrine inadequacies** A lowered metabolic rate due to suboptimal thyroid function and hypoglycaemia
- **Psychological factors** Depression, anxiety that causes muscle tension, and general "sickness" behaviour
- **Chronic infections** These may be viral, bacterial or parasitic infestation
- **Other factors** Miscellaneous factors including allergies, insomnia and chronic visceral disorders.

Diagnostic criteria

In arriving at a diagnosis of myofascial pain syndrome, characterised by active trigger points, the practitioner should be aware of the following criteria:

- history of onset and its causes

- distribution of pain
- restriction of movement
- mild, muscle specific weakness
- focal tenderness of a trigger point
- a palpable taut band of muscle in which the trigger point is located
- a local twitch response to snapping palpation
- reproduction of the referred pain with sustained mechanical pressure on the trigger point.

Examination for trigger points

Trigger points are located by careful digital palpation. Travell & Simons (1983) describe three types of palpation, viz flat, pincer and snapping:

Flat palpation "Examination by finger pressure that proceeds across the muscle fibres at a right angle to their length, while compressing them against a firm underlying structure, such as bone. It is used to detect taut bands and trigger points."

Pincer palpation "Examination of a part by holding it in a pincer grasp between the thumb and fingers. Groups of muscle fibres are rolled between the tips of the digits to detect taut bands of fibres, to identify tender points in the muscle, and to elicit local twitch responses."

Snapping palpation "A fingertip is placed against the tense band of muscle at right angles to the direction of the band and suddenly presses down while drawing the finger back so as to roll the underlying fibres under the finger."

It is useful to measure focal tenderness of the trigger point with a pressure algometer, the nature of which is described by Fischer (1987). An algometer is a pressure meter that is calibrated in kilograms per square centimetre. The trigger point is first located by digital palpation and the tip of the meter is placed directly over the trigger point. The patient is instructed to report the first feeling of pain as the tip is slowly pressed into the trigger point. This report gives a baseline measurement of tenderness and can be compared with subsequent measurements obtained after therapeutic intervention. Although an algometer goes some way in obtaining an objective measurement of tenderness, there is still a degree of subjectivity as the patient has to give the subjective report of the threshold of tenderness.

Frampton (1985) reported that electrical conductivity may be increased in skin overlying the trigger point and this can be detected by using an acupunctoscope*.

Treatment

Medical therapy

Treatment includes injection with local anaesthetic, preferably 0.5% procaine in isotonic saline, followed by physical therapy modalities (see below).

Physical therapy

Techniques of physical therapy for the management of myofascial pain include stretch and spray with an evaporative coolant, ice cube massage, stretch and active range of movement to ensure that the affected muscle reaches both its shortened and lengthened positions (Simons & Simons 1989), ischaemic compression, massage, heat, ultrasound, electrical stimulation and dry needling.

Stretch and spray

Travell & Simons (1983) describe this technique as the "workhorse" of myofascial therapy, indicating that it is particularly useful in single muscle syndromes and the treatment of trigger points in young children and babies. Stretch and spray is beneficial as a supplement after trigger point injection or dry needling.

The technique consists of placing the muscle in which the trigger point is situated on the stretch and then carrying out several sweeps with a coolant spray

(sprays are commercially available). The objective is to obtain rapid superficial cooling of the skin overlying the trigger point and the pain referral zone. Exact location of the trigger point is not necessary when cooling, but the taut band in the muscle should be identified and kept well stretched while applying the spray. The technique of spray and stretch is described in detail by Travell & Simons (1983).

Ice cube massage

If a coolant spray is not available ice cube massage may be substituted. The ice cube is stroked over the stretched muscle to produce rapid cooling of the skin overlying the trigger point and pain referral zone without chilling the muscle. This method of cooling, described as 'intermittent cold with stretch', is now preferred by Travell and Symons (1992).

Stretch

Stretch alone may be sufficient to deactivate trigger points if they are of recent onset and are only moderately irritable. The practitioner should slowly but firmly stretch the muscle until it reaches its fully lengthened position. This may be facilitated by the application of moist heat before applying the stretch.

Ischaemic compression

This is manual compression of a trigger point in order to deactivate it. The technique consists of pressure applied by digits, knuckle or elbow when the relaxed muscle, in which the trigger point lies, has been stretched to the point of discomfort. Moderate pressure is applied at first and, as the discomfort of the initial pressure subsides, the compression is increased. The total time of compression should be for 1 min with between 9 and 13 kg of pressure.

It has been postulated that ischaemic compression produces its effects by a combination of the following factors: (1) ischaemic nerve block – this implies that the pressure causes a temporary ischaemia thus depriving the area of oxygen. This causes a reduction in action potentials and blocks noxious sensory afferent input to the higher levels of the nervous system; (2) reflex vasodilation – pressure over the trigger point causes an initial blanching and

---

*An acupunctoscope is an electrical device which works on the principles of Wheatstone Bridge and Ohm's Law. It is used to detect small areas of low electrical resistance over acupuncture points and active trigger points.

when it is released the area undergoes reflex vasodilation and an active hyperaemia ensues. This probably produces a "washout" effect, removing the metabolic products responsible for the hyperirritability; (3) release of endogenous substances – the pressure can be regarded as a form of hyperstimulation analgesia, described by Melzack & Wall (1982). Analgesia is due to activation of descending inhibitory mechanisms, which results in the release of endogenous pain-relieving substances such as endorphins and enkephalin.

Massage

Massage for the treatment of trigger points is modified to what Travell & Simons (1983) call "stripping" massage. This consists of a stroking massage where a digit is slowly slid along the muscle to encroach upon the area of the trigger point so that the muscle is "milked" of its fluid content. Pressure should be slow at first but increased with each successive stroke. It is considered that this technique produces an initial ischaemia, which is followed by an active hyperaemia in the region of the trigger point.

Heat

Moist heat appears to be the most effective form of heat in myofascial therapy. It can be applied as a hot moist pack, by bathing or by spraying the affected area under a shower. Moist heat seems to be more penetrating than dry heat and relaxes the muscles better, thus reducing tension on the trigger point area.

Ultrasound

Travell & Simons (1983) describe how ultrasound can be used to diagnose the presence of trigger points, as well as its therapeutic use. Ultrasound should be used at a frequency of 1 MHz for deep penetration (up to 3 cm) for deeply situated muscles and 3 MHz for the more superficial muscles (penetration up to 1 cm). Ultrasound produces thermal and mechanical effects (acoustic streaming), and it is the opinion of Schneider (1994) that ultrasound affects trigger points mainly through the mechanical effects of

acoustic streaming, which alters membrane permeability and improves local microcirculation in the trigger point area.

Electrical stimulation

Many practitioners use transcutaneous electrical nerve stimulation (TENS) for the treatment of myofascial pain. Travell & Simons (1983) report that its use can effect temporary and, in some cases, more prolonged relief, though it is not regarded as a specific myofascial modality. Usually TENS electrodes are applied to acupuncture points or reference zones related to the pain. However care must be exercised not to cause vigorous muscle contractions as this can aggravate the symptoms. Frampton (1985) describes a study in which patients with chronic neck pain benefitted from the application of electrical current of up to 4 mA at a frequency of 1.4–2 Hz. The current was applied to tender trigger points in the neck muscles using a probe.

In recent years microcurrent electrical neuromuscular stimulation (MENS) has been used in preference to TENS (Schneider 1994). This employs a current in the microamperage range as opposed to milliamperes in TENS. Thus MENS is a much milder form of electrical treatment as the patient often does not feel any sensory stimulation and there is less possibility of the trigger point pain being aggravated.

In summary

There are several physiotherapeutic modalities that have proved effective in myofascial therapy. Stretch of the muscle in which the offending trigger point is situated is of paramount importance. Stretch may be used on its own, in conjunction with other modalities, for example spray and stretch, or following other procedures, such as ischaemic compression.

Attention to perpetuating factors is an essential component of management whatever therapeutic modalities are used.

The use of dry needling acupuncture of trigger points will be described in detail.

Dry needling of trigger points

Although it is a conventional form of treatment, injection of trigger points is not without its disadvantages. Certain deleterious effects such as muscle necrosis and allergy have been reported by Travell & Simons (1983). In addition, the local anaesthetic effect of the injected substance may spread to untreated adjacent trigger points thus "masking" their sensitivity, and making them difficult to locate for precise injection. However, Travell & Simons (1983) indicate that the use of 0.5% procaine does allow for effective treatment of the trigger point without causing the masking effect on nearby tender spots.

Dry needling is the insertion of acupuncture needles into trigger points in order to deactivate them. It is an effective therapy with good results and is ideal for use by physiotherapists.

The beneficial effects of dry needling have been reported in the literature. A paper by Travell & Rinzler (1952) reported that needling tender trigger points resulted in good relief of pain in myofascial syndromes. Other workers reported similar findings with either dry needling or the injection of isotonic saline. The effect of dry needling of trigger points was termed the "needle effect" by Lewit (1979). As a result of investigations Lewit concluded that relief of pain was more likely to be caused by the irritating effect of the needle than by any substance that is injected, and that for the best effects the needle must penetrate at the point of maximal pain. A double-blind study carried out by Frost, Jessen & Siggard-Andersen (1980), which compared the effects of mepivacaine and saline injection into myofascial trigger points, showed that patients who received saline injection had significantly more relief (80%) than those who were injected with the local anaesthetic (52%). In addition the relief in the saline group lasted six times longer than that in the local anaesthetic group. Frost and colleagues concluded that the saline was more effective because it irritated the tissue and that the local anaesthetic blocked this effect. Travell & Simons (1983) state that in their experience "precise dry needling of trigger points without injecting any solution approaches, but does not quite equal, the therapeutic effectiveness of injecting procaine into the trigger points".

Dry needling of tender trigger points has many advantages. The techniques are relatively easy to learn and fall well into the scope of use by physiotherapists, who, generally, are not permitted to use procedures involving injection. The insertion of the needle and its subsequent manipulation can produce sufficient stimulation to result in relief of pain and induce a curative effect on the trigger point by the generation of "currents of injury", Chan Gunn (1989). Also adverse autonomic phenomena associated with active trigger points can be normalized. Access to deeply situated trigger points (piriformis) can be obtained by the use of a needle of appropriate length.

Physiological mechanisms of dry needling

The thoughts on the exact mechanisms of working of dry needling may be speculative. For example Travell & Simons (1983) state: "The needle may mechanically disrupt abnormally functioning contractile elements, or nerve endings which are sensory and motor components of the feedback loop believed responsible for sustaining the trigger point activity. Cessation of the neuromuscular dysfunction relieves the tautness of the palpable band of muscle fibres and the hyperirritability of the sensory nerve that is responsible for both the referred phenomena and local tenderness." Furthermore: "Local release of the intracellular potassium due to damage to muscle fibres by the needle also could cause a depolarization block of nerve fibres in the area where extracellular potassium reached sufficient concentration".

Baldry (1989) indicates that the insertion of a needle into the "supersensitive nerve endings" (site of hyperirritability) in the tender trigger point gives rise to a short-lasting but "intense noxious stimulus". This exemplifies the notion of Melzack & Wall (1982) that dry needling is a form of counter-irritation, the modern term for which is "hyperstimulation analgesia". The three major features of hyperstimulation analgesia are as follows: (1) A moderate to intense sensory stimulus, the nature of which could be described as noxious, can relieve a pre-existing pain state. (2) The stimulus need not be applied to the site of pain as it can have beneficial effects when applied at distant sites. (3) A stimulus that is applied for short periods (few seconds to 30 min) is capable of relieving pain for appreciable periods of time or even permanently. Melzack & Wall (1982) offer convincing explanations of the three features and indicate that the noxious sensory stimulus activates areas in the brainstem that are responsible for initiating descending inhibitory control over neural mechanisms responsible for causing pain.

Chan Gunn (1989) explains that the microtrauma caused by needle insertion results in a current of injury, and that the insertion of a needle into a muscle can result in electrical activity that has been measured to be as high as 2 mV. Furthermore this current can be augmented by mechanically stimulating the needle. Pain relief and relaxation of muscle can ensue as a result of the current of injury and these effects are capable of spreading through the entire segment related to the painful area. This is probably due to reflex activity that initiates responses in spinal-modulating neural circuits. Chan Gunn also explains that dry needling areas of fibrosis causes microtrauma that results in local haemorrhage and the consequent delivery of growth factors to the injury site. One of these, the platelet-derived growth factor, attracts cells and facilitates DNA synthesis as well as stimulating collagen and protein formation, thus promoting healing.

Techniques of dry needling

Acupuncture needles Sterile stainless steel acupuncture needles are suitable for dry needling. The length of the needle should be in accordance with estimated depth of the trigger point. A 1″ or 1 $\frac{1}{2}$″ (25/38 mm) needle is suitable for the more superficially placed trigger points (trapezius) whereas a 3″ (75 mm) needle is required for appropriate penetration of deeper-placed structures (e.g. gluteus minimus). The thickness of the needle should ensure that it does not bend during insertion; 28 (0.35 mm) or 30 (0.30 mm) gauge are recommended.

Reusable acupuncture needles may be sterilized after use but nowadays most practitioners use sterile, disposable needles in the interest of the patient's well-being in respect of infectious diseases such as AIDS and hepatitis B.

Procedure The treatment should be explained to the patient, making it clear that this involves the penetration of the tissues with a needle. The nature of the sensation(s) that are likely to be experienced should be described, for example a slight prick as the needle penetrates the superficial skin layer and a very brief, sharp sensation with an accompanying muscle twitch as the tip of the needle locates the trigger point. This may be followed by one or other sensations described as throbbing, warmth, fullness (distension), heaviness, aching or numbness, and that these sensations may be slightly increased when the practitioner manually manipulates the needle while in situ. The patient is assured that sterile, disposable needles will be used and verbal consent for the procedure should be obtained.

The patient should be placed in an appropriate position to ensure comfort, relaxation and ease of access to the affected area for examination and treatment. The position should be one of recumbency with variations such as side lying, half lying, supine lying or prone lying with the neck comfortably positioned.

The trigger point should be carefully located by precise digital palpation and, if a pressure threshold meter is available, a baseline measurement should be obtained and recorded for comparison with the post-treatment measurement. The area over the point is cleaned with an antiseptic. The skin over the trigger point is held taut between the index and middle fingers of one hand; the needle is then inserted quickly with the other hand through the stretched skin. The depth of the needling should be increased carefully until a slight stiffening is felt; at this point the needle sensation described above and the muscle twitch response are usually obtained. If they are not obtained the needle should be withdrawn slightly, without being completely removed from the tissues, and then the depth increased again at a slightly different angle. This procedure is repeated until the required sensations are obtained.

While in situ the needles may be manually manipulated to increase the amount of stimulation; however, at the first treatment session the stimulation should be minimal until the patient's response to the needling has been determined. The manual stimulation consists of holding the needle handle between the index finger and thumb and then briefly rotating the needle through 180° one way and then the same amount in the opposite direction. When this is done the patient usually experiences an increase in the needling sensation. Often a circular area of erythema appears around the needle after insertion. It is likely that this is due to stimulation of the microcirculation around the needle and is a desired effect.

The length of time the needle should remain in situ has given rise to considerable debate. Some practitioners insert the needle, apply the manual stimulation vigorously for a few seconds and then remove the needle. Others leave the needle in situ for up to 10 to 20 min, applying periodic stimulation after the needle has been in place for a few minutes. Practical guidelines for the length of time the needle remains in the tissues can be determined by: (1) the sensation felt by the patient on rotation of the needle; if after initial increase in the needling sensation on rotation, the sensation diminishes considerably or does not occur, it is likely that the trigger point has been deactivated and the needle can be removed; (2) although the erythema does not occur in all patients, when it does the needle can be removed as it has probably produced the desired effect.

The depth of needling is another consideration. Some reports indicate that very shallow pricking of the skin over the trigger point without needle retention is sufficient to relieve pain (Mann 1983). An investigation carried out by MacDonald et al (1983) showed that it was possible to obtain relief of low back pain by insertion of needles to a depth of about 4 mm through the skin and into the subcutaneous tissue over the trigger point. Baldry (1989) describes his technique as follows: "My current practice with respect to deactivating a myofascial trigger point is firstly to hold the skin taut, and then to insert a needle either superficially into the substance of the muscle or as far as is necessary for it to penetrate the palpable band or fibrotic nodule, having first entrapped such structures between two fingers. After the needle has been inserted, it is my custom to leave the needle in situ, without any form of manipulation, usually for only about 1–3 minutes. The needle is then momentarily rotated between the thumb and finger in order to ascertain as to whether one or other of the sensations known as te chhi has

developed. If it has, the needle is withdrawn, but if not, it is left in place for as long as it is necessary to obtain this but never for more than 10 minutes."

On analysing the above procedures it is feasible that shallow and brief needling produces pain relief by stimulating the superficially placed A-delta nerve fibres, which in turn relay nociceptive information to ascending pathways to be subsequently perceived as pain (the prick of the needle), and en route stimulate central inhibitory processes for pain. However it may be necessary to give deeper needling to produce complete deactivation ("cure") of the trigger point. Thus needling to the fascia as suggested by the findings of Kawakita, Miura & Iwase (1991), or needling just into the muscle passing through the fascia to initiate currents of injury and the attraction of "healing" growth factors (Chan Gunn 1989) may produce longer-lasting effects.

The procedure is carried out for all the active trigger points that have been located by examination. Although it may seem to be a lengthy process, in practice several needles may be in situ at the same time, and the treatment session need not last longer than about 30 min. It may be necessary to give repeat treatments, in which case intervals of 3–4 days should be allowed between sessions.

After treatment After the needle has been withdrawn the muscle containing the trigger point(s) should be passively lengthened to its full range by the therapist, (if there is distinct muscle shortening then fascial release techniques can be employed). Then a hot moist pack should be applied to the area (after ensuring that the patient has normal sensory response to thermal stimuli). This is a preventative measure against the occurrence of local soreness, which may follow dry needling. After removal of the pack the patient should be encouraged to actively work the affected muscle(s) through full range of movement, both lengthening and shortening. Following this regimen the trigger points should be palpated. An absence or reduction in focal tenderness indicates a successful treatment. If a pressure threshold meter has been used in the initial examination it should be used again at this stage; the success of the treatment in respect of tenderness will be confirmed if a higher reading is recorded on the scale when the threshold of tenderness is elicited.

Advice on home therapy should also be given, emphasis being placed on muscle stretching procedures, activities that work muscles through their full range and simple methods of applying moist heat if soreness is experienced, particularly after the initial treatment. Where causative factors for the trigger points have been identified, appropriate instructions should be given. This may necessitate the patient making modifications to such factors as sleeping and sitting positions, and occupational, recreational and other postures, as well as giving consideration to any of the perpetuating factors previously mentioned.

References

Baldry P 1993 Acupuncture, trigger points and musculoskeletal pain, 2nd edn. Churchill Livingstone, New York

Chan Gunn C 1989 Treating myofascial pain: intramuscular stimulation (IMS) for myofascial pain syndromes. University of Washington, Seattle

Fischer A 1987 Pressure algometry over normal muscle–standard values, validity and reproducibility of pressure threshold. Pain 30: 115–126

Frampton V M 1985 A pilot study to evaluate myofascial or trigger point electroacupuncture in the treatment of neck and back pain. Physiotherapy 71: 1, 5–7

Frost F A, Jessen B, Siggard-Andersen J 1980 A control double blind comparison of mevipacaine injection versus saline injection for myofascial pain. Lancet March: 499–501

Kawakita K, Miura T, Iwase Y 1991 Deep pain measurement at tender points by pulse algometry with insulated needle electrodes. Pain 44: 235–239

Kellgren J H 1938 Observations on referred pain arising from muscle. Clinical Science 3: 175–190

Lewit K 1979 The needle effect in the relief of myofascial pain. Pain 6: 83–90

Liu Y K, Varela M, Oswald R 1975 The correspondence between some motor points and acupuncture loci. American Journal of Chinese Medicine 3: 347–358

MacDonald A J R, Macrae K D, Master B R, Rubin A P 1983 Superficial acupuncture in the relief of chronic low back pain. Annals of the Royal College of Surgeons of England 65: 44–46

Mann F 1983 Scientific aspects of acupuncture, 2nd edn. Heinemann Medical, London, pp 41–46

Melzack R, Stillwell D M, Fox E J 1977 Trigger points and acupuncture points for pain: correlations and implications. Pain 3: 3–23

Melzack R, Wall P 1982 The challenge of pain. Penguin, Harmondsworth, pp 324–331

Schneider M J 1994 Principles of manual trigger point therapy. Michael J Schneider, Pittsburgh, p. 86

Simons D, Simons L S 1989 Chronic myofascial pain syndrome. In: Tollison C D (ed) Handbook of chronic pain management. Williams & Wilkins, Baltimore, p. 518

Steindler A 1940 The interpretation of sciatic radiation and the syndrome of low back pain. Journal of Bone and Joint Surgery 22: 28–34

Travell J G, Rinzler S H 1952 The myofascial genesis of pain. Postgraduate Medicine 11: 425–434

Travell J G, Simons D G 1983 Myofascial pain and dysfunction: the trigger point manual. Vol 1. Williams & Wilkins, Baltimore

Travell J G, Simons D G 1992 Myofascial pain and dysfunction: the trigger point manual. Vol 2. The lower extremities, Williams & Wilkins, Baltimore

8

Moxibustion and cupping

Kim Ong

Principles of treatment using moxa and cupping

This chapter is based on the classical Chinese approach to the techniques of moxibustion and cupping, seeking to tonify Cold chronic conditions. The heat removes congestion from the blood vessels, and moves Qi and Blood, which ultimately removes pain. The aroma from the burning moxa and additional herbs can sedate the patient. Cupping is used for stagnation and to warm the body superficially. Currently heat lamps are sometimes used instead of moxa. This has a general vasodilatatory effect, increasing the circulation. Metabolic waste substances, such as substance P, are also removed with a resulting reduction in muscle spasm and hence a decrease in pain. However, if more specific effects are required, it is better to use heated needles inserted into the acupuncture points.

Physiological effects

The physiological effects of local body tissue heating lead to a complicated set of changes that produce further complex responses (Low & Reed 1994). The body will respond to heat by trying to maintain its own thermal homeostatic balance. Different forms of moxa treatments will produce different effects depending on the method of application and length of treatment time, for example:

- heat conduction down the needles
- skin warming
- reduction in inflammation
- pain reduction
- vasodilatation.

Therapeutic effects

Heat has been found to encourage healing by increasing metabolic rate, cell activity and local blood flow (Low 1987). A comparison of the effects of moxibustion and infrared, hot packs and steam indicates that moxa treatment over acupuncture points gives a conduction of heat directly into the deeper tissues via the needles. Other forms of moxa have probably a more superficial effect.

Pathways by which local heating from moxa and cupping may alleviate pain include the following:

1. Heating lowers the viscosity of blood, which leads to increased local blood flow leading to pain relief. The decreased viscosity also increases the collagen extensibility and therefore makes it easier to stretch fibrous tissues, thus resulting in pain relief.
2. Heat increases the metabolism and metabolic rate, which in turn leads to an increase in:
   (a) cellular activity; the process of tissue repair and healing has been found to be improved by this activity, therefore leading to pain relief;
   (b) the products of metabolism; this leads to dilatation of the small blood vessels and acceleration of circulation.
3. Neural effects. There are three mechanisms:
   (a) axon reflex, resulting in vasodilatation and increased blood flow;
   (b) proprioreceptors, decrease muscle spasm and therefore increase pain relief;

(c) cutaneous heat receptors, which are mediated by the hypothalamus, the heat-regulating system of the body situated in the brain, and which have an analgesic and sedative effect.

These effects are also seen when infrared and other forms of heat are used.

The origin and development of moxibustion

It is speculated that acupuncture and moxibustion had their beginnings in China amongst the Stone Age tribes. These primitive people lived in cold damp caves, and fought and killed wild animals for defence and food. Stone tools were used; in particular a sharpened stone called 'Bian' was developed to pierce the skin in order to treat disease. Several Bian stones were discovered during an archeological excavation in Anyang dating from 1700 BC.

Moxibustion derived from cauterization and was used about the same time as a development of the controlled use of fire. Primitive man discovered the warmth and comfort of a fire and others may have been fortuitously relieved of aches and pains after touching a burning stick. These incidences gradually led to deliberately applied cauterization for the treatment of diseases by burning combustible materials such as twigs and dry leaves. Later charcoal, chopsticks and the commonly distributed weed mugwort or Chinese wormwood (*Artemesia vulgaris*) were used. The last of these was sun dried and ground to the consistency of cotton wool; it became known as moxa. Moxa was used extensively as far back as the Zhou period (1066–221 BC). The plant was referred to in the book attributed to Mencius (290 BC) (Shanghai College of Medicine 1985): 'for a disease of seven years seek three years old Moxa'. From this statement, moxa must have been used extensively for many years. In ancient times direct cauterization was used whereby the ignited material was placed directly on to the skin, causing blistering and subsequent scarring. The moxa was shaped into large cones about the size of a

hazel nut and many applications were used for each treatment. During the Jing and Tan dynasties (AD 618–907) the indirect method of moxibustion was introduced. At that time the classical medical book the 'Thousand ducat prescriptions' gave details of placing moxa on top of other materials, such as ginger, salt, soy bean, garlic and beeswax. The moxa was ignited and the skin was heated indirectly through the intervening material (Shanghai College of Medicine 1985). During the Ming dynasty (AD 1368–1662), a branch of a mulberry or peach tree would be dipped in sesame oil, ignited and the flames put out, leaving a glowing stick. This was wrapped in soft paper and used on the affected area. Later the moxa stick or roll was made by packing moxa, or moxa plus a variety of other herbs, into a cigar-shaped stick. Today, moxa rolls are manufactured in different sizes of different density for different rates of burning. Mild moxibustion has a slower combustion rate and so the heat emitted is less intense. This method is used for children and the elderly. Smokeless moxa rolls also give off a gentle heat. Adhesive sticks can be used for direct application to the acupuncture points. An advantage of the moxa roll is that patients can be taught to use it themselves.

Moxa techniques

Direct moxibustion

Loose moxa is shaped into a small cone and placed on to the acupuncture point. The apex is then set alight, preferably using an incense or joss stick. This method reduces the risk of burns or scars. Incidentally, joss sticks can also be used to treat the acupuncture points directly as joss sticks contain moxa amongst other herbs. Cones vary in size from a rice grain to half a date-stone to the upper part of a thumb. Small cones are used at the Tsing points and small areas such as on the forehead. Larger cones are used on areas such as the back, thorax and abdomen. After ignition the cone remains in situ, burning slowly until the patient finds the heat intolerable. The cone is removed rapidly with forceps. Several cones can be applied in succession. According to one authority, the number of cones to apply is determined by the patient's age divided by seven if a woman and by eight if a man. These days it would seem more desirable to avoid burning the patient! Burns from the use of moxibustion can take a long time to heal and may leave scars.

Indirect moxibustion

In the first indirect method, a medium such as ginger or garlic is placed between the burning moxa and the skin. It is less painful than the direct method and reduces the risk of infection and hence scarring. When the patient feels the heat is intolerable the whole cone plus the medium is lifted off the skin. The procedure is repeated until the skin is red and moist. Care must be taken to avoid blistering. This method (with ginger) is frequently used on the face, particularly for facial paralysis, which is prevalent in people living in the northern provinces of China where it is extremely cold. Ginger probably adds to the warming effect of the moxa; it can be used for weaknesses of the stomach and spleen, such as abdominal pain and diarrhoea.

Salt is used only in the umbilicus. The umbilicus is filled with salt. A garlic or ginger slice may be placed on the salt if desired and the moxa cone placed on top. This method is effective in Xu (see p. 6) conditions of violent abdominal pain, diarrhoea and vomiting.

Moxibustion using the stick/roll

This is a more convenient method than using cones. The patient can be treated in any position. The end of the roll is ignited, giving an even red glow (Fig. 8.1). The paper wrapping and excess ash should be removed during burning. Various methods are used, especially in osteoarthritis of the knee and other chronic disorders.

In the first method, the lighted moxa stick is brought close to the skin (about 12 cm), the distance varying with the tolerance of the patient and the amount of thermal stimulation required. The stick is moved to and fro across the affected area until it becomes hot and pink, normally for about 5 to 10 minutes. This treatment is associated with blockage or obstruction disorders (analogous to arthritic pain).

In the second method, the 'sparrow pecking'

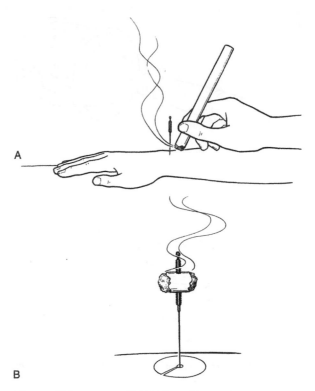

Fig. 8.1 *Using a moxa roll: (A) The pecking method. (B) A cut off a moxa roll, placed on a needle and heated.*

method, the moxa stick is brought rapidly to the acupuncture point without touching the skin. It is said that the heat is more penetrating using this method. The stimulation is strong and takes only 2–5 min. This method is used for tonification of Xu conditions.

Thirdly, the 'rotational/circular' method is used to spread the focus of thermal stimulation over large surface areas in the treatment of 'blockage' pain, soft tissue injuries and musculoskeletal problems encountered in knees, hips, shoulders and in the spine generally. It is also said to be effective in skin disorders. An interesting example of the application of the moxa stick is in the treatment of breach presentation.

Metal warming cylinders

Metal warming cylinders (Fig. 8.2) provide a relatively safe procedure for those who do not like

A

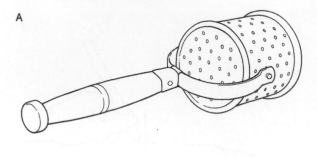

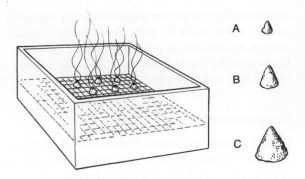

A

B

C

Fig. 8.3 *A moxa frame and moxa cones at various sizes: (A) rice grain (B) date stone (C) broad bean.*

B

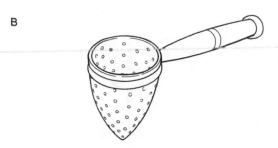

Fig. 8.2 *Metal warming cylinders: (A) For a flat surface. (B) For angular locations.*

Table 8.1 *Location of spinal points from vertebrae L2 to L5*

Level of vertebra	Lateral distance from the spine			
	3 Cun	1.5 Cun	0.5 Cun	0 Cun (spine)
L2	B-52	B-23	EX-21	GV-4
L3	—	B-24	EX-21	—
L4	—	B-25	EX-21	GV-3
L5	—	B-26	EX-21	—

cauterization. Its use is indicated for children. After the moxa has been ignited in the container it is placed briefly on the selected point, then removed, and then replaced until the skin becomes red. A recent innovation is to use a specially designed electric heating device instead of the moxa.

The moxa frame

The moxa frame (Fig. 8.3) is for use over larger areas incorporating several points since the frame is six inches square. It can be used for Cold chronic stomach or back conditions. In stomach and gynaecological conditions the wooden frame with its lighted moxa cones is centered over the umbilicus. In chronic low back conditions the frame is placed over the L2 to L5 vertebrae, which incorporate the points listed in Table 8.1 to the left of the spine. (There are similar points to the right.)

The points given in the table have the actions shown below:

- B-23 – Back Shu point of the Kidney, regulates Kidney Qi

- B-52 – augments action of B-23, tonifies Kidney Qi
- B-24 – strengthens Qi; local point for low back pain
- B-25 – Shu point of colon, stimulates function of colon
- B-26 – 'Shu point' of sacral area
- GV-3 – eliminates Cold-Damp and regulates Kidney Qi
- GV-4 – strengthens Kidney Qi, tonifies the Yang.

Note: diagrams showing the acupuncture points are to be found in Chapter 3 of this book or in other works of reference.

For a smaller area a perforated metal box with a hinged lid, lined top and bottom with fibreglass can be used. A moxa stick is lighted along one side and placed between the fibreglass. The box is then enclosed in a knitted cover and placed centrally over the acupuncture points such as CV-4 and CV-6 for abdominal pain and over B-23 to B-25 for low back pain.

Moxibustion with acupuncture

In this technique, the needle is inserted into the acupuncture point until Deqi is obtained. A piece of moxa roll or moxa punk is placed on top of the needle and ignited. When using moxa punk a paper guard is used to prevent the hot ash falling on to the skin.

Alternatively a moxa roll is ignited and the lighted end placed on top of the needle until the patient feels a spreading sensation of warmth.

Contraindications

1. Do not put moxa directly on to the face, as moxibustion could cause scarring.
2. It should not be used near any orifices or tender areas, such as eyes.
3. Points are forbidden near major or superficial blood vessels, the popliteal fossa, the axilla and the neck.
4. For safety reasons one would not treat with moxa over the front of the chest, nipples or over the umbilicus.
5. The ancient texts include points that are forbidden for the reasons listed above. They also include points that are forbidden because they would have too strong an effect, since moxibustion is said to reinforce the body's energy. Refer to the Further reading section for a list.
6. Areas of reduced sensation. Take extreme care over any area of sensitive skin. Skin sensation should be tested using two test tubes, one containing hot water, the other cold. The patient is asked to distinguish between them. If in doubt, do not use moxa.
7. Diabetes: moxa should be used only with the greatest care in this condition since diabetics often experience loss of sensation in their extremities due to neuropathy, and healing is poor.
8. Moxibustion is a treatment whereby heat energy is transferred in the acupuncture channels and blood vessels. It should not be used in Yang conditions such as high fever, or headaches from excess Liver Yang.
9. Avoid oedematous tissue because of poor healing quality and over varicose veins.

Precautions

1. When using moxa in conjunction with acupuncture, the sterilized needles must all be metal. The plastic-topped varieties are unsuitable for moxa heating. The needles must be thick enough to support the moxa (gauge 28 or 30).
2. Smoke from burning moxa tends to cling and some patients find the aroma overwhelming. Fortunately odourless and smokeless moxa rolls are available.

Moxa smoke can sometimes set off smoke alarms.

Cupping

In ancient times, animal horns and gourds were heated and applied to the body to dispel pus. Nowadays cupping involves the placing of an inverted, partially evacuated, warmed glass or bamboo cup over selected acupuncture points on the skin. A tight ball of cotton wool, held in long handled forceps, is dipped into alcohol and ignited. It is then rapidly placed into the cup for a few seconds, removed and the cup inverted over the selected point. The heated air expands and as it cools within the cup it produces a reduction of pressure with respect to the outside, thus causing a suction effect upon the skin beneath. The skin is raised, the heating causes the blood vessels to dilate and carbon dioxide is exuded. If the blood is impure the raised

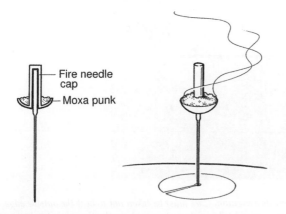

Fire needle cap
Moxa punk

Fig. 8.4 *Moxa used with an acupuncture needle.*

skin tends to be darkened; the darker the colour the greater is the degree of stagnation and impurity. Placing a cup over a Back Shu point of a related organ can show whether there is stagnant blood in that organ. This is obvious when using a glass cup. The cup is left in situ for 5–15 min and is then removed by pressing surrounding flesh to allow the air in and thus equalizing the pressure. Strong erythema and sometimes bruising occur. Cupping drains areas of congestion and rids the body of excess perverse energy. This is in contrast to the tonification of moxibustion, according to TCM theory. The two methods, cupping and moxibustion, are linked because of heating effect on the body. General indications are for arthritic pain, abdominal pain, indigestion, headache, hypotension, common cold, low back pain and painful menstruation.

Types of cup

These days cups are made of glass, bamboo and sometimes earthenware. The most commonly used cup is the glass cup as it is transparent and the practitioner can observe the degree of congestion so can time the treatment accurately. Any glass jar with a smooth mouth can be used, such as babyfood jars for small areas. The cups vary in diameter from 25 to 75 mm. They are applied to large, smooth areas such as the back, abdomen, thighs and shoulders.

Methods of creating a vacuum using heat

Use cotton wool on the end of a stick, dipped in alcohol and ignited, and plunged quickly into the base of the cup and removed. Several attempts may be required to create a vacuum.

An alternative is to use a barbeque lighter, which is a lighter on the end of a long stick. The method is the same as above.

Other methods of creating a vacuum

Cups are available with valves, so that the cups can be partially evacuated of air. The pump can be either mechanically or electrically driven. Alternatively, the cup can be attached to a strong rubber balloon. When the balloon is squeezed, the air is released

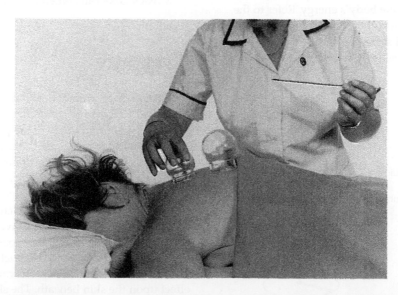

Fig. 8.5 *Cupping using a lit long taper to heat the inside of the cup to create a vacuum. Care must be taken not to heat the outside edge and with the speed of application for gaining contact. Cupping is used on an oiled back to reduce stagnation in the tissues and to improve circulation. It is also effective as a relaxant prior to needling.*

from the cup. Finally, interferential suction cups are simple and effective to use over local points. These three methods can be used in areas of congestion where the joint is red and swollen, such as knees, shoulders, necks and backs.

The heating method is not used much in England because of the possibility of marking the patient's skin. Vacuum suction is used in the physiotherapy department when using interferential vacuum suction.

Methods of application

1. Single cups can be placed over specific areas such as LI-15 for supraspinatous tendinitis.
2. Several cups can be placed on large areas such as the back, abdomen, front, and back of thighs.
3. Cups can also be placed over needles that have already been inserted, such as B-23 Shenshu and B-52 Zhishi.
4. To move the cup, the edge of the cup is lubricated with petroleum jelly or ultrasound gel so that it can move easily over the skin after application without breaking the air seal. The front of the cup is lifted slightly while pushing from the back, to ensure a smoother flow. Small cups can be used in this way for facial palsy, as used in China.

Contraindications

High fever, convulsions, cramps, allergic skin conditions and gravitational ulcers are contraindications for cupping.

Precautions

The following precautions should be observed:

- when using several cups avoid placing them too close together as this will pull the surrounding skin too tightly and cause pain
- when moving the cups extra lubrication may be necessary on the skin; bony prominences should be avoided
- if the cup leaves a continuing mark (a bruise) or a pronounced wheal, the cup should not be applied to that area a second time.

Applications of techniques in physical therapy

In what follows, some examples are given of the use of moxibustion and cupping which are by no means an exhaustive account of the treatment possibilities.

Musculoskeletal conditions

Rheumatic conditions in TCM, are referred to as Bi syndrome (see Chapter 1) – the obstruction of circulation of Qi and Blood due to external perverse influence of Wind, Cold and Damp. It can be transformed to Heat in the body, which can give rise to fever, accompanied by joints becoming red, hot and swollen with pain that moves around. In rheumatoid arthritis the tissues around the joints are affected. The disease burns itself out in due course, leaving the patient with painful, stiff joints. Here the treatment is to use needles to dispel the Wind and Heat generally and locally in the joints. GV-14 is an important point for reducing fever, Heat and the elimination of Wind. As mentioned in the precautions, care must be taken if the patient is hypertensive.

When the disease reaches the Cold, painful Bi stage the pain is static, stabbing and restricted to specific joints, such as the small joints of the hands and feet. This is a Cold Deficient stagnant condition. Heat, using a chunk of moxa on top of the needles, stimulates the Blood flow, tonifies the Yang and helps to remove Cold.

■ *Points used –*
   To regulate Qi and Blood, eliminate Wind and Damp: ST-36
   To invigorate Qi circulation to disperse Damp, especially if moxa is used: CV-6
   To help circulation and stimulate the blood: LI-11
   To eliminate stagnation of Qi and Damp-Heat: B-18
   Both the following points help in removing Damp and transforming Fluid: SP-6, 9

Bony Bi is due to the stagnation of Blood, the lack of movement leads to stagnant Phlegm which in time turns into bony osteophytes. The aim of the treatment is to tonify the Yang Qi using the influential points of bone and Marrow. This helps to disperse the Phlegm.

■ *Points used –*
The Influential point of bone: B-11
The Influential point of Marrow; dispels Wind and Damp (care – ankle skin could be very thin): GB-39
The Influential point of tendons and ligaments: GB-34
To dry up the Spleen and strengthen Wei Qi (defence energy); transforms Damp: ST-40

Osteoarthritis

Osteoarthritis (OA) is a Cold disease. It may be caused, originally, by an injury to the point or by a gradual trauma, which is often seen in overweight patients. Fundamentally any extra stress on the point can give rise to an obstruction of Blood and Qi that leads to osteophyte formation. The condition can be aggravated by Cold, Wind and Damp. Since OA is a Cold chronic condition, heat using moxibustion will boost the Yang, Qi and Blood circulation. Heat can also relax the patient and relieve pain.

The three times moxa technique This is used on OA and other Cold, chronic, stuck Qi conditions (see Table 8.2).

The technique, devised by Dr Royston Low, is taught at the British College of Acupuncture.

■ *Points used –*
TM joint: ST-7
Acromial joint: LI-16
Shoulder: LI-15, TB-10, 14
Elbow: LI-10, 11, 12, + LI-13
      (when contractures are present)

Table 8.2 *The 'three times moxa technique'*

Time (min)	Procedure
0	needle inserted giving Deqi sensation
5	light moxa punk, which has been placed on top of the needle, and allow to burn for 2 min, then allow to cool for 3 min and remove ash
10	repeat above process
15	repeat again
20	withdraw needle

Thumb: LI-5
Lumbar spine: GV-2, 3, 4
Wrist: TE-4, 5
Hip joint: GB-30, 39
Knee: 'eyes of the knee'
    ST-34, 35; GB-34
Ankle: ST-41
Dorsum of the foot: ST-42

Facial palsy

According to TCM, facial palsy is due to Wind and Cold. It is not recommended that moxibustion is applied directly to the face, because of the possibility of scarring. An example of its application to distal points is given in Case Study 8.1.

Low back pain

This is commonly experienced in cold, damp climates. The onset can be insidious, indicating that Cold is from within. An injury or trauma from lifting may cause acute back pain, which then becomes chronic, giving a stiff, painful back. A chronic weakness of Kidney energy tends to give chronic pain, especially in the elderly. Treatment with moxibustion strengthens the kidney Yin Xu. Since this is a musculoskeletal condition certain points are used as well as the local tender points in the Urinary Bladder meridian.

■ *Points used –*
GB-34, 39; B-11, 23, 47; K-3; GV-4

■ *Local tender points used in addition to some of the above are –*
For pain in L5/S1 to coccyx: B-28
For pain in the L4/L5 region: B-25
Sacroiliac joints: B-24

Local Huatuojiaji EX-21 points are also used. These are located half an inch (12 mm) either side of the spine extending from C1 to S4. Three to five of these points are used in one session.

Various moxibustion techniques can be used on the vertebral column, depending on the depth of heating required; these include moxa punk or piece of moxa roll placed on needle, moxa cones and moxa frame.

CASE STUDY 8.1 Facial palsy

Reason for referral Mrs A, a woman aged 24, presented with a facial palsy following childbirth. While in the labour ward, the patient felt very frightened and alone as well as being cold. She eventually plucked up enough courage to ask for a blanket. She gave birth to a baby girl 5 hours later. The facial palsy was noticed the following day.

Assessment finding On examination the right side of the mouth was drooping and she could not shut her right eye. The face felt cold and stiff. Mouth movements were limited to the right.

Treatment
1. Acupuncture stimulation was given on the Stomach meridian points on the face: ST-4, 5, 6, 7 and 8 and GB-14 on the right side. Used 1" (25 mm) needles inserted obliquely in the direction of the next point (i.e. ST-4 towards 5, towards 6, towards 7, towards 8). Needles were left in situ for 20 min, and stimulated manually every 5 min.
2. Face exercises are taught, using a mirror for feedback.
3. Heat, using a moxa stick on distal points: LI-4, 11; ST-44, 36. Pecking technique used (three times) for each point. Local heat was applied using a warm, wet flannel, and advised to use a baby-sized

insulated hot-water bottle locally between treatments.

Treatment was given twice a week for the first month, and once a week for the next 2 months. After this the patient's face returned to normal with full range of movement and normal sensation.

Treatment outcome On review, 1 1/2 years' later after the birth of her second child, the right side of her mouth tended to droop very slightly when the patient became tired. She was encouraged to do her face exercises and keep her face warm and protected by wearing a silk scarf round her neck and over her head in windy and cold conditions.

Discussion According to TCM, facial palsy is due to Wind and Cold. In this case, it was due to Cold and fear of the unknown and painful contractions, this being her first child. Moxa was applied to the distal points of Large Intestine and Stomach meridians, since the proximal points are found on the face.

LI-11 was used to dispel Wind and Cold. LI-4 and ST-36 to boost the immune system and to elevate the patient's energies. ST-44 is used as a distal point as the opposite end point on the Stomach meridian in order to transfer Heat energy to the face. The patient was recommended to apply a warm, wet flannel.

Cupping can be applied for chronic congestion and for superficial heating. If heating needs to be deeper (e.g. as in low back pain) then cupping can be done over needles inserted over the following points.

■ *Points used –*
B-23, 25, 28, 40, 47
For sciatica: GB-30; B-54
If pain is in the whole leg: add B-60

A moxa stick can be used along the entire Urinary Bladder meridian in the leg.

Cervical spine

The Small Intestine and Urinary Bladder channels run through this area of the spine and the relevant points are treated. These channels are very superficial and if the Wei Qi energy is weak then Cold, Wind and Damp can attack.

■ *Points used –*
Generally needled but a moxa stick can heat the point if extreme caution is taken: GV-20
To dispel Wind, stimulate the meridians: B-10
Special point for bones: B-11
To eliminate Wind and Cold: GV-13, 14
To eliminate Internal Wind: SI-3; SI-6
To eliminate all Wind: LI-4, Yuan point
To dispel all External Wind: LU-7

The Bladder meridian is the most superficial Yang channel, starting near the eye and ending near the little toe. In the neck area around the first four points the Fong Wind can easily penetrate the body, giving Wind-Cold. Warming the above points with moxa helps to eliminate the Wind-Cold.

Baxie points can be heated with a moxa roll. These are useful as local hand points as well as distal points for the neck.

If the neck is very stiff and cold, owing to the entry of the Fong Wind, heating with cups over GV-13 and 14 can be very beneficial.

Shoulder

For frozen shoulder or capsulitis due to stagnant Blood and stuck Qi, cupping over LI-15 is effective. If the shoulder is stiff and painful a heated needle in ST-38 while moving the shoulder gently will bring relief. Alternatively, cupping may be used over LI-15 and 16 while needling ST-38. For pain in the scapular area, cupping over SI-10 and 11 is used.

Respiratory conditions

Chronic bronchitis is due to Deficiency of the Lung function in dispersing and descending Qi. It is caused by Wind and Cold. The Spleen becomes Deficient in function so that Phlegm and Dampness collect in the Lungs, resulting in a coarse cough producing white sputum. The tongue is thin with a white coating. The pulse is tense and superficial. Prolonged coughing can also injure the Kidneys. The treatment principle is to eliminate Cold and Wind and transform the Phlegm.

■ *Points used –*
To expel Wind, help Qi to circulate, strengthen the dispersing action of the Lungs: B-12
To help to spread Lung Qi and hence relieve the wheezing symptoms: Dingchuan EX-B1
To help dispersing function of the Lung: B-13
The Point of intersection of the Yang channels: GV-14
For a sedative action on chronic cough: B-17

Moxa cones can be used on GV-14 and B-12 and 13. A moxa stick may be used and the patient's carer taught how to use it. Cupping can be used in conjunction with the needles on the above points. Moving cups may also be used on the upper sides of the thoracic area on either side of the spine. Treatment is every 3 to 5 days.

Miscellaneous conditions

For plantar fasciitis (stuck Qi and Blood with Yang Deficiency), moxa cones may be used on special points in the centre of the foot on the medial side. B-23 and 47 are used at the same time.

For torn medial ligament of the knee, heated needles over SP-5, 9 or 10 are used.

References

Low R 1987 The acupuncture treatment of musculo skeletal conditions. Thorsons, London, p. 99
Low J, Reed A 1994 Electrotherapy explained – principles and practice, 2nd edn. Butterworth & Heinemann, London, p. 195

Further reading

Anon 1975 An outline of Chinese acupuncture. Foreign Language Press, Beijing
Anon 1980 Essentials of Chinese acupuncture. Foreign Language Press, Beijing
Autoreche B, Gervaise G, Autoroche M, Navail P, Toui-Kam E 1992 Acupuncture and moxibustion: a guide to clinical practice. Churchill Livingstone, New York
Jayasuriya A 1977 Clinical acupuncture: medicine alternatives international, 7th edn. Sri Lanka
Nanjing College of TCM 1988 The acupuncture treatment of common diseases based upon differentiation of syndromes. People's Medical Publishing House, Beijing
Shanghai College of Medicine 1985 Acupuncture, a comprehensive text. Eastland Press, Seattle
Stux G, Pomeranz B 1988 Basics of acupuncture. Springer-Verlag, Berlin
Turner R N, Low R 1981 The principles and practice of moxibustion. Thorsons, London

9

Transcutaneous electrical nerve stimulation

Deirdre Walsh

Introduction

Transcutaneous electrical nerve stimulation (TENS) is the application of electrical stimulation to the skin via surface electrodes to stimulate afferent nerves for pain relief. Since the mid 1960s, our understanding of the neuropharmacology and neurophysiology of pain has developed rapidly with the discovery of endogenous opioids and the publication of the gate control theory of pain (Melzack & Wall 1965). This knowledge has greatly enhanced the application of electrical stimulation for the management of pain with the result that TENS is currently accepted as a popular non-pharmacological method of pain relief for a wide variety of conditions. However, despite the availability of TENS units since the early 1970s, there is still a deficiency of knowledge regarding the mechanisms of action and hypoalgesic potential of this modality.

Historical perspective

The first use of electricity as a therapeutic modality did not involve a portable stimulator with an array of diodes and resistors but rather certain species of fish that contained organs that produced an electric charge (e.g. Torpedo mamorata, Malopterurus electricus, Gymnotus electricus). Indeed, as far back as the Egyptian era, stone carvings in tombs from the Fifth Dynasty (about 2500 BC) depict the use of Malopterurus electricus (a species of catfish found in the Nile) for the treatment of painful conditions. So, even at this early stage our ancestors had realized

the potential of electricity in the management of pain. The earliest documentation of the use of electrotherapy involved the application of a torpedo ray for pain relief from headache and gout; Scribonius Largus AD 46, one of the first Roman physicians, advocated:

■ *For any type of gout a live black torpedo should, when the pain begins, be placed under the feet. The patients must stand on a moist shore washed by the sea and he should stay like this until his whole foot and leg up to the knee is numb. This takes away present pain and prevents pain from coming on if it has not already arisen* (KELLAWAY 1946).

The crude methodology of such treatment didn't really improve until the 1700s. The introduction of the Leyden jar in 1745 was a major milestone; this device could generate and store quantities of electric charge. However, the introduction of electroanaesthesia during the 1800s was met with a considerable degree of scepticism and this, combined with variable clinical results, led to a decline in interest towards the end of the 19th century. Melzack and Wall's gate control theory (Melzack & Wall 1965) provided a neurophysiological substrate for electrical stimulation analgesia that rekindled interest in electrotherapy; the publication of this theory subsequently acted as a catalyst to the commercial production of electrical stimulators. Wall & Sweet (1967) provided clinical evidence to support this theory when they reported the success of high frequency percutaneous electrical nerve stimulation for the relief of chronic neurogenic pain. At about the same time dorsal column stimulation was developed; this involved surgical implantation of electrodes in the dorsal column that were activated by an external battery-operated device (Shealy, Mortimer & Reswick 1967).

Shealy (1974) began using the Electreat, an early TENS device, as a screening method to establish patients' candidacy for dorsal column stimulation. Long devised the first modern TENS for screening such patients; preliminary results showed that some patients responded better to the transcutaneous stimulation than to dorsal column stimulation, and so a new era emerged (Long 1974). In the early 1970s, clinical reports began to emerge that reported the successful application of TENS for the relief of pain (Long 1973); the subsequent production of small portable devices greatly enhanced the application of electrical currents for the management of pain.

Clinical application of TENS

There is a tendency to believe that TENS should be used only for chronic painful conditions; this is a myth that has resulted in failure to realize the full potential of this modality. Low back pain, postoperative pain, arthrogenic pain and labour pain are examples of the range of applications of TENS (Harrison et al 1987, Ho et al 1987, Lampe & Dunn 1987, Lamperski 1986). In common with other modalities, not every patient will respond to TENS and each case demands a certain degree of 'trial and error' in establishing optimal treatment parameters and electrode sites. One of the main advantages of TENS over several other modalities is that it can be prescribed for home use (under guidance), which allows the patient a degree of desirable independence in their own treatment programme.

TENS modes

There are currently four TENS modes used in clinical

practice. Any commercially available unit should provide the necessary parameter ranges to allow all four modes to be set on the one unit (this requires variable frequency, pulse duration, intensity settings and burst versus continuous mode).

1. High frequency – low intensity TENS (conventional TENS)

Conventional or high frequency/low intensity TENS is the most commonly used mode. As the name suggests, the stimulation parameters are low intensity and high frequency, typically around 100 Hz. In addition, the pulse duration is usually short (50–80 μs). These parameters are required to stimulate the group II afferent fibres. The sensation experienced with conventional TENS is one of comfortable paraesthesia with no muscle contractions, although if the electrodes are placed over a motor point some contraction is visible with high intensities. As the group II fibres are stimulated, this TENS mode achieves its analgesia primarily by spinal segmental mechanisms (i.e. gating effects). Thus the analgesia is of relatively short onset because local neurophysiological mechanisms are responsible; the analgesia tends to be relatively short lasting, that is, a few hours post-treatment.

2. Low frequency – high intensity TENS (acupuncture-like TENS)

Acupuncture-like, or low frequency/high intensity TENS, primarily stimulates the group III and IV nociceptive fibres and small motor fibres. The stimulation parameters are low frequency (1–4 Hz), high intensity and long pulse duration (~ 200 μs). The electrodes should be placed over a myotome related to the painful area. The patient will experience paraesthesia and muscle contraction (twitching type) with this mode. It is desirable that the patient experiences motor contraction; therefore the intensity should be increased until the patient feels this. Some texts refer to the next mode of TENS (see below) as acupuncture-like TENS; the main difference in definition is that the burst train mode has high frequency trains of pulses delivered at a low frequency, whereas the mode described in this section has single pulses delivered at a low frequency.

3. Burst train TENS

This mode of TENS is really a mixture of conventional and acupuncture-like TENS, in which a baseline low frequency current is delivered that contains high frequency trains. This type of TENS was developed by Eriksson, Sjölund & Nielzén (1979) as a result of their experiences with Chinese electroacupuncture. They found that when high frequency trains of electrical stimuli were delivered at a low frequency via an acupuncture needle then patients could tolerate the stimulus intensity required to produce the desired strong muscle twitches much better than when single impulses were delivered through the needle (these authors consequently referred to this mode as acupuncture-like TENS). Typically, the frequency of the trains is 1–4 Hz with the internal frequency of the trains around 100 Hz. Some patients prefer this mode to acupuncture-like TENS because the pulse trains produce a more comfortable muscle contraction.

4. Brief, intense TENS

This mode of TENS uses a high frequency (100–150 Hz), long pulse duration (150–250 µs) and highest tolerable intensity for short periods (< 15 min). Mannheimer & Lampe (1984) recommend that this mode can be used for painful procedures such as skin debridement, suture removal, etc.

Typically, most TENS units will offer variable intensity, pulse duration and frequency settings. In addition, another control will allow the user to switch between continuous, burst and modulated outputs. The continuous and burst outputs are self-explanatory; the latter is used in burst train TENS as described above. The modulated output produces a cyclic amplitude modulation that increases from zero to a preset level then back to zero again; this has been included by manufacturers, apparently to overcome accommodation of nerve fibres and to provide more comfort to the patient.

Selection of TENS parameters

Once it has been ascertained from clinical assessment of a patient that TENS treatment is appropriate, the therapist is then faced with the dilemma of selecting a suitable treatment regime. When the therapist is presented with a wide range of stimulation parameters and modes, a number of factors must be taken into account before making a decision:

1. Has the patient responded to TENS before; if so, what were the parameters used? There is no point in 'reinventing the wheel' and if a patient has previously responded favourably to a set of parameters then the treatment should commence with the same combination.
2. What type of pain is involved? Both acute and chronic pain can be treated with TENS but quite often the patient's symptoms will dictate which frequency to use. For example, if a patient has sustained an acute soft tissue injury of the shoulder, there may not be a favourable response to a low frequency current, which would cause pulsing contractions in the already traumatized muscle.
3. Where is the electrode placement site? If you are treating a bony area devoid of muscle tissue, there is no point in using acupuncture-like TENS as the parameters indicate that some muscle must be present in order to produce desirable contractions (see Electrode placement sites below).

With any patient who has not used TENS before, it is advisable to commence treatment using conventional TENS. Most patients find the 'tingling, buzzing' sensation associated with this type of TENS more comfortable than the sensation and contractions experienced with acupuncture-like TENS. If pain relief is achieved with conventional TENS, acupuncture-like TENS should also be tried for at least one treatment and any variation in the length and amount of analgesia noted. It is a good habit to try out both conventional and acupuncture-like TENS because quite often dramatic differences can be noted in the same patient. The intensity of the TENS should be increased slowly and the patient asked to report the onset of any sensation under the electrodes. Once this is reported, ask the patient to describe what they feel; it is a useful tip to use the patient's mode of description when explaining that the intensity will be increased slowly until this sensation is 'strong but comfortable'. The patient should be warned that if the intensity is too high then the most beneficial effects will not be achieved.

In the application of acupuncture-like TENS the production of muscle contractions is desirable but the patient should be able to tolerate the intensity.

Treatment time

The first TENS trial should be kept short, less than 30 min. This treatment time will allow the patient to get used to the sensation but it also allows the therapist to monitor any adverse reactions, for example allergies to electrode tape or gel, or in some cases where the patient simply cannot tolerate the electrical stimulation. After the initial trial, the TENS treatment can be increased up to an hour at a time at subsequent visits to the therapist. Personal experience has led the author to advise a maximum period of 1 h per treatment; if the TENS is being used at home, the patient should be advised to use the TENS as often as required but only for an hour at a time. If a unit is worn for several consecutive hours, quite often the skin underneath the electrodes gets irritated, so even half-hour breaks between applications can reduce the likelihood of such skin irritation. With acupuncture-like TENS, remember that the patient will experience muscle contractions and therefore with prolonged stimulation they may experience muscle fatigue; this is another good reason for advising a maximum treatment time of only 1 hour at a time.

Electrode placement sites

One of the primary factors responsible for a poor response to TENS treatment is ineffective electrode placement. No conclusive evidence has emerged from the surprisingly few studies (clinical or experimental) that have investigated the effect of electrode placement upon the outcome of TENS treatment (Wheeler et al 1984, Wolf, Gersh & Rao 1981). The therapist must therefore be prepared to try several sites before deciding on an optimal placement site; thus some degree of 'trial and error' is involved in this aspect of the treatment regime. The optimal electrode site not only varies according to the condition to be treated but will also vary between individual patients. Consequently it should

be explained to patients that a few treatments are required initially to locate an effective electrode site for their symptoms and that this period of 'trial and error' will ultimately serve to provide a more successful treatment.

Essentially, there are four broad categories of anatomical site to which TENS electrodes can be applied – the painful area, the peripheral nerve, the spinal nerve roots and other specific points (acupuncture, trigger and motor points). Irrespective of the electrode site that is chosen, stimulation will ultimately result in the passage of afferent information into the central nervous system. In each of the four categories above, an appropriate degree of anatomical knowledge is essential in order to achieve effective stimulation.

Painful area

Probably the most commonly used electrode site, which is invariably the first choice of most clinicians, is that over or close to the painful site itself. In particular, as it is desirable with conventional TENS to achieve a sensation of paraesthesia over the affected area, this may involve placement of electrodes at proximal and distal ends of the painful area. Skin sensation must be assessed before TENS can be applied to ensure normal innervation of the affected area. This may apparently pose a potential problem in those patients where sensation is diminished or absent. However, in such cases the electrodes can be placed just proximal to this site (over normal innervated skin) in order to stimulate the afferent sensory nerves travelling to the spinal cord from the affected area; thus effective treatment can be given even where there is diminished sensation. There are also occasions when application of electrodes at the painful site would prove to be uncomfortable to the patient, for instance in a case of hypersensitivity after a peripheral nerve injury. In such situations, it may also be more appropriate to place the electrodes proximal to the area of hypersensitivity.

An example of TENS treatment applied to the painful area is given in Case study 9.1.

CASE STUDY 9.1

Reason for referral Mrs R, a 40-year-old woman, presented with a 4 to 6 week history of lumbar spine pain. The pain was worse first thing in the morning and on sudden movements. Degenerative changes at L4/L5 level were apparent on X-rays taken a few years previous to her visit. Mrs R reported that she had suffered from a few episodes of low back pain over recent years.

Assessment findings Examination of this patient revealed tenderness over the lumbar spine at L4/L5 level (centrally). Range of lumbar spine movement was normal with only slight discomfort on full extension.

Treatment Four TENS treatments were given. TENS was applied to the lumbar spine by two self-adhesive electrodes placed both sides of L4/L5 vertebral spines.

Stimulation parameters were: 200 μs pulse duration, strong but comfortable intensity and 110 Hz frequency. Initial treatment time was 30 min. Mrs R was also given routine back care advice and extension exercises. On the second attendance, Mrs R was instructed on home use of TENS; she was advised to wear it for 1 h periods as many times as was required to control her pain during the day.

Outcomes By the fourth attendance, which was 3 weeks after the initial assessment, Mrs R's symptoms of low back pain had almost resolved completely apart from a very slight ache at L5 level. She was so impressed with the pain relief from TENS that she purchased one for future management of her continuing back problem.

Peripheral nerve

The electrodes may also be placed over a peripheral nerve that has a cutaneous distribution in the painful area. A sound knowledge of surface marking and neuroanatomy is required to determine where the peripheral nerves are most superficial and therefore most easily accessible for stimulation. For example, pain experienced on the dorsum of the lateral aspect of the hand and the first and second digits can be treated with electrodes placed over the superficial radial nerve, which runs along the lateral aspect of the lower one-third of the forearm. Other examples of superficial points of peripheral nerves are the ulnar groove for the ulnar nerve and the head of the fibula for the peroneal nerve.

Spinal nerve roots

Thirty-one pairs of spinal nerves emerge from the vertebral column via the intervertebral foramina. Each spinal nerve is formed by the union of ventral (motor) and dorsal (sensory) roots, which unite in the intervertebral foramen to form a mixed spinal nerve. By placing the electrodes parallel to the vertebral column (paraspinal application) and over the intervertebral foramen this will allow for stimulation of the appropriate roots of spinal nerves that supply the affected dermatome – that is, the area of skin that receives its nerve supply from a specified spinal nerve. There is considerable overlap between adjacent dermatomes in a specified body part; therefore knowledge of the spinal nerve responsible for the dermatome in question is required in order to select accurately the correct spinal segment for stimulation.

Acupuncture, motor and trigger points

The final category for electrode placement is a group of points referred to as 'specific points', of which there are essentially three types: acupuncture, motor and trigger points. A motor point is the point of entry of a motor nerve into a muscle and is characterized by high electrical conductance and low skin resistance. Motor points are thus used for optimal stimulation of a muscle and therefore may be effectively employed as application sites when applying acupuncture-like TENS when muscle contraction is desirable. Trigger points and acupuncture points are also frequently used as sites for electrostimulation in experimental and clinical studies as well as routine clinical practice. Trigger points are areas characterized by tenderness on palpation and the production of referred pain; they are found in skeletal muscles, tendons, joint capsules, ligaments, the periosteum and the skin. In contrast, acupuncture points are well-defined specific points on meridians on the body that TCM asserts can be stimulated to treat disease; disease in this case is proposed to be due to the imbalance to Yin and Yang and stimulation of certain points can improve the flow of Qi energy and thus treat the disease. Fine metal needles are usually employed to stimulate such points; however, a variety of other techniques (electrical, laser, pressure) have been used to stimulate both trigger and acupuncture points for pain relief (see Chapters 6, 11). Many clinicians advocate the use of these points as they are easy to locate by palpation and patients' subjective reporting of local tenderness. Melzack, Stillwell & Fox (1977) compared the spatial distribution and associated pain patterns of trigger points and traditional acupuncture points using body maps compiled by several authors and concluded that there was a high degree of correspondence (71%) for both criteria.

Several clinical studies have reported the success of TENS application over these specific points (Fox & Melzack 1976, Laitinen 1976), all of which have some degree of decreased resistance to electrical currents, and thus represent ideal sites for electrical stimulation.

The ultimate choice of electrode site depends upon accurate assessment of the cause and location of the pain and also the type of TENS to be used. If conventional TENS is used, the desired sensation is that of a comfortable paraesthesia; therefore it follows that it is undesirable to place the electrodes over a bony prominence (e.g. the malleoli) as this would produce a rather uncomfortable sensation for the patient. In contrast, when acupuncture-like TENS is used, it is desirable to produce visible muscle contractions. Therefore placement of electrodes should be over a muscle.

Link between TENS and acupuncture

From the last section on electrode placement sites, the relationship between TENS and acupuncture has

---

CASE STUDY 9.2

Reason for referral Mrs K, a 32-year-old woman presented with a 2 year history of constant pain in her right shoulder, thoracic spine and rib cage. The patient thought that the onset of problems was related to a soft tissue injury of her right shoulder sustained while cutting a hedge. Several investigative tests were performed (blood tests, chest X-ray, bone scan) all of which showed nothing abnormal. The patient was clearly distressed with the lack of diagnosis and was showing signs of depression. She was very anxious and lack of sleep contributed to her distressed appearance.

Assessment findings Examination of this patient revealed marked tenderness medial to the right scapula and both trapezii. Palpation of the upper to mid right thoracic spine facet joints produced referred pain around the right rib cage.

Treatment Six treatments were given; they consisted of

posture correction, exercises, acupuncture and home TENS. Acupuncture was applied to LI-4 bilaterally and over the tender area medial to the right scapula. The patient responded very well to acupuncture, experiencing almost immediate relief and relaxation. TENS was applied by two self-adhesive electrodes placed over the painful area (medial scapular border). Stimulation parameters were 200 μs pulse duration, strong but comfortable intensity and variable frequency. Initially, the stimulation frequency was set at 120 Hz; then the patient was advised to switch to low frequency (4 Hz) to compare effects. Mrs K was told to wear the TENS for an hour at a time as often as required. She reported that the 'magic box' controlled her pain both at work and at home. While at work, the patient related that she had to keep away from a colleague who was wearing a hearing aid as he complained of unusual disturbances in the appliance whenever she was in close proximity.

CASE STUDY 9.2 Cont'd

Outcomes The patient's general appearance improved markedly, and she became much more confident about managing her condition. An important factor in the success of her treatment was that she was reassured that she was not imagining her symptoms and that she understood the concept of referred pain. Three months after the first treatment, examination revealed no tenderness over the thoracic spine and related area. The patient had occasional episodes of discomfort in the right shoulder region associated with increased activity but was able to manage this with her TENS, which she subsequently purchased. Mrs K's history is an example of how success can be achieved by combining TENS and acupuncture treatments.

emerged in that both can be applied over the same specific points with a high degree of success. Indeed, it was the success of acupuncture treatment for pain relief that resulted in the emergence of acupuncture-like TENS (Eriksson, Sjölund & Nielzén 1979). Both treatment techniques can be used successfully in combination for pain relief, an example of which is given in Case study 9.2.

Even though TENS has been used with a high degree of success in pain management for approximately 25 years, there is still considerable controversy regarding optimal treatment regimes. However, through continued research in both the laboratory and clinical fields, more information can be obtained about the precise mechanisms involved in electroanalgesia (Johnson, Ashton & Thompson 1991, Walsh et al 1995a). Such research will then provide the clinician with the necessary information to maximize the potential of this modality.

Summary

1. Electricity has been used in pain management since the Egyptian era.
2. TENS was initially developed as a screening device for dorsal column stimulation.
3. The four modes of TENS differ by their stimulation parameters.
4. Although TENS has wide applications for a range of acute and chronic conditions, there is still controversy regarding optimal treatment regimes.

References

Eriksson M B E, Sjölund B H, Nielzén S 1979 Long term results of peripheral conditioning stimulation as an analgesic measure in chronic pain. Pain 6: 335–347

Fox E J, Melzack R 1976 Transcutaneous electrical stimulation and acupuncture: comparison of treatment for low-back pain. Pain 2: 141–148

Harrison R F, Shore M, Woods T, Mathews G, Gardiner J, Unwin A 1987 A comparative study of transcutaneous electrical nerve stimulation (TENS), entonox, pethidine + promazine and lumbar epidural for pain relief in labor. Acta Obstetricia et Gynaecologica Scandinavica 66: 9–14

Ho A, Hui P W, Cheung J, Cheung C 1987 Effectiveness of transcutaneous electrical nerve stimulation in relieving pain following thoracotomy. Physiotherapy 73(1): 33–35

Johnson M I, Ashton C H, Thompson J W 1991 An in-depth study of long-term users of transcutaneous electrical nerve stimulation (TENS). Implications for clinical use of TENS. Pain 44: 221–229

Kellaway P 1946 The part played by electric fish in the early history of bioelectricity and electrotherapy. Bulletin of the History of Medicine 20: 112–137

Laitinen J 1976 Acupuncture and transcutaneous electric stimulation in the treatment of chronic sacrolumbalgia and ischialgia. American Journal of Chinese Medicine 4(2): 169–175

Lampe J, Dunn B 1987 Symmetrical and biphasic TENS waveform for treatment of back pain. Clinical Journal of Pain 3: 145–151

Lamperski C 1986 TENS in the management of rheumatoid arthritic wrist and hand pain. Physical Therapy 66(5): 788

Long D M 1973 Electrical stimulation for relief of pain from chronic nerve injury. Journal of Neurosurgery 39: 718–722

Long D M 1974 External electrical stimulation as a treatment of chronic pain. Minnesota Medicine 57: 195–198

Mannheimer J S, Lampe G N 1984 Clinical transcutaneous electrical nerve stimulation. F A Davis, Philadelphia.

Melzack R, Stillwell D M, Fox E J 1977 Trigger points and acupuncture points for pain: correlations and implications. Pain 3: 3–23

Melzack R, Wall P D 1965 Pain mechanisms: a new theory. Science 150: 971–979

Shealy C N 1974 Six years' experience with electrical stimulation for control of pain. Advances in Neurology 4: 775–782

Shealy C N, Mortimer J T, Reswick J B 1967 Electrical inhibition of pain by stimulation of the dorsal columns: preliminary clinical report. Anaesthesia and Analgesia 46(4): 489–491

Wall P D, Sweet W H 1967 Temporary abolition of pain in man. Science 155: 108–109

Walsh D M, Foster N E, Baxter G D, Allen J M 1995a Transcutaneous electrical nerve stimulation (TENS): relevance of stimulation parameters to neurophysiological and hypoalgesic effects. American Journal of Physical Medicine and Rehabilitation 74(3): 199–206

Walsh D M, Liggett C, Baxter G D, Allen J M 1995b A double-blind investigation of the hypoalgesic effects of transcutaneous electrical nerve stimulation upon experimentally induced ischaemic pain. Pain 61(1): 39–45

Wheeler J B, Doleys D M, Harden R S, Clelland J A 1984 Conventional TENS electrode placement and pain threshold. Physical Therapy 64(5): 745

Wolf S L, Gersh M R, Rao V R 1981 Examination of electrode placements and stimulating parameters in treating chronic pain with conventional transcutaneous electrical nerve stimulation (TENS). Pain 11: 37–47

Acupuncture: a peripheral sensory stimulus for the treatment of pain

Moolamanil Thomas and Thomas Lundeberg

General physiological background to treatment

There has been increasing interest in the neurophysiology of pain since Melzack & Wall's (1965) statement of the "gate control theory" of pain. The basis of this theory is that impulses in large diameter afferent fibres, conducting information about pressure, touch and vibration, inhibit the central excitation of cells at the dorsal horn of the spinal cord, evoked by nociceptive stimuli (Melzack & Wall 1965). Further neurophysiological research followed and the discovery of endogenous opioid systems led to improved methods for the management and treatment of pain. Directly related to these fundamental concepts is the use of techniques of peripheral stimulation such as TENS (Woolf & Thompson 1994) and vibratory stimulation (Lundeberg 1983) for pain alleviation. These instruments are developments of modern technology.

In contrast, acupuncture has not generally been accepted by Western Medicine. Several reasons for this can be suggested apart from prejudice. First, there is an understandable resistance to the theories of TCM of which acupuncture is a part. Second, while results of clinical research are available, criticisms are levelled about their methodologies. Lastly, the often contradictory results (ter Riet et al 1990) that are seen, particularly in the use of acupuncture for chronic pain, are cited as evidence that the better the study technique the less likely it is that results exceed that of placebo. The former criticisms will be dealt with later in this chapter, where we argue that the methodology of studies

with acupuncture must be adapted to account for the many variables involved in a hands-on method of treatment.

However, the last of the points above, the contradictory results of studies previously reported with acupuncture (ter Riet, Kleijnen & Knipschild 1990), or for that matter with TENS (Deyo et al 1990), can largely be accounted for because the pathophysiology of chronic pain, a patient variable, has been ignored in otherwise controlled studies.

If the parameters of acupuncture as a technique are related to pathophysiologically differentiated pain (Arnèr 1991, Williams & Spitzer 1982) it would provide considerable consistency when treating chronic pain (Thomas 1995). The ancient method of counter-irritation (acupuncture) as a technique therefore, is a modality of peripheral sensory stimulation (Table 10.1, Lundeberg 1984) and is available for use with various parameters, the validity of some of these confirmed by experimental and clinical evidence (Lundeberg et al 1987, 1988, 1989, 1991). It can as such be dependably based on neurophysiological developments and without necessary reference to the protoscience of TCM.

The pathophysiological differentiation of clinical pain as indication for the use of acupuncture

Pain is not merely a symptom of pathology nor a description for a problem in a region (i.e. pain of

Table 10.1 *Peripheral sensory stimulation*

Systems	Biological medicine	Alternative medicine
Theoretical basis	Peripheral afferent stimulation evoking segmental or descending inhibition of central neurons excited by pain	Traditional Chinese theory – a holistic tradition based on the five elements, Yin/Yang and the orbisiconography of meridians and classical acupuncture points
Techniques	Vibration TENS Acupuncture 1) Trigger points 2) Periosteal stimulation 3) Superficial stimulation 4) Classical Chinese points	Moxa Plum blossom needles Cupping Burning needles Acupuncture with Deqi at classical points

malignancy, low back pain, etc.). It must be differentiated on the basis of neurophysiological changes in the pain control systems following pathology and tissue damage. Its aetiology may be categorized as:

- nociceptive, with a substantially intact neural network; peripheral noxious stimuli evoke excitatory or inhibitory activity at synapses within this network and recruit endogenous pain modulatory circuits (Arnèr 1991)
- neuropathic, pathology or injury at some level of this neural network may modify activity at the periphery or at central neurons; such activity results in non-noxious sensory inputs

evoking or sustaining pain (Arnèr 1991)
- idiopathic, where pain does not relate to known neural anatomy nor does pathology, if present, account for its distribution or intensity; somatization disorders and headaches are excluded from this category (Williams & Spitzer 1982)
- psychogenic, when pain is associated with major psychiatric illness (Williams & Spitzer 1982).

The pathophysiological aetiology of pain is experimentally substantiated, and clinically by distinctive patient responses to opioids and other forms of treatment (Table 10.2).

Table 10.2 *Receptor number and response to modes of acupuncture in pathophysiological pain*

Pathophysio-logical pain	Opioid receptor number	Acupuncture modes		
		Per/man	Low frq. el	High frq. el
Nociceptive	↑	++	++	+
Neurogenic	↓	(+)	+	++
Idiopathic	(0)	(+)	(+)	(+)

Per/man = periosteal or manual mode of acupuncture stimulation; Low frq. el = low frequency electrical stimulation; High frq. el = high frequency electrical stimulation.

↑ = up-regulation; ↓ = down-regulation;
(0) = lack or malfunction of the endogenous opioid system.

++ = statistically significant improvement shown; + = responses seen but not significant; (+) = equivocal since not investigated as pathophysiological pain.

Because pain control systems are differentially activated by pathology or injury and acupuncture must necessarily function through these altered endogenous systems, the above distinctions provide a reference for response to acupuncture in patients with pain. As with other treatments, for example, response to morphine or other interventions (Arnèr 1991), more consistent and better responses are obtained if these indications are adhered to. This is not to say that acupuncture may be tried only if a prognostic indication suggests a good outcome.

The response of clinical conditions based on pain pathophysiology

Chronic nociceptive pain, musculoskeletal in origin, responds well to acupuncture. Conditions for which a reasonable response can be expected include (Thomas 1995, Thomas & Lundeberg 1994): tension headaches, cervical spondylosis lesions about the shoulder such as, periarthritis or frozen shoulder, tennis elbow (Haker & Lundeberg 1990, Haker 1993), low back pain without frank stenosis or nerve damage, osteoarthritis, bursitis particularly around the hip and possibly fibromyalgia.

Carefully diagnosed idiopathic and psychogenic pains are least responsive (Thomas 1995, Thomas et al 1992). Detailed studies on the different aetiological manifestations of neurogenic pain require to be done but the results so far are equivocal (Thomas 1995). There is some evidence that sympathetically maintained pain that is responsive to sympathetic blocks may also respond to acupuncture (Ghia et al 1976). Pain that is neurogenic in origin, but defined more by nociceptive mechanisms provoking neural patterns of distribution, must be distinguished from established nerve lesions (neuropathic). Examples of the former are the reversible root pains following a vertebral disc lesion or entrapment syndromes. These pains are responsive to acupuncture treatment (Thomas & Lundeberg 1994).

The parameters of acupuncture that influence outcome

Modes of stimulation

There is evidence that available parameters of acupuncture using differing intensities or sensory qualities of stimulation possibly evoke responses through different mechanisms and at different levels of the neural network responsible for pain modulation, that is, at segmental levels of the posterior horn of the spinal cord, at the trigeminal nucleus or at supraspinal levels (Andersson & Lundeberg 1995, LeBars, Dickenson & Besson 1979, Sjölund & Eriksson 1979). This is a network of pain modulation that is ordinarily functional or variably so in patients with chronic or acute pain. It is understandable, therefore, that the response to the available modes of acupuncture stimulation will depend on the functional state of the pain modulatory network at any given time and modifications of this network that such stimulation may provide (Thomas 1995, Sjölund & Eriksson 1979) (Fig. 10.1).

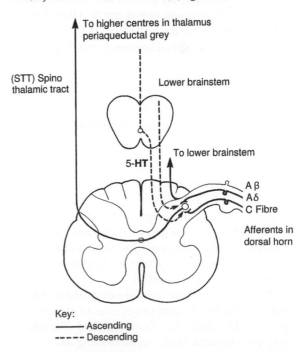

Fig. 10.1 *Spinal and supraspinal mechanisms in pain modulation.*

Manual (Deqi) stimulation at classical acupuncture points

The rationale for the use of classical acupuncture points is that they are on classical meridians (WHO terminology); therefore, they can be redefined by anatomical locations and morphology (Andersson et al 1993) since their sites have traditionally been specified. This is a factor of added safety for their use in the hands of those medical personnel with an acquaintance with anatomy. The specificity of location of classical acupuncture points is an invaluable requisite for communication, both in teaching and for the replication of studies. Further, they manifest intense responses (Deqi) to manual stimulation following insertion, a possible requisite for adequate treatment response. These qualities are not so easily forthcoming from non-acupuncture points or when their required depths of insertion are not maintained. Deqi sensations are possibly mediated through C-fibre and/or A-delta afferents (Andersson 1979). Yet another advantage is that their locations also specify innervation, allowing for a rational use of points (see Sites for needle insertion, below) as well as neuroanatomical explanations for effects. For example, an irritable hip with a flexion deformity due to psoas spasm can be relieved by needles in the lower back at points B-23 and 25, the peripheral field of spinal segments that innervate the psoas muscle.

Electrical stimulation using classical acupuncture points

Following the selection of acupuncture points (see Sites for needle insertion), inserted needles can be coupled to the electrodes of an electroacupuncture apparatus of specific design. TENS apparatus are designed to overcome greater tissue resistance before a range of nerve fibres are stimulated and their built in electrical parameters could be dangerous if adapted for use with needles.

Electroacupuncture units are designed to deliver variable amplitudes and frequencies of electrical pulses, while their waveforms are fixed. The latter may be symmetric biphasic, alternating or asymmetrical biphasic pulses of varying

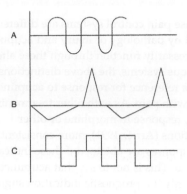

Fig. 10.2 *Patterns of alternating currents (note changes in magnitude of current and reversal of direction of flow; hence no positive or negative electrode): (A) Sine wave. (B) Original faradic (asymmetric). (C) Alternating square wave.*

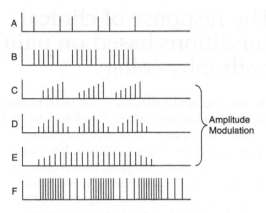

Fig. 10.3 *Pulse trains: (A) Individual spikes. (B–E) Different forms of pulse train. (F) Combination of low frequency spikes and high frequency trains (the combination used by Han et al 1984 – see text).*

configurations (Fig. 10.2). The pulse width is usually of fixed duration (0.2 or 0.4 ms).

Commercially available electroacupuncture units can deliver various trains of pulses at different intensities and frequencies (Fig. 10.3). These possibilities are shown in the elementary diagram of a model apparatus in Figure 10.4. Thus there exists, apart from the possibility of varying the current intensity (an individual requirement of appropriate perception), a facility for altering the amplitude of the current, either constant or modulated (CA/AM control in Fig. 10.4). Frequencies can be set at usually either continuous or intermittent (F_1 or F_2 in

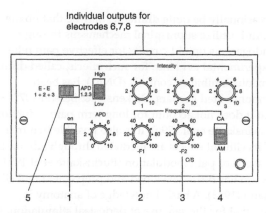

1. Power on/off switch
2. Frequency/constant pulses
3. Frequency/interrupted pulse trains
4. Control position for constant amplitude/amplitude modulation
5. Outputs (6,7,8) connected in series/separate

Fig. 10.4 *A model electroacupuncture apparatus showing available parameters.*

Fig. 10.4) and, of course, high or low frequencies within either. With this facility a combination of two frequencies of pulse delivery is possible, for instance a continuous 2 Hz frequency along with intervening but intermittent pulse trains of 15 Hz. Han et al (1984) have shown that this combination of frequencies (part F of Fig. 10.3) in experimental animals releases two different endogenous opioid peptides. Whether or not this combination occurs in the human subject is unknown, but when used for clinical conditions it is often a comfortable frequency combination.

Whether such electrical variety obtainable in an apparatus translates into the mobilization of different aspects of human physiological pain modulation is unknown; in any case the clinical benefits are largely unresearched. Parameters for which there is experimental or clinical evidence of effectiveness which are generally used in the clinic include the following.

Low frequency electroacupuncture To obtain pain relief a high intensity of stimulation, sufficient to produce muscle or muscle fibre contractions, is recommended. Intensities of a lesser magnitude, more tolerable for a patient, may also be effective. There is some evidence that ergoreceptors, receptors involved in the control of muscle metabolism

(Andersson & Lundeberg 1995), contribute to the mechanism of pain reduction. Frequencies of stimulation between 2 and 4 Hz are used. Such stimulation produces analgesia in normal subjects but its reported effective use for surgery has been contradicted. It is, however, an invaluable adjunct for the treatment of chronic nociceptive pain.

Low frequency pulse train This technique (Sjölund & Eriksson) is a mode of stimulation that delivers impulses of 2 Hz with an inner train frequency of about 80 Hz. Meeting the requirement of muscle fibre contraction is possibly more tolerable with this mode of stimulus.

High frequency electroacupuncture The large diameter sensory fibres, Aβ, are effectively stimulated when a frequency of 80–100 Hz is used at intensities sufficient to produce a comfortable degree of tingling (paraesthesia). There is experimental evidence that this mode of stimulation may depend largely on segmental mechanisms (Fig. 10.1) and that the pain reduction obtained may not be mediated by endogenous opioids since it is not reversible by naloxone, a specific opioid antagonist (Sjölund & Eriksson 1979). When muscle tension pain is present, as in the acute exacerbations of chronic pain, the mode is effective in obtaining muscle relaxation and pain reduction; it is not effective, when pre-emptively used, in the pain of dysmenorrhoea (Thomas et al 1995), but may provide some immediate relief, as with TENS, for some pains of neural origin (Woolf & Thompson 1994).

Superficial insertion of needles

This method of needle insertion, due to the minimal intensity of stimulation, has often been considered as a placebo control for the deep insertion of needles. However, there is evidence that it is a treatment mode comparable to other stimulation modes (Macdonald 1989, Thomas 1995). Macdonald has used this mode for the treatment of low back pain and recommends its use as a method of acupuncture treatment. However, superficial insertions need to be over underlying trigger points for the best effects. The mechanism for its effects are unknown.

Trigger point acupuncture

In this method, trigger points are identified and deactivated by the brief insertion of needles into them. This method of treatment is recommended by Baldry (1993). Unlike in superficial acupuncture, the stimulus may be painful. Trigger points may be widely distributed and while many are at specific locations, others are not. Some care is required during insertion especially when trigger points occur in areas overlying the pleura, pericardium or peritoneum or the larger vessels in the neck.

Periosteal acupuncture

This method utilizes brief bursts of painful stimuli at three to four locations in the vicinity of, or within, a peripheral field segmentally related to the area of pathology. Needles may be used simultaneously with stimulation at points distal to pathology. The mechanism for clinical pain reduction, which can occasionally be quite dramatic, may be that noxious stimuli utilize supraspinal mechanisms through endogenous opioid circuits for effective pain relief. Experimental evidence for such effects, called diffuse noxious inhibitory controls (DNIC), has been demonstrated (LeBars, Dickenson & Besson 1979). But it does not account for long term pain reduction (Bucinskaite et al 1996). It is also possible that many of its clinical effects are mediated through adrenergic systems of pain modulation (Bucinskaite et al 1994). Its use has been developed and propagated by Felix Mann (1983). A basic knowledge of anatomy is essential for the safe use of periosteal stimulation. It is an effective method of treatment for many conditions involving the musculoskeletal system. Visceral pain such as dysmenorrhoea (Thomas et al 1995) and some other problems pertaining to viscera (e.g. ulcerative colitis) appear to respond to such treatment.

A summary of acupuncture methods for treating pain is given in Table 10.3.

Table 10.3 *Summary of acupuncture methods for pain*

	Traditional	Using classical acupuncture points			Noxious stimuli Periost./trigger
		Manual	Low FRQ	High FRQ	
Methods	Deep insertion to prescribed depths and retained 20–30 min	Similar to traditional	Similar to 2–4 Hz electrical stimulation	Similar to 80 Hz electrical stimulation	Needles inserted, sensation elicited and withdrawn
Sensation	'Deqi' i.e. heaviness, soreness or radiating sensations	Deqi	Muscle contractions	Paraesthesia	Briefly painful
Tissues involved	Muscles, subcutaneous tissues or ligaments	Similar to the traditional			Needles into periosteum or trigger points
Theory	TCM	A peripheral sensory stimulus utilizing endogenous pain modulation mediated at spinal segmental and supraspinal levels			Similar mechanisms in addition to DNIC effects
Point selection	Combinations based on above theories	Classical acupuncture points selected on basis of above mechanisms: points local and distal			Specific noxious local and distal points
Safety	Fair	Fair	Fair	Fair	Requires greater anatomical precision

Further details of these methods are available within the text.
DNIC = diffuse noxious inhibitory controls (Thomas, Arnèr & Lundeberg 1992).
FRQ = frequency; Periost./trigger = periosteal point or trigger point stimulation.

Sites for needle insertion

Parameters of acupuncture other than the modes of stimulation also require consideration when treating pain. There is considerable experimental evidence suggesting the activation of differing mechanisms when parameters of stimulation are varied (Mayer 1988, Lundeberg et al 1989). Clinical studies support optimal selections for their use (Lundeberg et al 1988). In general the optimal selection for the number of needle insertions at classical acupuncture points is four to six, located with reference to the segmental innervation of tissues that produce pain. Joint pain derives from tissues within it, its surrounding capsule, or muscles that control its movement. Since the innervation of a functional unit like a joint involves, as a rule, confluent segments at the level of the spinal cord (segmental), needles inserted into muscles controlling joint movement will result in segmental reflex effects. Such points may be located either locally or distally. For example, a problem in the shoulder could be treated with three needles in the deltoid muscle in the vicinity of the joint (local) and two in the forearm or hand where the spinal segmental values of the muscles penetrated by the needle include or are sequential to those segments that innervate the shoulder joint (Cervical V, VI). Longer duration of pain reduction is obtained if such needle locations are combined with extrasegmental placement of needles (in this instance possibly two needles in the leg or foot). Segmental combined with extrasegmental locations obtains long term pain relief (6 months to 2 years) amongst those patients initially responding to treatment (Lundeberg et al 1988, Thomas & Lundeberg 1994, Thomas et al 1995).

Single extrasegmental locations alone need sometimes to be considered if pain is acute and results in intense muscle spasm. An acute torticollis, trismus of masticatory muscles, the onset of a frozen shoulder, an acute low back pain (break-back pain) or the acute, inflammatory pain resulting from a calcaneal spur can be relieved on the table by intense intermittent manual stimulation at distal sites. Points where such stimulation can be sustained without producing a haematoma require them to be in comparatively avascular tissue (e.g. ST-38, SI-5, or the periosteum located under LIV-3). The likely

explanation for this effect, again, relates to a mechanism akin to the phenomenon of DNIC. Later, routine interventions can be continued (see below).

Times for intervention

It is generally agreed, as with treatment with TENS, that acupuncture reduces present pain (Lundeberg 1984). Hence treatment may be initiated when pain is present and continued twice weekly, less or more often, depending on response. Occasionally overtreatment (overstimulation) can result in an exacerbation of pain; this can be controlled by adjusting treatment schedules or intensity of stimulation. Certain conditions, however, where pain is distinctly episodic, benefit most by treatment in the absence of pain. Migraine headaches and dysmenorrhoea (Thomas et al 1995) are two conditions where it is possible to pre-empt the onset of pain with acupuncture. Due consideration must be given to the optimal time of intervention as a requisite parameter for the use of acupuncture as it appears to relate to mechanisms that maintain chronic pain.

Contraindications and complications with acupuncture

Acupuncture with electrical stimulation should not be used when a patient has a pacemaker.

Low frequency electrical stimulation of points lying in the vicinity of the pleura, mediastinal structures or joints should be avoided because occasionally the depth of penetration is altered by repetitive muscle contractions.

Care should be exercised in the selection of points that lie in myofascial compartments. This is especially relevant when patients are on anticoagulants or in points where deep varicosities are likely to be present, such as in the soleus, gastrocnemius muscle complex.

Since no studies have been conducted on the effects of acupuncture on the fetus the technique must be used with due explanation and caution, especially during the first trimester. It is known that acupuncture has a pronounced effect on the reproductive system and hence abortions or miscarriages may result from strenuous stimulation.

It is always best to be informed of any pre-existing conditions in addition to those for which the patient has come for treatment. For example, a hypoglycaemic destabilization of an otherwise stable diabetes is possible following treatment with acupuncture.

Research

Considerations for the design of acupuncture studies

It has been shown that pain modulatory systems are activated by pain, by anxiety, by treatment or by placebo treatment cues. A placebo treatment cue designed to provide an inert variant or incidental ingredient (Grunbaum 1985) of the treatment modality is not possible for acupuncture since any needle insertion necessarily offers an afferent stimulus evoking a neural response. For acupuncture the neural response is the characteristic ingredient of treatment (Grunbaum 1985). The responses may, of course, differ. For example, when intradermal as against deep muscle needle insertions were compared a better response to the deep insertion of needles was seen (Thomas et al 1991). It does not follow that an intradermal needle is the placebo variant of deep muscle insertion (Grunbaum 1985, Thomas 1995, Richardson 1994). For the same reason neither can the use of 'sham' acupuncture points as opposed to 'true' points be considered a valid placebo.

It is necessary, therefore, to consider other designs that would provide information about the placebo component of acupuncture. Study designs involving randomized exposure to various acupuncture modes at trial sessions, then allowing the patients' experience at the trials to determine their choice of mode of continuing treatment (a naturalistic protocol) may provide some answers to study design. Such a procedure allows for both randomization and a naturalistic protocol (Richardson 1994), which may be one solution to the problems of controls in acupuncture studies. Patients' choice, a naturalistic protocol, heightens the expectation of benefit, a potent factor of placebo, and

it can be assumed that the least effective mode approximates closest to placebo within the context of the study. Greater confidence in the results may be obtained by comparing it with a separate untreated control group, or a group treated with a different modality (e.g. TENS) as well as the latter's more plausible design of placebo (Thomas et al 1995). Such an approach to methods, a departure from previous acupuncture studies, has recently been undertaken (Thomas et al 1995). Not only were the responses to treatment assessed but it was also important: (1) to account for inconsistent results of previous studies on acupuncture, (2) as discussed above, to treat differentiated pain and relate the results to these categories as well as to the parameters of acupuncture, (3) to study long term effects of treatment on chronic pain and (4) to use a methodology of study relevant to acupuncture, a hands-on method of treatment, where design should incorporate proper controls and account for placebo effects.

Cassidy (1995) comes close to the above formulations of methodology in a recent article. Her concern is that, for the scientific investigations of systems other than of biomedicine, for instance those involving such hands-on procedures as acupuncture, the paradigm of anthropological studies may be adaptively pursued. The studies of such systems involve far greater numbers of variables amongst patients and therapists, so the attempt to replicate the norms of pharmacological interventions in which a plausible inert placebo can be administered double blind is unreal and defeats the objective of obtaining relevant information. This position has considerable scientific validity.

Attitudes determining the use of acupuncture in the West

The following is a quotation from an editorial titled 'Many points to needle' in the *Lancet* (1990) following a brief review of a few recent studies and meta-analyses of acupuncture studies (ter Riet et al 1990): "This suggests that the better the study technique, the less likely that acupuncture treatment surpasses the placebo effect". This editorial concedes a possibility that there may be something in acupuncture although maintaining that many

Western researchers must conclude that this possibility asymptotically tends to zero.

The above is a position in certain scientific circles concerning placebo: an attitude of philosophical dualism, a mentalism dissected out from other organic aspects of the phenomenon of placebo, including its underlying physiology (Wall 1994). However, this stance rationalizes and sustains the bias against acupuncture. The rejection of the possibilities of acupuncture comes from a powerful quarter of the medical establishment.

Others would compromise by providing a lesser status for acupuncture within front line medical care, reasoning that it is a product of a protoscience, a system whose philosophy has nothing in common with the foundations of 'scientific' Western medicine. It is, therefore, not surprising that the practice of acupuncture is presently relegated to an alternative status (British Medical Association 1986), or seen as complementary (British Medical Association 1993) or folk medicine (Melzack 1994).

Is this position justifiable? Only to the extent that many of the disciplines that are now part and parcel of frontline medicine, such as surgery, psychiatry or anaesthesiology, commenced beyond the pale of established medical care. Each was in their time relegated, for different reasons, to a non-scientific status by the conservatism of established medicine.

A historical perspective of acupuncture

The use of a technique of acupuncture within the system of biomedicine (Table 10.1) (i.e. a technique of peripheral sensory stimulation that has as its basis experimentally known physiological responses modulating pain), is possibly an easier means of systematizing acupuncture studies. Certain areas of TCM must necessarily come into the picture but, in general, the holistic system of Chinese thought need not. That system, however, cannot be ignored nor discarded on the assumption that one system and method is wholly scientific and the other is not. We have been late – even, as in other fields, sometimes by centuries (Needham 1979) – in accepting the relevance of acupuncture as a therapeutic possibility because of such misconceptions. A brief survey of this extraordinary position may help.

Europe's contacts with other continents has provided access to ideas, scientific processes and techniques. Due acknowledgment would show that the forerunners of many sciences and inventions, for instance magnetism, mathematics and algebra, the technology of variolation, gunpowder and the mechanics that resulted in the clock, were possible in the sciences, philosophy and cultures beyond Europe's continental borders (Needham 1979). In medical science, for instance, while William Harvey can rightfully be credited for the discovery of the circulation of blood by experimental methods, it should not be forgotten that Chinese scientific observations had well before previously arrived at a figure of 28.8 minutes as the time for a complete circulation of the blood, a figure that is roughly 60 times too slow but initially far nearer to actuality than Harvey's assessments. "But let it be said that this does not take place in half an hour, but in an hour, or even in a day;" (William Harvey, de Motu Cordis 1628). Even more remarkable is that the fact that, 18 centuries earlier, the concept of a blood circulation had been apparent to Chinese science (Su Wên, 2 BC), while it took Harvey's experimental methods of the 17th century to shake the West from the quagmire of a mistaken concept of the tidal ebb and flow of blood, rather than its circulation (Lu & Needham 1980).

Again pertinent to the present discussion is the fact that methods of Chinese natural science had resulted in the conceptualization and categorization of observed acupuncture effects. For instance, sequential placement of needles on the back or front of the trunk were seen to effect changes on visceral functions. They were, therefore, named after these organs and placed on respective posterior (Bladder) and anterior meridians as their 'Back Shu' and 'Front Mu' points. These changes, as is now obvious from research in this century, were skin to organ reflexes mediated segmentally at the spinal cord. Further experimental work resulted in the charting of dermatomes, myotomes and sclerotomes.

A recent suggestion (see WHO nomenclature for meridians and acupuncture points) that the acupuncture points be numbered therefore loses the empirical rationale of TCM nomenclature. Hitherto, the names had suggested the viscera where needle effects would predominantly locate. There were other interesting insights that derived from point

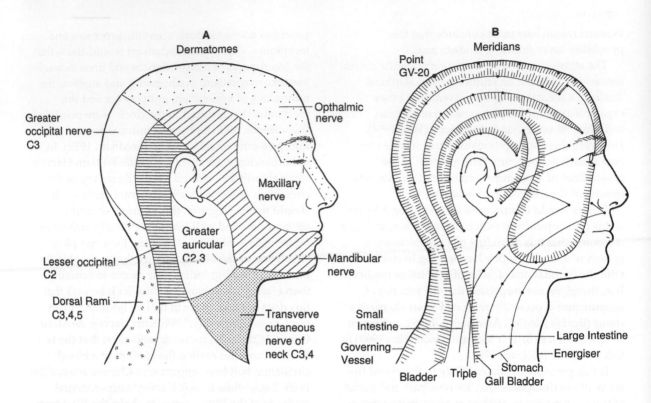

Fig. 10.5 *(A) Demarcations according to different nerve supply of the dermatomes. (B) Meridians in TCM, possibly drawn as a result of 'propagated sensation' from local or distal needle insert; the areas between, or enclosing, meridians are indicated.*

nomenclature that have not been investigated. For instance a confluence of six channels on the head is suggested to account for the potency of the point named Baihui (GV-20). The point is sagittally situated, and as we now know, at the meeting of two dermatomes; parietofrontally the innervation is from branches of the trigeminal, and occipitally it is from the cranial branches of the cervical nerves. It is an area richly innervated, in addition, by the autonomic nervous system via its rich vasculature and the facial nerve from its motor nerve supply. The hunt for the physical actuality of meridians would be as unproductive a pursuit as the very precise demarcation of dermatomes depicted in textbooks of anatomy. Both are concepts in the sense that they derive from empirical findings, although the latter's figurative patterns have better experimental substance (Fig. 10.5).

Ideas underlying dermatomes differ from those of meridians in TCM, in which, without the concept of a nervous system, observation of 'propagated

sensation' led to a charting of meridians as channels for the transfer of energy. Once the areas enclosed by, or sometimes within, channels are distinguished there is a notable correspondence between dermatomes and meridians. While the former concept has been experimentally verified, the latter was conjecture based on observation; the precision of the distinctions is figurative rather than real in both cases.

Discussion

Ideas that stem from TCM such as the manual control of intensities of stimulation, if proved, raise an interesting possibility as to whether peripheral sensory receptors relating to pain respond to specific stimuli or whether they differentially respond to gradations of stimulus intensity, or qualities of sensation ranging from local tension, cramp-like discomfort, or muscle contractions to frank pain. Are there then peripheral receptors that are not 'hard wired'? The possibility of 'propagated distant sensations' in TCM is worth following up in terms of present ideas of referred pain. TCM claims extraordinarily variable combinations for acupuncture points – techniques for treatment with a potential that may pertain to effects on the immunoneurohumoral systems.

It must be pointed out that, unless substantiated by research, the therapeutic range of acupuncture cannot be extended in the future with confidence (Andersson & Lundeberg 1995). The methodological rigour of scientific discipline should provide for the inclusion within disciplines of ideas derived from the natural sciences of other cultures. Their concepts may need to be re-examined, restored or transposed in terms of present knowledge but should not be discarded on the grounds that they are merely protoscientific and thus their bizarre formulations are unusable or without value for modern medical research. Conversely, without such research neither should extensions of clinical possibilities be attempted just because the treatment of deafness, infectious diseases and the control of serious illnesses like asthma have traditionally been within its field of usage. One must keep in mind that the use of acupuncture was promoted in the absence of the more reliable treatments and methods of management presently available. Iatrogenic complications of modern drug therapy are not sufficient reason for resorting to traditional therapies unless these can be shown to be a safe but also reliable substitute for drugs. This has been demonstrated for the treatment of certain types of chronic pain. No-one can recommend, in the state of present knowledge, that an infection such as tuberculosis, an asthenic condition described in TCM as a Xu syndrome, should be treated with acupuncture because of problems arising from the long term use of streptomycin.

Before comparisons of the efficacy of acupuncture as used respectively within two different systems of medical practice can be made, we need to recruit the help of personnel whose clinical concern and competence enable them to function within modern methods of investigation. This is especially pertinent to the treatment of disease. The methods of study may need adaptation to accommodate the two very different systems of thought. But an inclusive rather than exclusive position for the systems and methods of acupuncture would aid the recovery of relevant empirical information from TCM and, we venture to say, provide frontline medicine with some interesting insights. Otherwise entrenched positions will continue: the scientist maintaining that acupuncture is merely a technique to be used as a peripheral sensory stimulus without recourse to traditional insight; the clinician insisting on its being none other than trigger point stimulation whose anatomical locations are (or nearly are) trigger points anyway; the TCM buff arguing for its use according to the energy flows of Yin and Yang. The blind men of Indian legend disagreed, but each was convinced of the shape of the animal according to what he could feel, although none of them knew the elephant in question!

References

Andersson S A 1979 Pain control by sensory stimulation. In: Bonica J J , Liebeskind J C, Albe-Fessard D G (eds) Advances in pain research and therapy, Vol 3. Raven Press, New York, pp 569–585

Andersson S, Lundeberg T, Lund I, Stener-Victorin E, Thomas M 1993 Kompendium i Akupunktur. Vasastadens Bokbinderi AB, Göteborg

Andersson S A, Lundeberg T 1995 Acupuncture from empiricism to science: functional background to acupuncture effects in pain and disease. Medical Hypotheses 45: 271–281

Arnèr S 1991 Differentiation of pain and treatment efficacy. Thesis, Karolinska Institutet, Stockholm

Baldry P E 1993 Acupuncture, trigger points and musculoskeletal pain, 2nd edn. Churchill Livingstone, New York

British Medical Association 1986 Alternative therapy. Report of the Board of Science and Education, Chameleon Press, pp 93–105

British Medical Association 1993 Complementary medicine: new approaches to good practice. Policy document. BMA, London

Bucinskaite V, Crumpton K, Stenfors C, Ekblom A, Theodorsson E, Lundeberg T 1996 Effects of repeated sensory stimulation (electro-acupuncture) and physical exercise (running) on open-field behavior and concentrations of neuropeptides in the hippocampus in WKY and SHR rats. European Journal of Neuroscience 8: 382–387

Bucinskaite V, Lundeberg T, Stenfors C, Ekblom, Dahlin L, Theodorsson E 1994 Effects of electro-acupuncture and physical exercise on regional concentrations of neuropeptides in rat brain. Brain Research 666: 128–132

Cassidy C 1995 Social science theory and methods in the study of alternative and complementary medicine. Journal of Alternative and Complementary Medicine 1(1): 19–40

Deyo R A, Walsh N E, Donald M D, Schoenfeld L S, Ramamurthy S 1990 A controlled trial of transcutaneous electrical nerve stimulation (TENS) and exercise for chronic low back pain. New England Journal of Medicine 322(23): 1627–1634

Ghia J, Mao N, Toomey L, Tuuoling E, Gregg J 1976 Acupuncture and chronic pain mechanisms. Pain 2: 285–299

Grunbaum A 1985 Explication and implications of the placebo concept. In: White L, Tursky B, Schwartz G E (eds) Placebo theory, research and mechanisms. Guildford Press, New York, pp 9–36

Haker E, Lundeberg T 1990 Acupuncture treatment in epicondylalgia: A comparative study of two acupuncture techniques. Clinical Journal of Pain 6: 221–226

Haker E 1993 Lateral epicondylalgia: diagnosis, treatment and evaluation. Critical reviews in physical medicine and rehabilitation medicine 5(2): 129–154

Han J S, Xie G X, Ding H G, Fan S G 1984 High and low frequency electroacupuncture analgesia are mediated by different opioid peptides. Pain (suppl): 369–543

Harvey W M 1628 Exercitatio anatomica de motu cordis et sanguinis in animalbus. London – an anatomical disquisition on the motion of the heart and blood in animals. Translated by Robert Willis, Barnes, Surrey, England 1897. In: Willius F A, Keys T E (eds) Classics of cardiology. Vol 1, Dover Publications, New York 1961

Lancet (editorial) 1990 Many points to needle. Lancet 335: 20–21

LeBars S D, Dickenson A H, Besson J M 1979 Diffuse noxious inhibitory controls (DNIC) I. Effects on dorsal horn convergent neurons in the rat. II. Lack of effect on non convergent neurons, supraspinal involvement and theoretical implications. Pain 6: 283–327

Lu Gwei-Djen, Needham J 1980 Celestial lancets. A history and rationale of acupuncture and moxa. Cambridge University Press, Cambridge, pp 24–39

Lundeberg T 1983 Vibratory stimulation for the alleviation of chronic pain. Acta Physiologica Scandinavica (Suppl) 523, 1–98 Stockholm

Lundeberg T 1984 A comparative study of the pain reducing effect of vibratory stimulation, transcutaneous electrical nerve stimulation, electroacupuncture and placebo. American Journal of Chinese Medicine 12: 72–79

Lundeberg T, Eriksson S, Lundeberg S, Thomas M 1989 Acupuncture and sensory thresholds. American Journal of Chinese Medicine 18: 99–110

Lundeberg T, Hode L, Zhou J 1987 A comparative study of the pain relieving effect of laser treatment and acupuncture. Acta Physiologica Scandinavica 131: 161–162

Lundeberg T, Hurtig T, Lundeberg S, Thomas M 1988 Long-term results of acupuncture in chronic head and neck pain. The Pain Clinic 2(1): 15–31

Lundeberg T, Laurell G, Thomas M 1988 Effect of acupuncture on sinus pain and experimentally induced pain. Ear Nose and Throat Journal 67: 565–575

Macdonald A J R 1989 Acupuncture analgesia and therapy. In: Wall P D, Melzack R (eds) Textbook of pain. Churchill Livingstone, New York, pp 906–919

Mann F 1983 Scientific aspects of acupuncture. Heinemann, London, pp 89–97

Mayer D J 1988 Environmental activation of endogenous antinociceptive systems. In: Olesen J, Edvinsson L (eds) Basic mechanisms of headache. Elsevier, Amsterdam, pp 225–239

Melzack R, Wall P D 1965 Pain mechanisms: a new theory. Science 150: 971–979

Melzack R 1994 Folk medicine and the sensory modulation of pain. In: Wall P D, Melzack R (eds) Textbook of pain. Churchill Livingstone, New York, pp 337–351

Needham J 1979 The grand titration. Science and society in East and West. Allen & Unwin, London

Richardson P H 1994 Placebo effects in pain management. Pain Reviews 1: 15–32

Sjölund L, Eriksson M B E 1979 Endorphins and analgesia produced by peripheral conditioning stimulation. In: Bonica J J, Liebeskind J C, Albe-Fessard D G (eds) Advances in pain research and therapy, Vol 3. Raven Press, New York, pp 587–589

ter Riet G, Kleijnen J, Knipschild P 1990 Acupuncture and chronic pain: a criteria based meta-analysis. Journal of Clinical Epidemiology 43(11): 1191–1199

Thomas M 1995 Treatment of pain with acupuncture: factors influencing outcome. Thesis, Departments of Physiology and Pharmacology and Surgery KS III, Karolinska Institute, Karolinska Hospital, Stockholm, Sweden

Thomas M, Eriksson S V, Lundeberg T 1991 A comparative study of diazepam and acupuncture in patients with osteoarthritis pain: a placebo controlled study. American Journal of Chinese Medicine XIX(2): 95–100

Thomas M, Arnèr S, Lundeberg T 1992 Is acupuncture an alternative in idiopathic pain disorder? Acta Anaesthesiol Scandinavica 36: 637–642

Thomas M, Lundeberg T 1994 Importance of modes of acupuncture in the treatment of chronic nociceptive low back pain. Acta Anaesthesiol Scandinavica 38: 63–69

Thomas M, Lundeberg T, Björk G, Lundström-Lindstedt V 1995 Pain and discomfort in primary dysmenorrhea is reduced by preemptive acupuncture or low frequency TENS. European Journal of Physical Medicine and Rehabilitation 5(3): 71–76

Wall P D 1994 The placebo and the placebo response. In: Wall P D, Melzack R (eds) Textbook of pain. Churchill Livingstone, New York, pp 1297–1308

Williams J B W, Spitzer R L 1982 Idiopathic pain disorder: a critique of pain-prone disorder and a proposal for revision of the DSM-III category psychogenic pain disorder. Journal of Nervous and Mental Diseases 170: 415–419

Woolf C J, Thompson J W 1994 Stimulation induced analgesia: transcutaneous electrical stimulation (TENS) and vibration. In: Wall P D, Melzack R (eds) Textbook of pain. Churchill Livingstone, New York, pp 1191–1208

Laser acupuncture

G. David Baxter

Background

Laser is an acronym for Light Amplification by Stimulated Emission of Radiation, the principles for which were proposed in the early 1900s by Albert Einstein. The first operational laser was produced by Theodore Maiman in 1960, based upon a ruby crystal that produced (visible) red light at 694 nm. The ensuing decade saw the development of a range of laser devices employing alternative lasing materials that allowed the production of laser radiation at different wavelengths. This new technology rapidly found applications in a variety of fields, but particularly in medicine, where the potential for laser devices, particularly as a surgical tool, was quickly recognized. Lasers have subsequently found applications in ophthalmology, for welding detached retinas, as an alternative to metal scalpels in plastic and general surgery and for the removal of tattoos and port-wine stains in dermatology. This list is not meant to be exhaustive, merely illustrative; however, all such applications rely to a greater or lesser degree on the thermal and ablative light–tissue interactions of high power lasers producing relatively high incident intensities (> 100 W/cm^2).

In contrast, laser devices typically operating at much lower output powers and thus producing relatively lower power densities (< 5 W/cm^2) have also found medical application since the early 1970s, largely based upon the early work of Professor Endre Mester (Mester, Mester & Mester 1985), which demonstrated the potential of such irradiation to stimulate certain biological processes and thus wound healing. This so-called laser photobiostimulation rapidly found application for the treatment of various types of open wounds and ulcers in a number of countries, particularly in Eastern Europe and the former Soviet Union; for such therapy, the output of a helium neon (He-Ne) laser device was directed onto the surface of the wound bed typically using a fibre-optic system to deliver radiant exposures of up to 4 J/cm^2.

The use of lasers in this way to affect treatment, which has come to be termed 'low intensity laser therapy' (LILT) (Baxter 1994) or 'low level laser therapy' (Ohshiro & Calderhead 1988), subsequently spread during the late 1970s and particularly the 1980s to Western Europe, Asia and the Americas (excluding the USA), where, in addition to the use of gaseous (and therefore somewhat cumbersome) He-Ne units, small diode-based laser units operating in the red and near infrared spectra were quickly exploited as therapeutic units. Apart from open wounds, the applications of this therapy also extended to include the treatment of soft tissue injuries, arthritic conditions and the management of pain of various aetiologies. In addition to the direct application of diode-based probes to the appropriate lesion (e.g. a wound), therapeutic units have been applied to other sites such as nerve roots or trunks, as well as lymphatic vessels and nodes. In addition, and most importantly for the current text, laser units have also been applied directly to acupuncture or trigger points as a non-invasive alternative to metal needles, based upon the work of Dr Friedrich Plog of Canada and others (see Baxter 1989). Two examples are given in Case studies 11.1 and 11.2. This application of therapeutic lasers to perform acupuncture treatment is termed simply 'laser acupuncture' to

CASE STUDY 11.1

History This 48-year-old housewife had attended for treatment for musculoskeletal injuries sustained during a road traffic accident some 12 months before her first appointment; these were principally associated with shoulder and neck pain and dysfunction. In addition to these symptoms, she also complained of bouts of severe nausea coupled with sensations of "bloating", which had developed in the period since the accident; as a result (in conjunction with her musculoskeletal injuries) she had started to become depressed. The patient was on long term sick leave when she first attended for treatment.

Examination Apart from a full physical assessment for neck, back and shoulders, the patient was also referred by her General Practitioner for a variety of investigations because of her consistent complaints of emesis. Nothing adverse was detected by such specialist investigations.

Treatment In addition to a comprehensive regimen of physical therapy for her back and shoulder problems,

the patient also received laser acupuncture treatments of the PE-6 point on the ventral forearm using a 30 mW single diode 830 nm probe. This was initiated at a dosage of 1.5 J/cm^2 (~ 0.15 J per point) and progressed to 10 J/cm^2 (~ 1 J per point) by the end of treatment some 6 weeks later. In this case laser acupuncture was the method of choice as the lady was especially nervous of needles.

Outcome The patient's emesis resolved well with laser acupuncture, although frequent treatments (two per week) were necessary to maintain the beneficial antiemetic effects of treatment. In order to attempt to increase the effects of treatment, the patient was also advised on TENS as an alternative method of stimulation for home use; unfortunately the patient was typically non-compliant, which adversely affected this progression of treatment. At the time of discharge, the beneficial effects of treatment were still evident, although these remained short term (~ 48–72 h).

CASE STUDY 11.2

History A 44-year-old male sales representative had developed a painful neck and right trapezius one evening after a day spent carrying heavy loads to and from an exhibition stand. The patient was right handed and had reported no previous problems with his neck or right shoulder.

Examination On examination, the patient's cervical range of movements was found to be complete with the sole exception of right rotation, which was slightly limited ($\sim 25\%$). In addition a number of easily identified (i.e. extremely tender) trigger points were palpable in the patient's trapezius; the shoulder and neck appeared to be otherwise clear.

Treatment The patient's trigger points were irradiated

using a 200 mW single diode 820 nm probe pulsed at 16 Hz; such treatment was delivered at a dosage of 60 J/cm^2 (i.e. ~ 6 J per point). During treatment, the patient reported a distinct tingling sensation underneath the probe head, which left an area of "warmth" post-treatment; treatment was provided on two occasions approximately 12 h apart (i.e. late evening and early the subsequent morning).

Outcome The initial treatment effectively desensitized the trigger points to palpation; the patient reported a numb sensation by 10 min post-treatment. While some residual tenderness was obvious the following morning, the single further treatment completely resolved this problem.

distinguish it from LILT, which relies upon the principal desired effect of photobiostimulation.

The rest of this chapter will concentrate on the practical basis and rationale for the use of laser in acupuncture and will conclude with a brief overview of research findings to date.

Laser treatment devices: biophysical principles

Components (see Fig. 11.1)

All laser treatment devices may be thought of as comprising three essential components:

- a *lasing medium*, either contained in a chamber with reflecting surfaces mounted at either end if the medium is gaseous, or a simple diode that is highly polished to allow the light to resonate within the diode before "escaping" as the output of the unit
- an *electrical supply unit* or *battery*

- some form of *control unit* (which in terms of complexity varies from a simple on/off switch to panels that would not look out of place in the cockpit of an aircraft).

Characteristics of laser radiation

Monochromaticity and wavelength

Laser devices produce highly monochromatic (single-coloured) light, typically in the visible red or near infrared spectrum (i.e. wavelengths 630–950 nm); it should be noted that wavelength is not a user-defined radiation parameter on those devices used in laser acupuncture treatments. Absorption of laser radiation by target tissue is wavelength specific, and several studies have been completed at the cellular and clinical level that would suggest that this represents an important parameter in the biological and clinical effects of LILT (e.g. see Shields & O'Kane 1994). In contrast, for laser acupuncture treatments, it would appear that a range of wavelengths have been employed with little indication of the benefits of one wavelength over another.

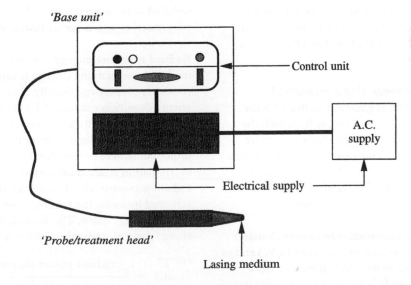

Fig. 11.1 *Component parts of a laser treatment device.*

Collimation/divergence

Unlike conventional light sources, the output (light) from laser units is essentially parallel (highly collimated), with virtually no divergence. This means that all the energy of the unit is "bundled" into a small cross-sectional beam area and thus laser–tissue interaction occurs in a highly localized area of tissue directly under the treatment head.

Coherence

The term 'coherence' essentially refers to the synchronicity of the rays or photons within the light beam. Normal light sources produce radiation that is non-coherent, radiating in all directions and out of phase; in contrast, laser sources produce parallel rays that are in sequence or "in step" over both distance and time. The importance of this characteristic of laser sources is not entirely clear; debate continues over the precise relevance of coherence to the biological and clinical effects of these devices.

Laser irradiation parameters

Laser irradiation (or stimulation of acupuncture points) is determined by a number of parameters, some of which are defined by the machine used for treatment, and others that are defined by the user. These are as follows.

Wavelength (see above) This is measured in nanometres (nm) and is generally defined by the diode fitted in the treatment probe, for which the wavelength is fixed during manufacture. Longer wavelengths (e.g. > 830 nm) are typically associated with greater depths of penetration; thus for some acupuncture treatments this parameter might be a critical factor in the success of treatment.

Radiant power output/irradiance (power density) Power output is measured in milliwatts (mW) and is again dependent upon the diode used; as already indicated, recent trends have been towards the use of higher power outputs (i.e. at least 30 mW). Power density, or irradiance, is specified in mW/cm² and is determined by dividing the incident radiant power by the area of irradiation; this parameter should be

maximized by use of a "contact" technique (i.e. with the applicator/diode held firmly against the target tissue). In the majority of cases, for a given unit used "in contact" the irradiance is essentially fixed; for a system based upon a 30 mW diode this should be in the region of 300 mW/cm².

Energy This is typically employed as a simple measure of dosage and is specified in Joules (J) or sometimes millijoules (mJ). Energy delivered during a treatment is defined by the operator and is essentially a function of the irradiation time, as for a given unit the longer the time of irradiation the greater is the dosage. The calculation of energy delivered during a treatment is simply:

energy (J) = radiant power output (W) × time (s)

Where the output is specified in milliwatts (mW), the calculated figure for energy will be in millijoules (mJ).

Based upon published accounts and current clinical practice, dosage in joules can range from 0.01 to 5 J per point for routine acupuncture treatments. Unless there are specific reasons to exercise special caution (e.g. suspected sensitivity to sunlight, or to acupuncture treatments), treatments can safely be initiated at between 0.1 and 1 J per point and progressed over a series or course of treatments.

Radiant exposure/energy density A more precise method for specifying dosage is radiant exposure or (more simply) energy density. As its name implies, energy density is calculated by taking the total energy delivered during a treatment and dividing it by the area of irradiation; its units are therefore Joules per square centimetre (J/cm²). Where the area of irradiation is small for a given energy level, the radiant exposure will be maximized; this is usually achieved by using the treatment head in firm contact with the target tissue. The formula for calculation of energy density/radiant exposure is:

$$\frac{\text{energy}}{\text{density}} = \frac{\text{radiant power output (W)} \times \text{time (s)}}{\text{time (s)}}$$
$$(\text{J/cm}^2)$$

Where radiant power output is specified in milliwatts (mW), energy density will be in millijoules per square centimetre (mJ/cm²). For the types of diodes typically used in laser therapy devices, a useful working estimate of spot size during in contact treatments (see below) will be 0.1–0.125 cm^2.

For laser acupuncture, current clinical practice and review of the literature indicates that dosages may range from less than 0.1 J/cm^{+2} (~ 0.01 J) to over 50 J/cm^{+2} (~ 5 J). For routine laser acupuncture applications, treatment may be initiated safely at radiant exposures of between 1 and 10 J/cm^{+2} and steadily progressed over the course of treatments.

Pulse repetition rate An increasing number of manufacturers provide the option of pulsing the output of their units, based upon the premise that such pulsing enhances the biological and thus clinical effects of irradiation. Where pulsing of output is provided, it is important to check the effect that this has upon the radiant output of the laser treatment device; in some units this can significantly alter the output, for example a unit delivering 30 mW as a continuous wave (non-pulsed) may deliver only 10 mW when pulsed. A variety of pulse repetition rates have been used during laser acupuncture treatments, from continuous wave (not pulsing) to pulsing frequencies in the megahertz range.

Principles of application

Selection of unit

A unit comprising a single diode unit is the most appropriate device for laser acupuncture treatments. While a variety of units have been cited in the literature as effective means of performing laser acupuncture treatments, the trend in recent years has been towards relatively higher power devices with radiant outputs of between 30 and 200 mW rather than the 1 mW or less that was typically recommended for acupuncture applications for up to 10 years ago.

Use of contact technique

The inverse square law applies to radiant light from a laser treatment unit, despite its having minimal divergence; as a consequence, the further the treatment head is from the target tissue, the greater will be the spot size, and the lower the density of photons on the tissue surface. For a given irradiation time, the further the head is from the tissue, the lower will be the radiant exposure (i.e. the lower the dosage). Therapeutic laser units are designed to be used in (firm) contact, which not only keeps the spot size small but also lowers the reflection from the surface of the skin and (with firm pressure) helps combine a manual "pressure" treatment with the laser irradiation. At centres in some countries, and particularly in Japan, contact technique is combined with vigorous manipulation of the treatment head to enhance the stimulation given during treatments. The potential benefits of such additional pressure or manipulations applied during acupuncture treatments are obvious.

Indications for treatment

Contraindications notwithstanding (see below), in theory laser stimulation may be used to affect any acupuncture treatment for which metal needles are typically used. Laser stimulation is particularly suited:

- for the treatment of nervous patients or children
- for the treatment of especially sensitive points (e.g. CV-1, GV-1)
- for the treatment of auricular points
- as an alternative to invasive procedures in patients infected with (e.g.) HIV or hepatitis.

Safety and good treatment practice

Safety considerations

Laser treatment units, like any other electrotherapy device, should be maintained in a good state of repair in line with the manufacturer's recommendations and as required by local health and safety arrangements. Safety arrangements for laser therapy devices are essentially those for any class 3B laser unit. In the first instance, the laser should be kept in a designated area, preferably with access restricted to trained personnel. The security key should be held separately and access to this should be similarly limited to designated, trained personnel, all of whom should receive a standard briefing on the operation of the laser device, including safety features, dangers and contraindications.

Dangers and contraindications

The standard precautions and dangers associated with acupuncture (e.g. forbidden points, etc.) apply to laser acupuncture, with the obvious exception of those precautions/dangers arising from puncture (e.g. dangers inherent in poor sterilization procedures/aseptic techniques). Details of these can be found elsewhere in this text (Chapter 4).

The major danger associated with laser treatment is the potential eye hazard through accidental intrabeam viewing, where the highly collimated output of the laser is focused on to a single (small) spot on the retina, thus causing (irreparable) damage to the eye. It is because of these attendant risks that caution is recommended when irradiating points near the eye, and direct irradiation of the eye for whatever reason is contraindicated. However, it must be stressed that the risk of such injury while using therapeutic laser units is essentially negligible, especially when the laser is used in contact with the irradiated area (as during laser acupuncture treatments) and where approved laser safety goggles are worn.

Contraindications to laser treatment principally include the following.

Laser treatment in cases of active or suspected carcinoma This is due to the biostimulatory potential of these devices which might exacerbate the growth and spread of tumourous cells.

Irradiation over the pregnant uterus This is a well-recognized contraindication that is common to most electrotherapeutic modalities.

Irradiation over areas of haemorrhage This is proposed as an absolute contraindication because of the potential exacerbation of blood loss through laser-mediated increases in blood flow.

Other contraindications These have been identified

by the Chartered Society of Physiotherapy's Safety of Electrotherapy Equipment Working Group (1991) and have been discussed elsewhere (Baxter 1994); these include treatment over areas of hypoaesthesia, infected open wounds and the gonads.

Overview of published findings

A detailed review of current findings is beyond the scope of the current text; however, the following provides an overview of work to date in this area. The most commonly reported trials of laser acupuncture treatments are for the relief of pain of various aetiologies, for example musculoskeletal and neurogenic pain (Choi, Srikantha & Wu 1986, Kreczi & Klinger 1986, Shiroto, Ono & Ohshiro 1989), as well as as an alternative anaesthetic for minor surgical procedures (Qin 1987, Zhou Yo Cheng 1984). Results from such studies on pain management are generally (although not exclusively) positive and reflect the popularity of the technique at certain centres (Baxter 1989). Despite such advocacy, it is interesting to note that, in at least one condition, the treatment of lateral epicondylalgia, careful controlled comparison of laser and conventional acupuncture found the latter to be significantly superior to treatment with laser (Haker 1991). However, other studies detail apparently successful treatment of a variety of other conditions such as pelvic inflammation and exophthalmic hyperthyroidism (e.g. Qin 1987, Wei 1981, Wu 1983). Although (again) such studies invariably report positive results, they are typically limited because of lack of blinding and inadequate controls. Thus further clinically based research is indicated to establish definitively the degree of efficacy of these techniques in the management of the conditions indicated and the benefits (if indeed any) over conventional (needle) acupuncture treatment.

As a precursor to such clinical studies, laboratory investigations using experimental models of pain in healthy human volunteers represent a useful means of assessment of the hypoalgesic effects of laser acupuncture under carefully controlled conditions. However, despite the potential advantages in this approach, only a few studies have been completed in this area to date, and these have been based exclusively upon threshold models of experimental pain, with variable results (e.g. Brockhaus & Elger 1990, Martin 1988, King et al 1990). Martin's early study at this centre (Martin 1988, unpublished dissertation University of Ulster) found significant increases in mechanical pain threshold after a single dose of laser acupuncture treatment in the lower limb; similarly, laser acupuncture of four auricular points (0.03 J per point) in the study of King et al (1990) was found to produce significant increases in electrical pain threshold compared with non-irradiated controls. In contrast, Brockhaus and Elger failed to find any significant effect upon thermal pain threshold after bilateral irradiation of the LI-4 Hegu and EX-37 Jianqian acupuncture points (0.6 J per point), whilst subjects receiving needle acupuncture in this study showed significant increases in pain threshold (Brockhaus & Elger 1990). Given such contradictory findings, additional research is necessary to establish definitively the hypoalgesic potential of laser acupuncture techniques in the laboratory.

References

Baxter G D 1989 Laser acupuncture analgesia: an overview. Acupuncture in Medicine 6: 57–60

Baxter G D 1994 Therapeutic lasers: theory and practice. Churchill Livingstone, Edinburgh, pp 58–62

Brockhaus A, Elger C E 1990 Hypoalgesic efficacy of acupuncture on experimental pain in man. Comparison of laser acupuncture and needle acupuncture. Pain 43: 181–186

Chartered Society of Physiotherapy; Safety of Electrotherapy Equipment Working Group 1991 Guidelines for the safe use of lasers in physiotherapy. Physiotherapy 77: 169–170

Choi J J, Srikantha K, Wu K-H 1986 A comparison of electroacupuncture, transcutaneous electrical nerve stimulation and laser photobiostimulation on pain relief and glucocorticoid excretion. International Journal of Acupuncture and Electrotherapeutics Research 11: 45–51

Haker E 1991 Lateral epicondylalgia (tennis elbow): a diagnostic and therapeutic challenge. Doctoral Thesis, Karolinska Institute, Stockholm

King C E, Clelland J A, Knowles C J et al 1990 Effect of helium neon laser auriculotherapy on experimental pain threshold. Physical Therapy 70: 24–30

Kreczi T, Klinger D 1986 A comparison of laser acupuncture versus placebo in radicular and pseudo-radicular pain syndromes as recorded by subjective responses to pain. International Journal of Acupuncture and Electrotherapeutics Research 11: 207–216

Mester E, Mester A F, Mester A 1985 The biomedical effects of laser application. Lasers in Surgery and Medicine 5: 31–39

Ohshiro T, Calderhead R G 1988 Low level laser therapy: a practical introduction. Wiley, Chichester

Qin J N 1987 Laser acupuncture anaesthesia and therapy in the People's Republic of China. Annals of the Academy of Medicine of Singapore 16: 261–263

Shields T D, O'Kane S 1994 Laser photobiomodulation of wound healing. In: Baxter G D (ed) Therapeutic lasers: theory and practice. Churchill Livingstone, New York, pp 89–138

Shiroto C, Ono K, Ohshiro T 1989 Retrospective study of diode laser therapy for pain attenuation in 3635 patients: detailed analysis by questionnaire. Laser Therapy 1: 41–48

Wei X 1981 Laser treatment of common diseases in surgery and acupuncture in the People's Republic of China: preliminary report. International Journal of Acupuncture and Electrotherapeutics Research 6: 19–31

Wu W 1983 Recent advances in laserpuncture. In: Atsumi K (ed) New frontiers in laser medicine and surgery. Elsevier, Amsterdam

Zhou Yo Cheng 1984 An advanced clinical trial with laser acupuncture anaesthesia for minor operations in the oromaxillo-facial region. Lasers in Surgery and Medicine 4: 297–303

A simple approach to ear acupuncture

Michael Anderson

The approach taken in this chapter is to view ear acupuncture (EA) as one of the microsystems; as such EA can be used as a treatment system in its own right, or as an adjunct to whole-body acupuncture.

Historical perspective

EA was first recognized as a reflex system by Paul Nogier in the 1950s. TCM has long described channels that passed through or around the regions of the ear, for example, the Yellow Emperor's Classic of Internal Medicine refers to Yang channels and the ear. However, even the Chinese give the credit of discovery of EA as a microsystem to Nogier (1983).

Dale (1984) described the microsystems in detail, but most importantly: "all neuro-points ... are bi-directional patterns; they are both organ-cutaneous and cutaneous-organ reflexes. The organ-cutaneous is a diagnostic indicator when the patient feels tenderness at the locus. Conversely, the cutaneous-organ reflex is a therapeutic trigger."

Nogier gradually built up the concept of "the man in the ear" – in this, a homunculus in the form of an inverted fetus was conceived with the head in the lobe region of the ear and the limbs towards the top of the ear. If there is change in the body system due to pathology then a corresponding change can be shown on the ear, in an appropriate region.

When treating the pathology, using body acupuncture points as well as ear points, deal with the ear points first as these may change after body acupuncture. (This is due to the organ-cutaneous and cutaneous-organ reflex response mentioned before.)

Note that this is a *reflex system* and as such should not be expected to have correspondences similar to those found in TCM. For example, a bone problem – say a painful metacarpal bone following a fracture – would show a change in the organ-cutaneous reflex in the zone where the metacarpal was represented. No change would be expected in the zone representing the Kidney (Kidney influences bone in TCM) unless there was Kidney pathology from another cause.

Principles

The indicators of pathology can include:

- changes in the appearance of the skin
- changes in the skin resistance
- changes in tenderness or sensitivity of the skin overlying the representative point.

This was demonstrated in a blinded trial by Oleson, Kroening & Bresler (1980) and published in the Western, peer-refereed, journal Pain. They demonstrated that by looking at the ear, testing for tenderness and measuring changes in electrical resistance of the skin, they could diagnose pathology in patients with 74% accuracy. This was statistically highly significant. As the method also picked up old pathology that the patients had forgotten about until reminded after the study, the results could have been even better if this was taken into account. Kroening (personal communication, 1993) points out that no-one so far has challenged the findings or reproduced this work.

The embryological work described by Bourdiol (1982) gives an explanation for EA based on the innervation of the ear, which results in nerves V_3, VII, IX, X and branches of the superficial cervical plexus (SCP) being incorporated into the ear. These nerves travel from the ear (only a short distance) to the cranial nerve inputs and the reticular formation of the brainstem.

To apply EA successfully it is essential to learn some basic anatomy of the external ear (Fig. 12.1). It can be broadly divided into four areas (see Fig. 12.2) depending on the appearances of the surfaces of the ear:

- raised
- hollow (depressed)
- flat
- hidden.

Oleson and Kroening (1983a) suggested nomenclature that can quickly and easily identify

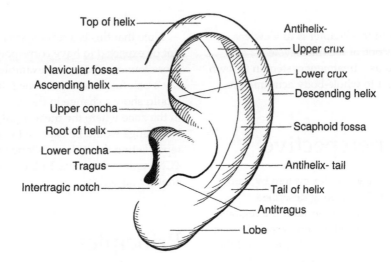

Fig. 12.1 *The anatomy of the external ear.*

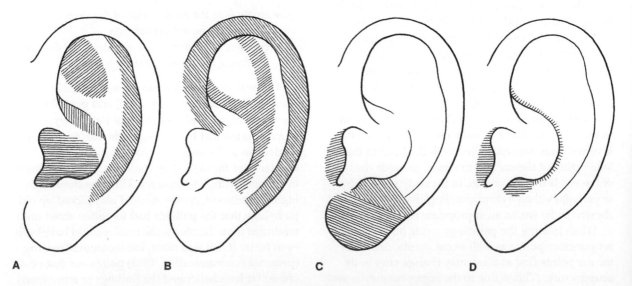

Fig. 12.2 *Areas of the ear: (A) Hollow surfaces (B) Raised surfaces (C) Flat surfaces. (D) Hidden surfaces.*

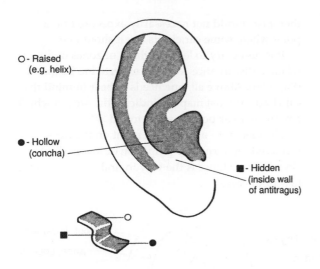

O - Raised
(e.g. helix)

● - Hollow
(concha)

■ - Hidden
(inside wall
of antitragus)

Fig. 12.3 *Raised, depressed and hidden regions of the ear (Oleson & Kroening 1983a).*

whether the region required is in a zone that is raised, depressed or hidden (Fig. 12.3). They also looked at some of the discrepancies between the Nogier school and the Chinese ear charts, (Oleson & Kroening 1983b). There are disparities in point positions between different charts obtained from China, i.e. they do not agree with each other. Some reasons for this can be understood by reference to the concept of zones rather than points, and stimulation of nerve supply to, rather than stimulation of the

organ per se. This leads to the concept of *structure* versus *function*.

Histology of the ear

Histology

The areas of interest from the perspective of acupuncture are the neurovascular bundles. Histologically they form three separate types: small, medium, and very large (over helix and lobule).

These correspond anatomically to three innervations:

- third division of the trigeminal nerve (V_3)
- the vagus nerve (X)
- the SCP (C1 and C2).

Territory (Fig. 12.4)

The above classification gives rise to a notion of territory in which areas are grouped according to:

- anatomical location
- origin in the embryo
- innervation
- autonomic polarity (i.e. sympathetic or parasympathetic)

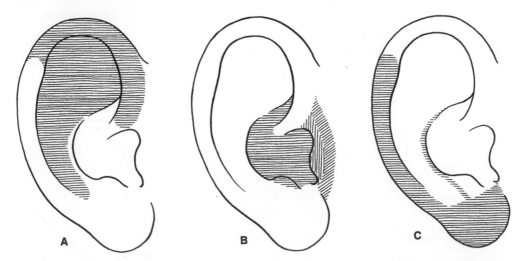

A   B   C

Fig. 12.4 *Ear territories according to embryological origin: (A) Territory one (T1) – mesodermal. (B) Territory two (T2) – endodermal. (C) Territory three (T3) – ectodermal.*

- structures and organs mapped in this area coming from the same embryological leaf e.g. mesoderm, endoderm, or ectoderm.

Finding the points

It is easy to learn where the expected zone of disturbance will be found if the picture of the inverted fetus is kept in mind (Fig. 12.5).

A quick look at several different ears will show that all ears are not made equal and consequently the therapist should not necessarily expect to find a point where some ear charts say it should be.

It is necessary to learn to think of zones of the ear where a disturbance could be expected to be found (Fig. 12.6). Above all, one needs to bear in mind that ear charts are just maps to indicate the area in which a particular ear point may be found.

The reactivity of a specific point on the ear – increased tenderness to palpation or lowered electrical resistance is the way to find the exact point to acupuncture.

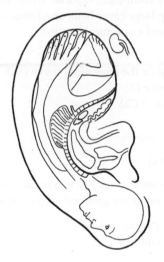

Fig. 12.5 *The 'inverted fetus' concept of the ear.*

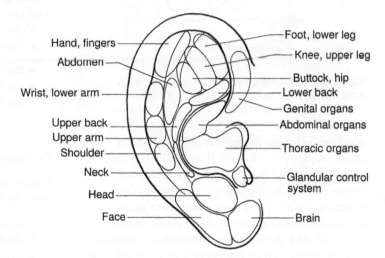

Fig. 12.6 *Organ zones.*

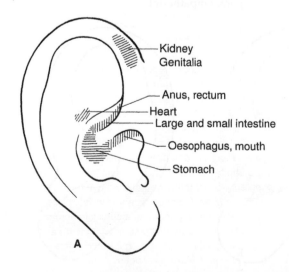

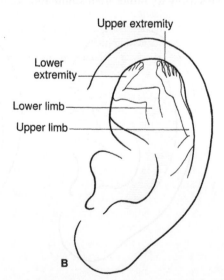

Fig. 12.7 *Examples of specific zones: (A) Internal organs. (B) Musculoskeletal.*

Procedure

First, the most tender area needs to be found by gently palpating the ear lobe with a steady pressure (250 g). There are spring-loaded pressure palpators available, but the handle end of the needle can also be used, or the end of a matchstick. The important factor is the constant pressure. When the most tender spot becomes apparent (and it may take up to 30 s of gentle probing) then this is the site for needle insertion.

The ear should then be cleaned, using alcohol to remove the natural oils from the skin. The needle is inserted through the skin and through the cartilage (there are points on the back of the ear). A small needle is satisfactory (e.g. 0.22 × 15 mm). There is little risk of infection if the skin has been cleaned and then sterilized with 2% iodine in 70% alcohol, and left on the skin for at least 2 min, and sterile disposable needles are used.

The needles are usually left in for the duration of the treatment session (15–20 min) but can be left in for longer.

Semipermanent needles are designed to sit in the ear and stimulate the point for several days. They are retained longer if the area is treated with iodine or alcohol and then sprayed with plastic dressing (e.g. Opsite™).

Patients may be exquisitely tender over the reactive points and respond well to semipermanent ionic beads. These are small ballbearing-like objects that are struck over the site with an adhesive tape patch, and can be stimulated by the patient by pressing the bead. It is considered to be a form of acupressure of the point.

The ear points also respond to the energy from low level lasers, and this method can be used as an alternative to needles.

Electrical point finders

A word of caution regarding the use of electrical point finders must be given: the point must not be too sharp and the pressure must be constant (usually a spring-loaded point) to prevent damage to the stratum corneum of the ear. Once the skin is damaged by excessive pressure a lower skin resistance is recorded consequently, giving a "false positive" acupuncture point.

Similarly, if the point finder allows a current that is too high to flow across the stratum corneum, a low resistance pathway is burnt through, and this also gives false results.

Summary

- Ear acupuncture is a reflex system using organ-cutaneous and cutaneous-organ reflexes.
- Its discovery as a reflex system is attributed to Paul Nogier.
- Charts are often inaccurate and must be seen only as maps to guide to zones.
- Look for the region required by memorizing the somatic zones.
- Look for indicators of pathology.
- Indicators of pathology include:
    changes in appearances
    changes in sensitivity
    changes in skin resistance.
- Find the appropriate points and sterilize the skin.
- Needle the point using small needles.
- Consider the use of "semipermanent" beads or needles.

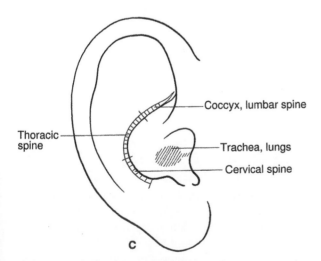

Fig. 12.7 *(C) Specific zones of spinal tenderness.*

- Laser treatment of the points may be tried.
- If combining body acupuncture with ear acupuncture, look for the points on the ear first, as they can alter as a response to body acupuncture (organ-cutaneous reflex).

References

Bourdiol R J (ed) 1982 Elements of auriculotherapy. Maisonnerve Editions

Dale R 1984 Principles and systems of micro-acupuncture. International Journal of Chinese Medicine 1(4): 1–28

Nogier P F M (ed) 1983 From auriculotherapy to auriculomedicine. Maisonneuve Editions, Paris, p. 32

Oleson T D, Kroening R J 1983a A new nomenclature for identifying Chinese and Nogier auricular acupuncture points. American Journal of Acupuncture 11(4): 325–344

Oleson T D, Kroening R J 1983b A comparison of Chinese and Nogier auricular acupuncture points. American Journal of Acupuncture 11(3): 205–223

Oleson T D, Kroening R J, Bresler D E 1980 An experimental evaluation of auricular diagnosis: the somatotopic mapping of musculoskeletal pain at ear acupuncture points. Pain 8: 217–229

SECTION THREE

Developments

13

Integration of acupuncture with physiotherapy

Maureen Lovesey, Carol Taylor, Nadia Ellis, Charles Liggins and Sara Mokone

A selection of viewpoints from around the world of particular aspects of clinical practice is given in the following sections.

Outpatients – private practice

UK (Maureen Lovesey)

Physiotherapists are increasingly using acupuncture in clinical practice and finding it a very useful modality of treatment. Its use depends on the training of the therapist concerned. Therapists who have undergone a basic training in acupuncture use it to help pain relief whilst those who have undertaken more advanced training use it to help a wide range of conditions as well.

In the early 1980s I undertook a 2 year part-time intensive course in acupuncture in London. My reasons for training in acupuncture were unclear as at the time I had no real in-depth interest or belief in the subject. However, it was becoming clear that the public were becoming increasingly interested in alternative therapies. My attention was drawn to a course that was designed and aimed particularly at physical therapists. One of the teachers on this course had fractured his wrist a few years previously and having previously taken an acupuncture course was able to treat patients using acupuncture during that period when he could not do manual therapy. This seemed to be a useful fallback position for someone in private practice.

The course was based on TCM. When approaching this system, it must be remembered that the Chinese at the time did not have any knowledge of anatomy or physiology but instead very carefully and systematically recorded clinical observations, from which they gradually built up a pattern that was fairly logical in its approach. Unfortunately, where they did not have an explanation for something they appeared to me to elaborate a story around the area concerned, and I found that I was not able to embrace the Chinese philosophy very well.

However, once we started seeing patients in the clinic it became clear to me that there appeared to be marked benefits from the acupuncture treatments. Most of these patients were at the end of the road and had sought help from many other sources before coming to acupuncture. Although most of them were not "cured" the majority seemed to be greatly helped by acupuncture. I had long realized that the actions of many medicines and therapies were outside current knowledge and it was not possible to put these into neat little boxes with labelled explanations, however much one desired to have full scientific understanding of the underlying mechanisms. Having seen the beneficial effects demonstrated and that there appeared to be potentially very few side-effects, and that these were rare provided that the treatment was skilfully given, I decided to carry on with my studies and have since had no regrets on that front.

Learning is a continual process and I am delighted that acupuncture continues to be a fascinating subject that one learns more and more about as one delves into it. This is in contrast to learning some new technique or modality which appears to be the "flavour of the year" and then fades out. I am pleased to report that as one learns more over the years and applies the modality better the results seem to improve. Not only is this beneficial to patients but also gives the therapist increased personal satisfaction. Physiotherapists are particularly suited to give acupuncture, with their background knowledge of anatomy and neurophysiology, and they find it very complementary to their other skills; the majority of treatments are carried out in conjunction with other modalities such as lifestyle advice and counselling, manual therapy, etc. (Alltree 1993). The effects that have been noted by the Chinese have gradually been validated by scientific research around the world.

When I first started using acupuncture in my practice I had some difficulty at first with "assessment procedures" as to whether to use a Western-based approach or a Chinese one. It was relatively easy with external/superficial/channel/musculoskeletal problems where I continued to use a Western assessment adapted from a "Cyriax" type assessment (Cyriax 1975) (see Chapter 5) and with more internal problems such as asthma and irritable bladder where it was more obvious to me to use traditional type assessment. The problem came over which assessment route to choose when, as commonly happens, the patient presented with mixed pathology. An example of this might be a patient with low back pain that was worse at times of menstrual periods, although not necessarily only associated with them, who also had dysmenorrhoea. Ideally with this sort of case it would probably be useful to follow both types of assessment fully but this is not always possible; although I allow quite a long time to assess patients on the first occasion the time frame did not allow for this in the early days and I was left unsure as to which route to choose at first. Gradually this problem solved itself and I now find it relatively easy to combine the best from both worlds according to the patient presenting, although sometimes following up with a more intensive assessment using one of the routes on the second session.

The initial problems with the assessment procedures soon settled down and I found I was able to move reasonably comfortably from one system to another. Acupuncture works well with other therapies and I was easily able to assimilate in into my practice.

In my practice I have two associates working with me; we treat a wide range of patients with ages ranging between 4–90 plus years. Many of the patients have multiple, complex problems. The largest groups of problems include: musculoskeletal (spinal, injuries, joint and muscle problems, etc.), stress-related problems (including headaches, depression, anxiety attacks and some patients with chronic fatigue states), women's problems (PMT, dysmenorrhoea, irregular periods, menopausal problems, incontinence and obstetric complications). We also treat quite a few patients with respiratory problems (sinusitis, asthma, hayfever and bronchitis), some bladder and bowel problems and a few neurological and skin conditions. About 75% of patients attending the practice receive acupuncture or acupuncture-related techniques in one form or another. All patients attending the practice also have lifestyle advice, which is usually accompanied by some simple exercises. Many patients have acupuncture or related techniques in conjunction with other physiotherapy techniques that we offer such as electrotherapy, manual therapy and massage.

As a migraine sufferer myself I have a particular interest in the treatment of this condition and treat quite a large number of migraine and tension headache sufferers. A number of research studies (Lundeberg et al 1988, Vincent 1989) have shown that acupuncture can help reduce the severity and frequency of attacks. I use a combination of treatments tailored to suit the patient; these might include acupuncture, electrotherapy, exercises, food testing, lifestyle counselling and training, manual therapy, massage and relaxation training. Most of the patients have acupuncture and the other treatments seem to enhance the effects so that, as with the research trials above, the frequency and severity of attacks and need for medication are much reduced. After a course of treatment the majority of patients are able to manage themselves with the help of occasional medication; often a simple analgesic will suffice whereas previously they needed prescription drugs. Some patients need periodic treatment.

Some of the ways in which we utilize acupuncture in the practice for simpler situations, include the following. After a careful assessment of the problem, a possible treatment programme to help this would be discussed with the patient. In formulating a treatment programme it must be remembered that, although public opinion has moved greatly in recent years and many people are actually requesting acupuncture, for some it will remain an alien method of treatment and this will obviously vary between cultural groups. If acupuncture would seem to be the treatment of choice it may be possible to persuade the patient to try a few sessions but clearly one must not go against their wishes. For those patients who have needle phobia, acupressure and laser acupuncture are other suitable methods.

For sports injuries, laser acupuncture is a helpful adjunct to perhaps more local treatment with something like interferential and/or laser cluster to the damaged area. With spinal problems I would normally start with more conventional physiotherapy such as manual therapy, heat and interferential, traction, etc. unless the patient had complex problems or had not responded to treatment given elsewhere. I would then move on to using acupuncture if they were not getting better after a few sessions.

Some of the patients coming to the practice have had more conventional treatments elsewhere and have not responded but often respond well when treated with acupuncture. Many patients report after having a few sessions of acupuncture that they feel much better in themselves and ask whether acupuncture could be having an effect on other parts of the body that they had not previously mentioned. This phenomenon has been noticed and reported by many others using acupuncture. Mrs Nadia Ellis, who is currently Chairman of the Acupuncture Association of Chartered Physiotherapists (AACP) noticed when treating her patients for musculoskeletal problems such as arthritis that many of them were reporting that they were not getting up at night to go to the toilet. She utilized this observation in a private research project that she did as part of an MSc at Southampton University, where she studied night frequency in the elderly (Ellis 1993). The results of her pilot study showed a statistically significant reduction in night frequency in this group of patients after 2 weeks' treatment. The example given in Case study 13.1 illustrates how two problems may be eased at the same time.

CASE STUDY 13.1

Reason for referral Mrs H S, aged 41, with low back and right sciatica.

Assessment findings Mrs S reported that she had had some mild intermittent low back pain for about 5 years but it had not necessitated any treatment. About 6 months previously she experienced a sudden onset of acute right-sided low back pain and sciatica. She had had a minor road traffic accident 2 years previously, which had increased weakness on the left side. She also reported frequency and urgency on urination and was getting up two to three times at night. Upon examination flexion was moderately limited, in extension there was major loss, side flexion was reasonable, and she was sore at right lumbar 5. Her tongue was slightly pale, swollen and wet. Her pulse was slippery and the Kidney pulse was depleted.

Treatment I started her on some acupuncture. The points I used included B-23 as a general point for back pain and to promote the function of the Kidneys, B-40 as distil point for pain and to promote urination, SP-6 to help urination, right Huatuojiaji EX-21 point lumbar 5 (facet joint L5), the trigger point on the right sacral iliac joint and right G-30 and 34 as distal points and points along the affected channel.

Outcomes The following day she reported that she had slept much better and she had felt better for several hours. I started her on some simple exercises and on the third session included some manual therapy on L5–S1, a sustained grade 4 to the left. After the third treatment she reported that she was feeling generally much better and the pain was becoming intermittent and also that she was only getting up once at night to pass urine. She continued to improve and after a total of nine treatments was pain free. Her bladder was reasonably normally controlled and she seemed to be walking better. I continued to see her at monthly intervals for about the following 6 or 7 months to give her boosters. On the last occasion her MS had deteriorated and she had been given a dropfoot splint to use when tired. The toes on her left foot were slightly purplish so I added LIV-3 to the previous points and also gave her a Nordic bed, which is a vibratory-type treatment for her feet, and this session seemed to help her circulatory problems.

Canada (Carol Taylor)

I have included acupuncture in my physiotherapy practice since 1991 after passing examinations from The World Natural Medicine Foundation and The Acupuncture Foundations of Canada. I treat a wide variety of complaints; some of these are relatively simple and others seemingly complex, for instance patients with multiple problems and those who have sometimes been seen by many other practitioners. Many people arrive with one problem and then say: "by the way I have had ... for years. Can you help with this?" Sometimes I am able to help with a combination of modalities that may include acupuncture, craniosacral therapy and a variety of other physiotherapy techniques.

Musculoskeletal problems respond well to the use of local and distal points for pain control and to increase the Qi in the channel passing over the injury or because they are influential or other important points. These acupuncture points can be followed by other physiotherapy techniques to aid healing and restore function.

The type of acupuncture used for patients who come to a physiotherapy clinic will depend on the knowledge and training of the practitioner, but also on the level of disease or injury to be treated. It can be noted that clinics vary in the type of conditions treated by practitioners. This will usually depend on the practitioner, as with increased knowledge they will develop a reputation for treating more complicated conditions with acupuncture.

Reaching the level of disease to be treated is important. Treatment for a superficial injury, that is, at the body level, with acupuncture and physiotherapy may include:

- cardinal points
- confluent points
- influential points
- very acute Xi cleft alarm points
- Jing well point for emergencies.

Modalities may be used for decreasing inflammation and increasing healing locally whilst acupuncture is given for increasing the Qi in the related meridian and organs or for local pain relief. After needling to increase the Qi flow to the area of injury so that healing can take place it is then valuable to give appropriate physiotherapy treatment for stretching, mobility or strengthening.

An example of a simple treatment is the following:

Tennis elbow: laser locally to the inflamed, painful area at the appropriate frequency for the state of the injury. Acupuncture to local and distal points (i.e. Ah

---

CASE STUDY 13.2

Reason for referral A 47-year-old woman who had bitten into a nut and found that her jaw had locked. The temperomandibular joint stayed locked for 5 months and she could only sip soup through a straw.

Assessment On observation there was 1 mm opening of the jaw and acute pain of the left TMJ. X-ray reported a probable but not definite, dislocation of the disc. The patient had severe muscle spasms and jaw pain. Headaches were in the left temporal region radiating to the vertex.

Treatment The first three treatments were with a laser to acupuncture points. There was no significant relief. Acupuncture was then given using needles to points: TE-21; SI-19: G-2 (using one needle through all these points together), also ST-7, 6; TE-17 unilaterally; LI-4 bilaterally. Auricular points used bilaterally were: Kidney, Gall Bladder, Shenmen and jaw. One treatment improved the opening to 2–3 mm. Five more acupuncture treatments were given, with the addition of craniosacral therapy, and after the third treatment the jaw opened sufficiently to allow craniosacral therapy work inside the mouth. View of the tongue showed a red tip and alternate treatments included needles to H-7 to treat stress and promote relaxation.

Outcomes A total of seven acupuncture treatments were given, making 12 visits in all over 2–3 months. Upon discharge the patient had a full range of movement and no pain. She was given jaw exercises using Rocabado techniques. When seen 3 months and 6 months later the jaw was a little stiff but responded after laser treatment to acupuncture points.

Shi, LI-10, 11, TE-5), stretching and exercises to gradually increase strength.

I often use a Five Element approach to acupuncture and frequently use it with craniosacral therapy as I find that acupuncture facilitates craniosacral therapy (see Case study 13.2 for an example). During craniosacral therapy use is often made of the energy flow from therapist through the patient. Dr Upledger (1983) refers to this as a 'vee spread' technique. A technique to increase meridian Qi flow is also taught. I find that the use of acupuncture needles speeds up this process, reduces the work of the therapist and creates an enhanced effect.

Incorporating acupuncture in the physiotherapy treatment of patients in hospital

UK (Nadia Ellis)

Acupuncture was not an accepted modality for physiotherapists to use in the UK until 1982, when it was permissible only for relief of pain. Having successfully completed a 2 year course in acupuncture in 1980, I was anxious to include it in my clinical practice as soon as the Chartered Society of Physiotherapists (CSP) permitted me to do so. I was unfortunate in my hospital in that the consultant rheumatologist did not approve of physiotherapists doing acupuncture. She persuaded the Health Authority that legally they should not take 'vicarious' responsibility for my practice of acupuncture as an integral part of clinical practice, the argument being that I was employed as a physiotherapist and not as an acupuncturist. Massage, however, has been an accepted modality since the CSP was founded in 1894. I therefore adapted my acupuncture knowledge and manual skills by massaging acupoints where piercing of skin was not permitted.

I am happy to say that the first objections to my use of needles were eventually overcome; by the time I left this hospital I was helping the consultant above with acupuncture in her outpatients clinic and she was complaining that she would have difficulty replacing me. I am pleased to say that in my subsequent position as superintendent of a much larger hospital I experienced no difficulty in continuing with acupuncture practice.

The conditions addressed in the following sections are those that I have found can be effectively treated by combining the principles of acupuncture with those of standard physiotherapy practice.

Orthopaedic problems

It has been observed on visits to China that moxabustion, is frequently used to heat acupoints when a patient presents with chronic joint pain. In TCM the Kidney controls bones and joints, and loss of Kidney Qi could be the underlying cause of pain. A treatment for low back pain, for instance, would include applying heat by holding lighted moxa sticks over Shenshu (B-23) situated 1.5 Cun lateral to the spine at L2/3 level, which is the Associated Affect point of the Kidney. Heat over B-23 reinforces Kidney Yang energy and addresses the underlying energy problem. The application of heat with moxa over the lumbar spine is not that different to applying hot packs or infrared, as is used in many physiotherapy departments prior to more active treatment. Western theory would state that heat improves the circulation and sedates the area to relieve pain enabling the active treatment to be done more effectively. If one accepts the TCM theory heat may be applied over B-23 as an adjunct to treat any joint problem as it has a profound effect on the body as a whole through the Kidney organ. Some examples follow.

Osteoarthritic knees

A patient with painful osteoarthritic knees will be treated using local acupressure or acupuncture, mobilization and exercise, while half-lying on a heat pack placed over the lumbar spine. Local points could include: Yinlinquan (SP-9), Dubi (S-35), Xiyan (EX-42), Heding (EX-41), Weiyang (B-39), Ququan (LIV-8) and Zusanli (S-36). Other modalities used could be interferential or TENS, positioning the electrodes over the relevant acupoints.

Low back pain

Low back pain is a major problem met in clinical practice. It is a complex condition that can arise from both musculotendinous and skeletal involvement. The Gall Bladder controls muscles and tendons according to TCM theory and Yanglingquan (G-34) is the Influential point for these tissues. Thus a typical treatment for low back pain could include heat to the lumbar spine (reinforcing Kidney Yang Qi) and acupressure and acupuncture to G-34 (the Influential point for muscles and tendons), followed by Maitland mobilizations or Mackenzie exercises, effectively combining TCM theory with physiotherapy according to Western techniques and possibly avoiding piercing the skin. Other acupoints that could be treated might include those positioned over the sciatic nerve that are tender (e.g. Weizhong (B-40), Heyang (B-55), Kunlun (B-60) and Huantiao (G-30)).

Nocturia

There are few randomized controlled trials addressing the effects of acupuncture. In a pilot study (Ellis 1993) the stimulation by needles of SP-6 and S-36 bilaterally was shown to have a significant effect on this problem. Those patients who present with joint pain and who have nocturia can be treated for both conditions by using local and systemic acupoints. For example, presenting symptoms include painful knee joints plus having to void the bladder several times during the night then local knee points including those described above plus SP-6 may well address both sets of symptoms simultaneously.

Respiratory conditions met in surgical/medical wards

Postoperative chest care

There are two important acupoints that can be stimulated to assist patients who have difficulties postoperatively:

1. Shanzhong (CV-17) located on the sternum at a point midway between the nipples, can be gently massaged to relieve tightness in the chest and facilitate expectoration.

2. Feishu (B-13) the Associated Effect point of the Lung, positioned 1.5 Cun either side of the thoracic spine at the level of the lower border of T3, can also benefit patients who have developed postoperative chest problems. Combining local massage treatment to these points with huffing techniques (short expiratory breathing) greatly limits the discomfort of prolonged efforts to clear phlegm. Massage of the upper thoracic spine can aid relaxation of the accessory muscles of respiration (Western medicine) as well as stimulate Feishu (B-13) (TCM). Patients can be shown how to massage CV-17 gently during the day when the physiotherapist is not present.

Medical chests

Acute on chronic chest conditions are a common cause of hospital admission.

There are two aims of treatment: first, relief of the acute chest problem; second, instruction in continuing home care.

Combining the use of Feishu (B-13) with other acupoints can be very effective. Following the examination of a patient suffering with a respiratory problem, the use of heat to support the Qi in the Lung organ is often the treatment of choice. In the ward situation this is not always practical so massage to acupoint B-13 can be substituted. Shanzhong (CV-17) may be used as in postoperative chest care. There are other acupoints (depending on the presenting symptoms) that are effective in addition to those mentioned above. These include Fenglong (S-40) if there is a productive cough, Lieque (LU-7) for supporting Lung Qi, and Quchi (LI-11) if there is pathogenic Heat, which would be indicated if there were a yellow fur on the tongue. If needles are used they should be inserted to gain Deqi and then left for 20 min.

On discharge When patients are discharged after an acute respiratory episode, they can be instructed in home application of a hot water bottle or a heat pad when needed. Placing the heat source over the upper thoracic spine mimics the heat produced by burning moxa held over the acupoints. Acupressure can also be shown. Massage either side of the upper four thoracic vertebrae is demonstrated as this area includes Feishu (B-13). Other acupressure points could include Fenglong (S-40); this is a specific point both for treating a productive cough and to eliminate Damp from the Lung. Patients are advised to press gently or massage the points for approximately 1 min and to repeat this twice a day. Lieque (LU-7) can be used in addition or alternatively to Fenglong (S-40). Evidence that chronic and acute respiratory problems benefit from simple acupressure and heat described above is at present only experiential; there have not as yet been any controlled trials undertaken to prove the effectiveness of this approach.

Asthma

The full acupuncture treatment of asthma can be carried out only by an experienced acupuncturist. However, breathlessness can in many cases be alleviated by putting some heat over the upper thoracic spine while doing relaxation and diaphragmatic breathing.

Gynaecology

Following gynaecological surgery, abdominal 'wind' is sometimes an extremely uncomfortable experience. Acupressure on Zusanli (S-36) and/or Gongsun (SP-4) sometimes gives immediate relief. Weakness of the pelvic floor is also a cause of distress, and stimulation of Sanyinjiao (SP-6) combined with GV-20 is beneficial when added to active pelvic floor exercises. These points are especially useful following pelvic floor repair as these points are said to effect the support of the abdomen. Using needles is most effective, but acupressure can be beneficial.

Obstetrics

Early morning sickness is a common complication of pregnancy and is very unpleasant at its best and severely debilitating at its worst. Some practitioners advocate non-invasive treatment particularly in the first 12 weeks of pregnancy, and acupressure can be used safely. Neiguan (P-6) is the most effective acupoint as it calms the spirit, but others can also be used, for example Zusanli (S-36), the He Sea point of the Stomach channel, Zhongwan (CV-12), local point

to the Stomach, or Xingjian (LIV-2), which calms Liver Fire and draws energy down.

In some hospitals physiotherapists and midwives are using acupuncture and related techniques to turn breech babies and assist with deliveries. TENS is of course widely used to assist with pain relief.

Conclusion

There is much that can be done in hospital using acupressure and acupuncture to treat a wide variety of conditions met by physiotherapists in their clinical practice. However, a great deal of research needs to be undertaken to validate what is up to now only experiential practice.

An acupressure approach in primary health care and oncology
South Africa (Charles Liggins)

Primary care

When I first learnt acupuncture in 1983 I considered it would be a useful adjunct to my practice of physiotherapy and that it would extend my armamentarium of modalities for the management of chronic pain, my major interest in physiotherapy. Little did I know the big influence the newly gained knowledge would have on my career and the "adventures" I would have.

A few years ago while carrying out fieldwork for a study in the remote Mseleni/Manguzi area of Northern Kwa Zulu, South Africa, I was treating patients in the shade of some trees when I was approached by two of the local inhabitants. One introduced himself as the 'induna' (headman) of the area and he "told me that he had brought the other person to see me as he had heard that I could do ... magic things" with small needles. The second person was the district school teacher and he explained to me that his wife had fainted earlier that morning and was "still fainted". As it was now after 11 o'clock the situation sounded quite serious so I quickly finished what I was doing, then packed up my equipment and accompanied the two back to their homestead. On arriving I saw the wife lying on the ground outside the family 'kraal' (hut). She was motionless and unresponsive. On examination I noted that her skin was pale, cold and damp. The respiration was very shallow and slow, while the pulse was faint but quick. I asked the husband if she had ever experienced a similar attack and he told me that it had happened once before and that she had been admitted to a hospital, where she responded very quickly to treatment but no diagnosis had been ascertained. I estimated that she had been "fainted" for over 3 hours and, as the local hospital was over 2 hours' journey away and over very rough terrain, I decided to try some first aid acupuncture.

I inserted a 30 mm × 0.30 stainless steel needle in GV-26 and rapidly rotated it through 180° clockwise and then anticlockwise. Within a few seconds she started to move her head from side to side each time I rotated the needle. I then placed needles in KI-1 bilaterally and gave very strong manual stimulation. This resulted in her moaning, opening her eyes and moving her legs. I continued for a short while and the patient then attempted to sit up. All needles were then removed and after a short while she was able to stand with assistance and was taken into her hut. I considered that she was probably a diabetic and she was given a cup of sweetened tea and some bread to eat, after which she said she felt better but very weak. I suggested to her husband that he should take his wife to the local hospital on the following day and request a full medical check. Then, with grateful thanks from him and stares of wonderment from the neighbours who had witnessed the proceedings, I went back to my research work.

While I was in the area I was asked to treat several patients. Most of the patients treated had pain related to degenerative joint disease, Mseleni joint disease (which was endemic in the area) and trauma including amputation, stump and phantom pain. A considerable number of the patients responded well to acupuncture and it was probably as a result of this that I was "commanded" to visit the kraal of the local chief. This necessitated a cross-country trip in a four-wheel drive vehicle to the chief's kraal, where I was met by an induna and ushered into the presence of the chief. The chief, who was suffering with the effects of severe osteoarthritis of the knees and hips, was lying on a settee in a courtyard. After exchanging pleasantries and

partaking of beer, which is traditional under such circumstances, I examined the chief and considered that his condition would probably respond well to acupuncture. The appropriate treatment was given and the chief volunteered the information that he felt better, though the next day I learned that he had an exacerbation of his pain. Unfortunately it was not possible to continue with the treatment as I had to return to Durban.

Some time later, while I was participating in the training of physiotherapy assistants and community rehabilitation assistants in the same remote area, a suggestion was made that I incorporate acupressure into their training programme. One of the reasons for this was that analgesic drugs were not readily available as the Mission Hospital often ran short or the inhabitants could not afford proprietary preparations from the local trading store.

The assistants and community health workers had a knowledge of anatomy and physiology equivalent to the level of enrolled auxiliary nurses. Without teaching the underlying concepts of TCM it was explained that there were specific points on the body that could be stimulated by finger pressure and other means to bring about pain relief and resolution of common complaints such as nausea, constipation and muscle cramps. Thus it was possible, with their knowledge of anatomy and the fact that they had already learned Swedish massage, to teach the principles of acupressure, which included techniques, indications and contraindications. Each participant was given a chart showing the anatomical location of the acupuncture points to be learned and the clinical uses of the points. The charts were in diagrammatic form and the text had been translated into Zulu.

The "formulary" method of acupressure was taught and the following conditions were included: non-specific headache (LI-4; GB-20; EX-1, 2); shoulder pain (LI-4, 11, 15; TE-5, 14; G-21); elbow pain (LI-11; H-3; TE-10); hand pain (LI-4; Baxie points), neck pain (GV-14; GB-20, 21); low back pain (B-23, 31, 36, 40); hip pain (GB-29, 30, 31); knee pain (ST-35; Xiyan of the knee; SP-9, 10; ST-36) and menstrual pain (ST-36; SP-6). In addition to specific acupoint treatment the participants were shown how to look for and identify tender spots (trigger points) and how to treat them with sustained pressure (ischaemic compression).

The method of teaching was very simple. Initially the chart and its terminology was explained with the assistance of a Zulu interpreter. Then the various techniques of acupressure were demonstrated. Each area was then shown individually and time allowed for the class members to practise on each other. This practise was supervised by two physiotherapists and when performance was considered to be satisfactory then progress was made to another area. In this way it was possible to teach groups of eight to 10 all the common pain areas and conditions in one day. As the assistants and community personnel were working in the mission hospital or in the community they were encouraged to use the techniques of acupressure whenever appropriate.

Oncology

During 1994 I was invited by the head of a private oncology clinic to give a talk on acupuncture. The audience consisted of the oncologists of the clinic, nursing staff and personnel from oncology departments of public hospitals in and around the city of Durban. The talk, which was liberally illustrated by colour slides, consisted of the traditional Chinese concepts of acupuncture, an historical perspective of its use in the physiological mechanisms based on recent research findings and clinical applications and variants of acupuncture.

During the section on traditional concepts I noticed many smiles of amusement in the audience. However, when I presented the Western explanations, there was serious attention and at the end of the talk I was asked many questions about modern developments in acupuncture. As a result of the talk I received several patients from the centre for acupuncture treatment to assist in pain control.

A few weeks later I was asked to repeat the talk to the nursing sisters of the clinic and enlarge on the section on the variants of acupuncture, with emphasis on acupressure. I was requested to concentrate on the applications of acupressure that were pertinent to the needs of oncology patients. The audience consisted of 12 nursing sisters. After the talk I demonstrated the use of acupressure for headache, nausea (P-6), vomiting (P-6; ST-36), respiratory wheezing (CV-17, 22), constipation (ST-25; TE-6), diarrhoea (ST-25; SP-4), leg cramps (B-57),

anxiety and insomnia (P-6; H-7). The sisters showed great interest in the proceedings and they practised on each other with enthusiasm.

One of the responsibilities of the nursing staff of the clinic is to organize the patient support groups. These groups, consisting of patients, relatives, friends and other carers, meet periodically to discuss the various aspects of self-care, pain management, diet and other matters associated with the patient's condition. The sister responsible for the Breast Support Group asked if I could teach acupressure to her group and this was done in a similar way to the teaching carried out with the physiotherapy assistants and community health workers. This service has been greatly appreciated and the reporting back has been very encouraging. At present the teaching of acupressure to the other support groups is being carried out by the nursing staff who attended the original session.

Acupressure is a very useful procedure for self-care. It can be easily taught to professional and lay persons alike. Professionals appreciate the physiological explanations of acupressure and lay persons are comfortable with simplified explanations and the use of the term "energy". Physiotherapists who practice acupuncture are able to teach their patients self-administration for home therapy. It is the author's contention that a wide use of the procedure could be employed for the management of many common ailments, at all levels of society, but particularly in communities where medical services are limited or non-affordable.

Acupuncture in a community setting in the UK

UK (Sara Mokone)

There has been a community physiotherapy service in Britain for 45 years. The development of physiotherapy service expanded with the support of the MacMillan Report in 1974 (HMSO 1983).

Over the past 10 years there has been further reorganization of health delivery, the major one being the National Health Service and Community Care Act (HMSO 1990). This latest Act has introduced market economy into the health service. It led to the establishment of NHS Trusts and makes provision for direct financing of the practices of medical practitioners. In part 4 of the act it states that "a contract will be made whereby one NHS body (purchaser) arranges for the provision to it by another NHS body (provider) of goods and services which it reasonably requires" the contracts system has opened a door for other professional groups to enter the health service. Primary health care, previously the domain of the general practitioner and nurse, now requires a much larger team of staff to deliver public health provision, some organized as multidisciplinary teams, some as part of the social service and other in specific health teams providing services for clients in elderly care, mental health, children services or disability groups. Treatment is provided outside of hospital – in patients' own homes, social service settings, and day centres or residential homes, whether for the elderly, the mentally ill, or people with a learning difficulty. This includes adult training centres, educational establishments, mainstream schools and special schools, occupational settings, industry and, of course, health centres (Gibson 1988).

The type of service delivered will depend on how the service has been developed. Some services are funded only to give an advisory service (Gibson 1988). Others have expanded from an outpatient setting; physiotherapists make home visits and inform their hospital counterparts on the nature and conditions found in the home setting.

In Britain, physiotherapists have been using acupuncture to complement their skills in patient management since about the early 1980s. A special interest group of the CSP was established in 1984 and it has been instrumental in acupuncture being accepted as a regular modality to be used as part of physiotherapy treatment.

Problem solving

Many of the health problems found in a community setting require holistic methods of assessment and treatment planning. A community physiotherapist needs to be aware of the social, emotional and medical needs of patients and their families, and wide-ranging skills and abilities are required for maintaining health. Skills as an educator and adviser come to the fore. Problem-solving techniques may be required, with rehabilitation using counselling skills and goals setting. The approach is one of collaboration and participation, working with and empowering both carers and those who may be disadvantaged to appreciate their own abilities to solve problems (Egan 1985).

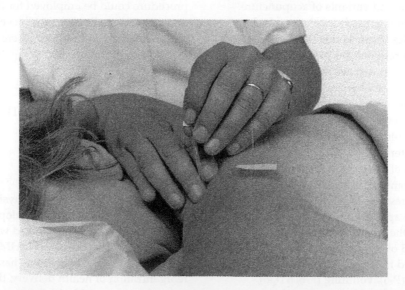

Fig. 13.1 *Treatment of shoulder pain needling Ah Shi points and GB-21. Note direction of needle: angle forward.*

A

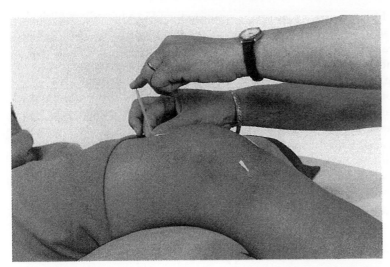

B

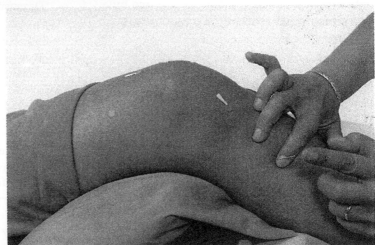

C

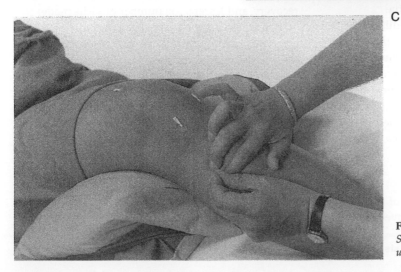

Fig. 13.2 A, B, C *Arthritis in the knee, needling ST-36. Eyes of the knee marked. Other points used: ST-34 and SP-10.*

Acupuncture is a means of treatment which can be easily used in any of these community settings. In Traditional Chinese Medicine, acupuncture is a part of the holistic health approach, which combines herbal medicine, exercise, massage, qikong, and moxibustion. The use of acupuncture is not simply for the alleviation of symptoms as it appears to help in regulating the body and promotes the homeostatic mechanisms (Bensoussan 1991). In combination with the non-invasive methods of working, which are part of the physiotherapist armoury, there appears to be a cumulative effect to acupuncture, which assists in the promotion of tissue healing and recovery (see Chapter 2).

Introduction of acupuncture in practice by a physiotherapist working in a community setting

Management

When I first introduced acupuncture into the practice, it was necessary for me to gain the support of the physiotherapy service manager. I did this by writing a report that demonstrated the effectiveness of the use of these techniques in a sufficient number of cases, and by producing research evidence, with the Acupuncture Association of Chartered Physiotherapists' safety standards and guide to clinical practice to back this up.

I had in addition, to show that I had adequate training in the use of acupuncture techniques. My requests to the service manager to buy the equipment needed to carry out safe needling were granted, and a contract was arranged for the regular supply of repacked sterile needles, and the collection boxes needed. Other forms of electrical equipment to back up treatments, such as TENS machines, and interferential and laser apparatus, had been in use before this. TENS machines could be loaned for an initial loan period of 6 weeks to 2 months.

Uses

A description follows of my experience of the application of acupuncture techniques over the past 6 years.

Increasing numbers of physiotherapists are

practising acupuncture and in a recently published study acceptance for the treatment of elderly people was high amongst both professionals and the target client group (Keys 1995). In inner city areas, large numbers of isolated elderly people live with little social support. They are the group who will be found to be in need of services, including both health and social care (Gibson 1988).

Clients who have benefited include older people experiencing pain due to arthritis, either rheumatoid or osteoarthritis, (see Case study 3.3) recent strokes or old strokes. I have also used acupuncture in oncology where pain relief is the main need, or dealing with the side-effects of medication, such as the dizziness and nausea experienced with chemotherapy and radiotherapy.

Degenerative conditions, such as multiple sclerosis, muscular dystrophy, motor neuron disease, terminal disorders, HIV and AIDS can also be helped. In my experience, moxibustion can be a beneficial treatment to use for boosting immune system in people with debility, and, Tai Chi and Qigong appear to be of benefit. The list is quite extensive.

Patients have reported alleviation of symptoms such as incontinence, other bowel and bladder problems, anxiety and stress (Ellis 1993). These benefits have occurred when using straightforward local and distal point needling, with the aim of alleviating pain. In a number of cases, a person unable to leave home has an acute problem from which they need immediate relief. Using acupuncture appears to increase the speed of recovery, and lessens the number of visits made.

In the past 2 years I have been introducing acupuncture into my work as part of a community team for learning difficulties. The consultant psychiatrist has referred young people with anxiety and agitation, and a trial is planned to look at the benefits for those with mixed psychological as well as physical difficulties. In these instances, a combination of ear acupuncture points with acupressure to the Back Shu points has been tried. The usual pain management problems met in any outpatient department are frequently referred.

Strengths

The strengths of acupuncture include shorter

CASE STUDY 13.3

Mrs M aged 73 had been discharged from hospital, following bilateral total knee replacements. She was referred by the District Nurses for physiotherapy assessment.

Reason for referral Requires intensive nursing care as she is not coping since discharge from hospital. History of present condition: lives alone and cannot cope with independent living. Needs help of two people to get off the bed and cannot stand or weight-bear at the moment due to pain in her right knee. Findings on first visit: Mrs M has generalized rheumatoid arthritis, with an osteoarthritic component. She has had some hypertension, but has not been given any treatment for this. At the moment she is experiencing oedema in both lower limbs. While in hospital, her son who had been caring for her had a coronary and was hospitalized. She had lost her husband within the past year.

As equipment; she had a wheelchair for outdoor use, and had been using two sticks before the operation, but at that time required a walking frame. She had been discharged with guidance on walking with crutches, but was far too anxious and inhibited to be able to understand how to do this.

Objective assessment Assessment of knee function, and general condition, indicated that her skin was very pale and thin, while her tongue had a yellow coating. Both lower limbs were oedematous, and she had some breathlessness. Her right knee was warm to the touch and inflamed; the range of movement was limited to 32° of flexion on the left but only 20° on the right. Neither knee could lock in full extension. There was weakness of the quadriceps; on the straight leg test, it was just able to lift against gravity on the left but not on the right.

The following needs were identified together with the patient. She had been housebound before the surgery, so her goals were to return to independence in her own home. She did not want to move to sheltered housing. She needed to be able to reach the toilet, get on and off the bed independently, reach the light switch and walk into the sitting room.

The nurses were at the time considering that she would need nursing home care, as she would not achieve any of the above.

Treatment plan The object was to reduce knee pain and, together with rest of the team, look at her environment and living circumstances, to see if her living

conditions can be made as easy as possible for her to remain living independently and comfortably. The supply of a commode was primary, as was a walking frame for temporary convenience, and bathroom adaptations. A possibility was a regular social service care worker to assist with basic care needs.

Acupuncture was used daily for a week, with points ST-36 bilaterally, eyes of the knee, ST-34, 35; SP-9. No moxa was used because of the heat in the knee, the hypertension and the yellow tongue. Distal points were ST-43, and/or ST-44. The rationale was that of ST-36 to boost the body energy and the circulation of Qi, and SP-9 Ho point of the Spleen, recommended for use with Damp and swelling. Other knee points were local points for stimulation for pain relief. The distal points on the Stomach channel are both antipyretic and as a distal point, to help energy flowing through the channel. Both knees were treated, on the principle that the nerve pathways cross, and treating the opposite side can augment the treatment.

This was combined with interferential two pad, through and through knee, 10–100 Hz for 20 minutes twice a week. A programme was given of strengthening exercises, gentle circulatory exercise and reminders to stand-up and sit as an exercise every few hours. She was provided with a TENS electrostimulation with low and high frequency modulation to use in between the treatments.

Outcomes Within 2 days she was able to weight-bear and transfer to a commode, which was provided by medical loans. She had been expected to use crutches, but she was safer mobilizing with a frame. Her knee range had increased, and the pain level was down to 50%. She continued to progress very rapidly once the inflammation in knee had settled. Arrangements were made to attend a day hospital to continue with the rehabilitation and physiotherapy. Both she and the district nurses felt that the response to the acupuncture had been quite dramatic. There followed a number of referrals from the district nursing team.

Discussion This treatment for osteoarthritis can be used with very basic knowledge of the theory of Chinese medicine. Problems of osteoarthritis causing immobility are frequently referred to community physiotherapy. A full study of the effectiveness of treatment is worth doing, as the usual treatment for arthritis is the use of anti-inflammatory medication, which may have consequences of secondary gastrointestinal damage. This woman's treatment, following an orthopaedic procedure, was provided on a special scheme known as "Hospital at Home", which allows for acute care in the community and more frequent visits than is usually available. Therefore daily treatment could be offered, which was unusual, owing to the limited access to community physiotherapists as treatment resources.

In this case, it was done as an experiment to test out the treatment. I had had initial training on a short course for pain management, and a weekend course on the Bi syndrome, musculoskeletal approach. The use of a much deeper TCM approach to the assessment and

diagnosis of this woman's problems may have combined a more systemic treatment on metabolic points, and using the parasympathetic pathways, which correspond with what are known as the Back Shu points on the outside of the spinal column for use as pain relief. According to TCM, and through knowledge also of segmental neurodevelopment, the spinal levels connect with internal organs, L-1,2,3,4,5 with Liver, Spleen, Triple Burner, Stomach, Large Intestine and Kidney and womb respectively. For metabolic problems, one would use the higher thoracic Back Shu and EX-21 Huatuojiaji points (named for the physician who identified them).

recovery times and a cumulative effect of treatment. In a study of 10 patients with arthritis that I conducted, treating patients with osteoarthritic knees, those being treated with acupuncture and exercise did better than those having home programme of exercise to use at home. There was a significant increase in the range of movement and diminishment of pain. Acupuncture equipment is easy to carry, and more transportable than is the standard electrical equipment available in outpatient departments.

There are few precautions, and if they are followed the treatment is safe. Discharge from treatment is generally earlier, and re-referral less frequent. Many patients are willing and eager to try this form of treatment.

Weaknesses

There was insufficient time to do a proper longitudinal study, and therefore I had to rely on finding suitable research evidence. A recent study on osteoarthritis in the knee indicated that there was no significant difference between the use of sham and real acupuncture (Takeda & Wessels 1994). However, both groups of patients had significant reduction both in pain, stiffness and physical disability.

Obstacles I found 10 years ago that few other physiotherapists with whom I was working in community settings had wanted to take up

acupuncture training, as they tended to see themselves in an advisory role, and had not taken up the challenge of using their very strong hands-on skills for more intensive treatments. Another obstacle to the use of acupuncture is lack of sufficient manpower and a great pressure from referrals for very specific mobility problems, which require simply some form of gait re-education and the use of mobility equipment. This has been partially overcome by employing more physiotherapy assistants, who can provide the necessary back-up and administrative support to allow for more specialist work to take place, and for these hands-on skills in acupressure to be shared and taught to these staff themselves.

Measures of validity

Patient satisfaction questionnaires indicate that more than 60% of those who answered felt that they had had an effective treatment, in which the goals they had set had been met.

Quality assurance studies have shown an increase in the number of people treated, and since through-put is of significance, this has been seen as a positive outcome of introducing this holistic approach, in which acupuncture has been combined with the teaching of basic massage and acupressure techniques to a wide number of different community groups.

References

Altree J 1993 Physiotherapy and acupuncture practice in the UK. Complementary Therapies in Medicine 1(1): 34–41

Bensousan A 1991 The vital meridian. A modern exploration of acupuncture. Churchill Livingstone, New York

Cyriax J 1975 Textbook of orthopaedic medicine. Balliére Tindall, London

Egan G 1985 The skilled helper. Brookes/Cole, Monteray, California

Ellis N 1993 The effect of acupuncture on nocturnal frequency and incontinence in the elderly. Complementary Therapies in Medicine 1(3): 168–170

Gibson A (ed) 1988 Physiotherapy in the community physical therapy services in Britain. Woodhead & Faulkner

Keys S 1995 Acupuncture in treatment of elderly people. Complementary Therapies in Medicine 7(3)

Lundeberg T et al 1988 Long term results of acupuncture in chronic head and neck pain. Pain Clinic 2(1): 15–31

National Health Service and Community Care Act 1990 HMSO, London

Takeda W, Wessel J 1994 Acupuncture in the treatment of pain in osteo-arthritic knees. Arthritis Care and Research 7(3): 118–122

Vincent C A 1989 A controlled trial of the treatment of migraine by acupuncture. Clinical Journal of Pain 5(4): 305–312

Working party of the Secretary of State for Social Services 1983 The remedial professions. HMSO, London

Further reading

Ellis N 1994 Acupuncture in clinical practice. A guide for health professionals. Chapman & Hall, London

Hopwood V 1993 Acupuncture in physiotherapy. Complementary Therapies in Medicine 1(2): 100–104

Jayasuriya A 1984 Clinical acupuncture. Sri Lanka

Lovesey M 1994 Acupuncture and physiotherapy: an international perspective. Complementary Therapies in Medicine 2: 99–103

Upledger J E 1983 CranioSacral Therapy. Eastland, Seattle, WA

Upledger J E 1987 CranioSacral Therapy II – Beyond the Dura. Eastland, Seattle, WA

Upledger J E 1990 Somato Emotional Release and Beyond. Eastland, Seattle, WA

Upledger J E 1991 Your Inner Physician and You. Eastland, Seattle, WA

Stewart G 1985 Counselling in Rehabilitation. Croom Helm, London

14

Introduction of acupuncture into some countries

Linda Rapson, Nadia Ellis, Diana Turnbull, Helen Madzokere, Eva Haker, Ana Maria Carballo

This chapter gives the reader some insight into how acupuncture has been introduced into six countries, particularly from the viewpoint of physiotherapists. As will be seen from the accounts, many common problems have occurred.

Medical acupuncture in Canada – a brief overview

Linda Rapson

Acupuncture has no doubt been used in Canada since the first Chinese immigrants came to our shores in the 19th century. None the less, most of us had never heard of this ancient oriental art until President Richard Nixon made his famous trip to China in 1971. After James Reston of the New York Times passed gas in response to the insertion of a needle, the whole world heard about acupuncture.

The earliest Canadian accounts of acupuncture come from Quebec, our Canadian province that is primarily French speaking. Acupuncture's introduction to Quebec probably came earlier than to English-speaking Canada since it has been practised in France for so long.

Canada is a vast country of 10 provinces and two northern territories, with very disparate mixes of ethnic groups in the various regions of the country. While acupuncture seems to have been accepted earlier and more readily on the west coast than the east, today it is used by more physiotherapists in our Atlantic provinces than in British Columbia, if membership rates and attendance at Acupuncture

Foundation of Canada (AFC) courses are any indication. In one large teaching hospital in Halifax, the Victoria General Hospital, virtually all the physiotherapists in the department are trained by the AFC and utilize acupuncture on a regular basis.

Health is administered provincially in Canada, and rules regarding acupuncture vary among the provinces. As of 1995, acupuncture was unregulated in all provinces except Quebec and Alberta. Regulation is pending in British Columbia and should be in place by early 1996. "Regulation" in this context pertains to the licensing and disciplining of acupuncturists who are not members of any other regulated group, such as physiotherapists, physicians, dentists, naturopaths or veterinarians, all of whom can use acupuncture within their practices. The direction in which regulation is going in Canada is towards either government or self-regulation of acupuncturists and the simultaneous integration of acupuncture into their practices by the above-mentioned regulated practitioners.

Self-regulation in Quebec began in mid 1995, following 7 or 8 years of government regulation. Medical doctors continue to require 300 hours' training in acupuncture, but physiotherapists are currently required to take 1000 hours of training prior to using acupuncture, since there were no regulations in place for physiotherapists at the time the new regulatory body for acupuncturists was created.

The AFC and others are protesting over this regulation as being inappropriate, since physiotherapists are not acting as acupuncturists, but are restricting their practices to their scope of practice. The AFC, founded in 1974, has become the medical acupuncture group that has the most influence throughout the country. An Ontario-based charitable organization, it was founded by seven physicians who had learned acupuncture in various parts of the world. They set out to design courses for medical practitioners and to lobby for the restriction of acupuncture to use by medical practitioners. From 1974 until the introduction of the Regulated Health Professions Act (RHPA) in 1991, the Health Disciplines Act in Ontario stated that acupuncture was a "medical act". However, a court case in 1981 effectively left the door wide open for acupuncturists to practice. The RHPA exempted acupuncture from the "controlled act" of inserting an instrument below the dermis, and this is the status quo until regulation is introduced. That process will take upwards of 2 years to initiate.

The AFC initially restricted courses to physicians alone. Dentists were included in late 1974, but it was not until 1982 that physiotherapists were admitted to the teaching programme. The initial plan was to teach them only to use TENS, but the teaching faculty unanimously agreed that it would be more appropriate to teach needle insertion. This was not acceptable to the Board of Directors, to say the least. This clash of opinions occurred a few weeks before the 1982 Annual General Meeting, precipitated a "coup d'état", and a new Board of Directors who supported the teaching of physiotherapists was elected.

The introduction of acupuncture to physiotherapists in Canada cannot be underestimated in terms of its positive impact on the dissemination of needle treatment throughout the country. It did not take long for therapists to recognize the value of this potent tool, particularly since they were being taught the AFC's unique anatomical approach to acupuncture. Students learned 20 important points in a 3 day introductory course, went back to their practices and saw immediate results in treating musculoskeletal pain.

Administrative roadblocks to practice have been many and varied. In some provinces, it has become mandatory for both physiotherapists and doctors to pass the AFC examination, or another exam given through the University of Alberta Medical Acupuncture programme, prior to using acupuncture. The AFC examination is open to students who have completed the first three parts of a nine-part curriculum. It is meant to be an examination that tests safety and good basic knowledge in the anatomical approach to acupuncture. It does not guarantee that the practitioner is a classical "acupuncturist", however. In fact, the AFC's position is that the title "acupuncturist" should be reserved for those who have met the standards for acupuncturists in those jurisdictions where there is regulation and members are told to not refer to themselves as "acupuncturists".

International relations

Besides belonging to the World Federation of Acupuncture Societies, the AFC is involved internationally with the NAFTA Acupuncture Commission and the Pan Pacific Medical Acupuncture Forum. NAFTA is the acronym for the North American Free Trade Agreement, an agreement among the USA, Mexico and Canada with respect to the flow of trade among our countries. The agreement contains provision for the free flow of professionals as well as goods, although there is no requirement for each country to recognize the others' professionals unless standards are equivalent.

USA regulation

Through the NAFTA Acupuncture Commission we have learned a great deal about acupuncture in the USA. Regulation of acupuncturists is in place in about 20 states. Currently 32 states plus Washington DC recognize acupuncture: 29 by statute and four by other means. There are about 40 schools of Acupuncture and Oriental Medicine in the USA and they are organized to the extent of having a Council of Colleges of Acupuncture and Oriental Medicine (CCAOM), which began in 1982 and sets standards for curriculum content. CCAOM in turn created the National Accreditation Commission for Schools and Colleges of Acupuncture and Oriental Medicine (NACSCAOM), which is recognized by the US Department of Education for accreditation of acupuncture programmes at the professional master's degree level and by the prestigious Council on Post Secondary Accreditation.

The National Commission for the Certification of Acupuncturists (NCCA) is a non-profit-making organization incorporated in the early 1980s to establish standards of competence for the safe and effective practice of Acupuncture and Oriental Medicine and to set and administer National Board Examinations. The NCCA set up an examination through an elaborate and expensive process (about $400 000 US) in order to ensure it is fair, reliable and valid. This was necessary in order to make it litigation proof, since disgruntled people who had failed exams had already sued successfully in some states, alleging unfairness of the process.

At the moment there are no states where physical therapists are allowed to do acupuncture within their scope of practice. A physical therapist can, of course, become an acupuncturist.

Pan Pacific Medical Acupuncture Forum

The Pan Pacific Medical Acupuncture Forum (PPMAF) is a group of four Pacific rim medical acupuncture groups (from New Zealand, Australia, USA and Canada), which was established in 1988 at a joint meeting of the AFC and the Medical Acupuncture Society of New Zealand in Queenstown, NZ. The first PPMAF meeting was hosted by the AFC in Vancouver, Canada in 1992 and the next meeting will be in Australia in 1996. The purpose of the alliance is to provide a forum for sharing knowledge and for promoting friendship among members.

The AFC has taken a firm position with this group in regard to physiotherapists, since none of the other groups admit them as members. The Australian Medical Acupuncture Society is particularly strong on the issue, but has agreed that AFC physiotherapist members are welcome at the meeting in Brisbane. We hope to convince our medical acupuncture colleagues that the alliance of medics and physiotherapists who have a keen interest in acupuncture can only enrich the knowledge of both groups. That has been the Canadian experience.

The future

If all practitioners can cooperate towards a goal of

integrating acupuncture into the fabric of Western society and the health care system, many problems that exist today in our high tech, pharmaceutically driven medical system will be solved. Some of us in Canada are working toward that goal.

Physiotherapy and acupuncture in the UK

Nadia Ellis

Until 1982, piercing skin with acupuncture needles did not form a part of a physiotherapist's clinical practice and was not in use in the National Health Service, other than by medical practitioners or dentists.

There were some physiotherapists who had learned acupuncture in the various colleges that existed in the UK providing traditional Chinese-based courses for a wide spectrum of medical and non-medical personnel. Others had attended short courses that were based on Western concepts of acupuncture and instruction in pain relief only.

The Acupuncture Association of Chartered Physiotherapists

In 1984, as a result of an enterprising advert by two physiotherapists in the Physiotherapy journal, there was a large meeting of physiotherapists interested in forming a clinical interest group in acupuncture. The Acupuncture Association of Chartered Physiotherapists (AACP) was founded and a committee elected consisting of representatives from throughout the UK, who were set the task of writing a constitution.

The first priority of the AACP was to be recognized by the Chartered Society of Physiotherapy (CSP) as a clinical interest group. We submitted our constitution to the CSP and were in fact the first clinical interest group to be formally registered with it. We then had to demonstrate our determination to establish a standard of good practice throughout our membership. A subcommittee was asked to write a code of practice, which was submitted and approved by the

Professional Practice Committee of the CSP and then distributed to all AACP members. The code of practice was also included in the CSP standards folder which all physiotherapy departments have for reference in their libraries.

Membership of AACP

When the AACP was originally formed all physiotherapists interested in acupuncture were invited to join. Practice of acupuncture was not a requirement. The membership consisted of a core of physiotherapists who had undertaken substantial courses in acupuncture in UK, China and Sri Lanka. Others had attended shorter courses of one or two weekends. Some had not as yet embarked on any training and were looking to the AACP to advise on the best course to take. Associate membership was given to those physiotherapists who were not members of the CSP or interested members of other professions. Many physiotherapists who were practising acupuncture did not opt to join the association. AACP could distribute information only to members of AACP or communicate with the CSP membership as a whole through the Physiotherapy journal.

At our 10th AGM it was decided to close membership and establish new criteria. Full membership is now granted only if evidence is given of having completed at least 20 hours of training on approved courses. Physiotherapists who have a minimum of 200 hours of training are awarded advanced membership of AACP, this status being achieved either by attending an extended course approved by the Education Committee of the AACP or by accumulated practical and theoretical experience through a series of shorter modules. This enables those who wish to concentrate on the Western approach to acupuncture to achieve advanced status. We hope that these requirements will result in an association which is not factional or elitist. Both full and advanced members now have to give evidence of 10 hours of further training every 2 years in order to maintain their membership status.

The supervision of the education register is of great importance in assuring standards. The National Blood Transfusion Service have agreed that donors treated by AACP members will be able to give blood

without having to wait a mandatory year to do so, as had previously been the case.

Education

We set ourselves the task of designing an acupuncture course that would be validated by the CSP. We felt that such a course should take into account the traditional Chinese teaching, which forms the basis of acupuncture, as well as the Western concepts of neurophysiology. We were also aware that our members were using acupuncture alongside other modalities in a variety of conditions, following a questionnaire survey of one of our members (Alltree 1993).

The validation of the course was suspended pending our convincing the Professional Practice Committee that acupuncture should be included in all aspects of clinical practice. Our representations for a revision in practice were accepted and the course was successfully resubmitted for postgraduate accreditation.

The first accredited course began in January 1993 and is based at the Nottingham School of Physiotherapy. The content and assessments for this course were approved by a joint panel of educationalists from the CSP and Greenwich University, giving it postgraduate status. After two very successful intakes this course is now being resubmitted for reassessment at 'M' level which will give credit points towards a Master's degree.

Insurance

The insurance situation prior to 1982

Before 1982, physiotherapists who wished to use their acupuncture in private practice had to take out a separate insurance policy in addition to that of the CSP and could not claim that this skill formed part of the recognized 'core of physiotherapy practice'.

The insurance situation 1982–1988

In 1982 the CSP, responding to growing demands by their members who were successfully using acupuncture in their clinical practice, decided to include acupuncture as a permissible modality for pain relief only. There were two main reasons that led to this decision:

1. There was a precedent as regards piercing skin in the UK as at one time physiotherapists had been taught the techniques of electrolysis, which involved skin piercing. There was therefore no great barrier to reinstating skin-piercing techniques.
2. The medical profession were using acupuncture as a modality for pain relief and at that time the logical conclusion was to do the same as regards physiotherapy practice. It also limited the scope of practice, making a more acceptable package for the CSP insurers.

By the mid 1980s it became evident that many AACP members were using acupuncture for a wide range of conditions. A questionnaire to members established that 55% of members were using acupuncture for conditions that were not necessarily painful, such as respiratory conditions. Following representations in 1987 to the Professional Practice Committee of the CSP it was agreed that physiotherapists who had been suitably trained could include acupuncture in treating any condition that came within the scope of physiotherapy practice.

The insurance situation 1988–1990

Having gained the CSP's approval for full integration of acupuncture within physiotherapy practice, the scope of practice became a problem. There were various conditions, such as addictive smoking and eating, that in themselves did not strictly conform to the range of conditions treated by physiotherapists, but had a profound effect on patients with many conditions treated by physiotherapists. The CSP advised that we were not covered to treat addictions; AACP therefore organized separate insurance for those physiotherapists who wished to treat addictions or other conditions that did not strictly conform to the current scope of practice.

The current insurance situation

In 1990 a revised Rule 1 of professional conduct was

issued. This stated that: 'Chartered Physiotherapists shall confine themselves to clinical diagnosis and practice in those fields of physiotherapy in which they have been trained which are recognized by the profession to be beneficial'.

There was acceptance that the role of physiotherapists was constantly evolving and that the clinical interest groups should monitor the range of clinical practice among their members insuring that their practice conformed to Rule 1 of professional conduct. AACP decided that their members no longer needed the extra insurance cover.

Relationship with medical practitioners

There was great opposition from our medical colleagues to the practice of acupuncture by physiotherapists. The doctors had formed their own association, the British Medical Acupuncture Society (BMAS). Moves were made at the highest level to restrict the practice of acupuncture to doctors and dentists only within the National Health Service. In some hospitals physiotherapists who had trained in acupuncture were unable to include this modality in their treatment programmes. Slowly but surely, however, a dialogue was developed between the BMAS and AACP. One of the misconceptions that BMAS members had was that physiotherapists would be primarily treating patient with internal medical problems, which do not come directly within the scope of physiotherapy practice. Once the senior members of BMAS were assured of our intention of practising primarily within the scope of physiotherapy and not as alternative medical practitioners, the basis for improved communication was established.

Conclusion

There have been many difficulties to overcome in establishing acupuncture as a legitimate modality in clinical practice. We have in the UK many physiotherapists who are including acupuncture in their clinical practice but who do not belong to AACP. This makes the task of ensuring the highest standards of practice very difficult. The way forward for the future is to establish training in acupuncture at an undergraduate level. Plans are already in the pipeline and several universities have expressed interest in including an elective module in their curriculae for undergraduates.

A history of the Physiotherapy, Acupuncture and Pain Modulation Association (PAPMA) a special interest group of the NZ Society of Physiotherapists Incorporated

Diana Turnbull

In 1972 a member of the New Zealand Society of Physiotherapists (NZSP) had a complaint laid against him for practising acupuncture as well as physiotherapy. The rules and ethics of the Society gave the Ethical Committee of the day no grounds to censure his acupuncture. However, he was censured for the implicit physiotherapy advertising relating to his promotion of the acupuncture side of his practice. In 1982 this same physiotherapist was elected as the Inaugural President of PAPMA.

The sad part of this tale is that our profession was so unbearably restrictive in its thinking. The good part is that at least it does respond to changing times in a positive and hopefully proactive way.

In the middle of the late 1970s this same person ran some weekends and then week-long courses for physiotherapists who showed any interest. This built a small nucleus of converted devotees who quietly pursued their interest with no official knowledge or backing of their activity. Of course, acupuncture was becoming more of an "in" thing following President Nixon's visit to China in 1973 leading to subsequent visits to China. The Director General of Health at that time was a member of one of those tours, and wrote a long and interesting report on his trip, which portrayed acupuncture and TCM in a very positive light. (He is on record as saying that acupuncture might reduce New Zealand's high drug bill!)

It was with this background that acupuncture in New Zealand entered the 1980s. Early in 1980, several New Zealand physiotherapists went to Australia to study acupuncture, where there was a more established acupuncture programme. These physiotherapists were keen to set up an acupuncture group in New Zealand. The numbers of physiotherapists in New Zealand practising acupuncture was growing and in 1982 a special interest group of physiotherapists practising acupuncture was formed in New Zealand. A name Physiotherapy Acupuncture and Pain Modulation Association (PAPMA), was chosen after a little discussion; it was felt that using the term "pain modulation" in the title would broaden the scope of the group to reasonably cover other pain techniques like TENS/laser and leave the way open for any new technology that might eventuate.

Constitutions were rapidly drawn up and approved. The most important work was seen to be the running of courses in New Zealand, thereby eliminating the need for the expensive trans-Tasman trips. Acupuncture courses for physiotherapists in New Zealand began in 1982 with doctors and physiotherapists teaching short programmes. In 1983, PAPMA ran its first programme with three 2 day weekends. This course was oversubscribed. It was only the beginning.

Acupuncture was accepted as a physiotherapy modality by the New Zealand Physiotherapy Board in 1984 and formal recognition by the NZSP followed later that year.

Two other groups were beginning to use Acupuncture in New Zealand also. These are the Medical Acupuncture Society, comprising doctors and dentists, and the "lay" acupuncture group called the "Register of Acupuncturists" whose members have non-medical backgrounds. Both these groups also began practising acupuncture and formalizing their Association in New Zealand at about the same time as PAPMA. Again, their members at this stage were trained overseas.

Education

There was (and still is) divided opinion amongst the groups as to who should be allowed to use acupuncture in New Zealand, and what qualifications and training are necessary to ensure competent acupuncturists. Over the last 12 years PAPMA's education programme has evolved by a process of continual re-evaluation and modification.

Today (1995) we have a 2 year programme of structured "units". The first year is our introductory course programme, which comprises 12 days tuition in four 3 day blocks, with self-learning components, a revision day and a base level examination (2 $\frac{1}{2}$ hour paper plus a 15 minute oral/practical). The second year sees more specialized units, extending the basic knowledge level in four individual units. We are in the planning stages of a diploma/degree level qualification in acupuncture for physiotherapists in New Zealand. We have a standard course text and participant and tutor course manuals. All PAPMA tutors attend teacher-training programmes. We have a teaching team of 10, primarily physiotherapists, but we also have two to three doctors teaching for us.

A Physiotherapy Acupuncture Register has been set up. This Register is the first step in an evolving mechanism of professional audit in the field on acupuncture. There are specific requirements to be admitted to this register – for example, sufficient educational hours, and an examination pass level of 75% are requirements to remain on this register. PAPMA has a membership of 300, with 97 members on this register.

Relationship with medical practitioners

PAPMA now has a reasonable relationship with our medical counterparts, the Medical Acupuncture Society NZ, (MASNZ). However, this has not always been so; until 1988, physiotherapists were required to present a CV to MASNZ in order to attend their annual conference. Times have changed for the better; PAPMA and MASNZ now run joint conferences on an annual basis, and have some interchange of tutors on courses.

The closer ties between the MASNZ and PAPMA have been useful as we look towards a National Qualification for Acupuncture in New Zealand. The government wishes to have one qualification in acupuncture for medical, paramedical and lay acupuncture groups. They wish these groups to formulate this qualification together under the National Education Framework. This is a very slow process because of the different backgrounds of the acupuncture groups. The main issues are the content (traditional and scientific approaches) and the level

of the eventual qualification. We have come a long way in this development, but there is still much work to be done to complete this process. At present (1995) all groups continue to run their own training programmes appropriate to their members.

Conclusion

In conclusion, acupuncture practice is alive and flourishing in New Zealand today with approximately 50 physiotherapists entering PAPMA's programme each year; over 100 members have attained register level, with these numbers growing every year. Acupuncture is practised by physiotherapists both in hospitals and in private practice as primary health care givers. It is my belief that the future will see increased numbers of acupuncture practitioners, both medical and non-medical in New Zealand and that the country will become more involved internationally with the establishment of internationally recognized levels of study, especially for physiotherapists and medical practitioners.

History of acupuncture in Zimbabwe

Helen Madzokere

Zimbabwe, like other African countries, has its own traditional medicine practices. After attaining independence in 1980, the government officially recognized the importance of traditional medicine with the formation of an organization for the registration of traditional healers. The challenge of the WHO Health for All by the year 2000 encouraged the Ministry of Health to utilize all possible means aimed at the Health for All goal. In addition to recognizing the local traditional medicine, the government employed expatriate Chinese doctors at the then newest hospital in the country, Chitungwiza General Hospital, which serves a population of nearly two million people.

The three Chinese doctors, led by Dr Lee, came to Zimbabwe in 1983. They were authorized by the government to practice TCM, which included acupuncture. I had taken a course in acupuncture in Southampton and on returning home in 1985 had the pleasure of finding the Chinese doctors practising in the country. I took an opportunity to work with these doctors for 2 weeks in 1987. I observed that their practice was well patronized, with an average of 150 patients per day presenting with various diagnoses from hypertension to mild sprains. The patients were very impressed with the results obtained from acupuncture. The popularity of the Chinese doctors spread fast and they were soon treating patients from bigger centres like Harare, Gweru and Bulawayo. The contract with the Chinese doctors ended in 1992 and the administrator of Chitungwiza Hospital tells me that the community misses them a lot.

When I got back home in 1985, the physiotherapy community in Zimbabwe were (like all other medical personnel) sceptical about the efficacy of acupuncture. I therefore did not have a chance to practise acupuncture until my visit to Chitungwiza when Dr Lee started referring patients from Gweru and Bulawayo to me for acupuncture. In 1990, the Zimbabwe Physiotherapy Association (ZPA) invited Dorothy Sweetman from South Africa to teach them trigger point massage. She included the concept of dry needling in her course. It was this course that generated the physiotherapists' interest in acupuncture.

In May 1990, the Harare branch of the ZPA invited Dr Lee to give a series of theoretical lectures on Saturday mornings from which the members obtained a fair understanding of acupuncture principles.

The first acupuncture course to be organized by the Continuing Education Committee of the ZPA was held in 1991 and it was presented by Charles Liggins from South Africa. He continued with modules two and three the following 2 years.

Dorothy Barker, the President of ZPA, and her husband participated in the IAAPT tour of China in 1992 and were kind enough to pay the subscriptions to IAAPT for 1993/4. The acupuncture interest group was recognized as part of the ZPA in 1992. The association has shown its support for the interest group by paying the IAAPT subscriptions for 1995/6.

I taught the introductory course to physiotherapists in both Harare and Bulawayo.

Physiotherapists in Zimbabwe are now enjoying practising acupuncture and those who have done courses with both Charles Liggins and myself are incorporating it well into pain control aspects of physiotherapy. There is a lot of interest in continuing education in the field of acupuncture. As an on-going programme the ZPA plans to run at least one introductory course every year to cater for new members and others.

As far as the future of acupuncture is concerned, I am confident that acupuncture is gaining more and more popularity with both the patients and practitioners. Zimbabwe stands to benefit a lot from its membership to IAAPT as the proposed continuing education programme will standardize training in acupuncture.

Acupuncture in Sweden

Eva Haker

In 1984 acupuncture was accepted as a treatment of pain by the Swedish National Board of Health and Welfare, and today it is completely integrated in the medical treatment arsenal. Acknowledged groups qualified to deal with acupuncture are registered physicians, physiotherapists, dentists and nurses with special training in acupuncture. The background for the acceptance was extensive basic physiological studies and a literature survey by Professor Sven Andersson.

To some the discussion of TCM is controversial. We do have colleagues trained according to the TCM theory. However, we find it difficult to communicate as we represent two different way of thinkings and we must also keep in mind that TCM was not the background for its official approval in Sweden.

The Swedish Association of Acupuncture for Physical Therapists (SALS) was formed in 1985; a few years later interest groups were formed among physicians and nurses. Today we have a good and close collaboration between the associations and together we publish The Swedish Journal of Medical Acupuncture four times a year. In January 1995 SALS had 1600 members, which represents 16% of all physiotherapists in Sweden. Since 1990 an acupuncture congress has been arranged every second year and the interest in these congresses has been enormous.

In 1993 acupuncture was extended to include diseases provided enough scientific evidence was presented and provided the physiotherapist has enough knowledge of that special condition to be treated. SALS recommends a close collaboration with the physician in charge.

Education

The SALS acupuncture training programme for physical therapists in Sweden includes 80 hours of theory and practice within a period of 1 year. The training programme includes the history of pain, neuroanatomy, neurophysiology, functional background to acupuncture classification of pain, localization of points, principles of treatment, indications, contraindication, electroacupuncture, interactions of acupuncture and drugs, legal aspects, etc. TCM theory is used just as an introduction. The main purpose of these courses is an understanding of the neurophysiology required to be able to approach the acupuncture field.

Advanced courses are also arranged, including further points and clinical discussions. In 1994 the first course including acupuncture and diseases was arranged. Since then it has been repeated four times a year. The intention of this course is to present research findings, to discuss the role of the autonomic nervous system and to present points that may be useful, including ear acupuncture.

From 1996 the basic physiotherapy training programme has been extended by 6 months to 3 years. The last period will include an elective basic acupuncture training programme for the students. This means that once they get their licence, they are also licensed for acupuncture treatment. Parallel to the elective course they do research project with a credit 10 points (over 10 weeks).

Some of the acupuncture courses are also taught to nurses at the university (postgraduate students). These courses involves a smaller project, mostly a literature survey within special areas (credit two to three points) at an academic level.

Research

Several theses have been presented in the field of acupuncture during the last years. In one dissertation, facial pain was studied and the pain-relieving effect of acupuncture and a bite-splint was compared. Acupuncture was found as good as a bite-splint with respect to relief of pain and muscle tension after 1 year (List 1992), although stress has been found to reverse the pain-relieving effect of acupuncture (Wiederstrorn 1993). Acupuncture produces more pain relief than ultrasound, low energy laser, steroids, elbow band and splintage in lateral epicondylalgia (Haker 1993). Different modes of acupuncture have also been studied (Thomas 1995).

Conclusion

For the moment the future of acupuncture seems favourable; we are slowly getting real approval by the physicians. The only way we will finally succeed, however, is by increasing our knowledge about the mechanisms of acupuncture by a critical evaluation of what we are doing. This is already happening as there is a great interest in the subject and it is often chosen for research projects for postgraduate degrees. We should not, however, forget that acupuncture should be considered as complementary to other modes of treatment.

Acupuncture in Argentina

Ana Maria Carballo

In Argentina, acupuncture as a part of TCM has been developed by important professionals in health care and is currently a common practice for the treatment of many types of illnesses. Although it is widely used and in many cases requested by the patients themselves, it has not yet been officially recognized as a medical practice and no university in the country acknowledges it as such.

As in many other countries, acupuncture has been considered until very recently, as a kind of non-scientific or magical practice. The fact that today it is an openly recognized therapeutic aid leads to the assumption that it has surfaced somehow all of a sudden. The truth is that the path followed by this knowledge moved along a sort of 'invisible undercurrent', very tiny at its beginning but with a sustained growth rate over the last decades, so that by now it cannot be ignored any longer.

In Argentina, the development of acupuncture was marked by the following highlights:

1948: The undercurrent was started with work on acupuncture by Dr José Rebuelto. Thus, Argentina became one of the pioneers, worldwide, and certainly the first Latin American country, to integrate these practices with the knowledge of scientific medicine.

1955: Dr David Sussman and Dr José Rebuelto created the Argentine Society of Acupuncture (ASA).

1960: Dr Floreal Carballo founded the Argentine Medical Institute of Acupuncture (IMADA).

These were the first public appearances of the undercurrent. Both institutions are currently working developing courses and activities to promote the practice of acupuncture. The activities of the ASA are aimed exclusively at physicians, while the objective of the IMADA is to propagate acupuncture among physiotherapists, medical doctors and odontologists.

1973: First official appearance of the undercurrent: a round-table discussion on acupuncture and its therapeutical possibilities is held at the Medical School of the University of Buenos Aires, sponsored by the Embassy of the Republic of China. Among the attendants, there were renowned Argentine physicians, like Dr Raul Matera, Dr Floreal Carballo and Dr Florencio Escardo.

1974: The Latin American Association of Acupuncture and Auriculotherapy was formed. At the same time, under the leadership of Dr Floreal Carballo, the training in acupuncture of physiotherapists began. These professionals started to work towards joining with physicians in the integration of physiotherapy, acupuncture and TCM. This work of integration was later continued in the medical offices of the Social Bank Services

Institute, at the headquarters of the National Bank, with the support of Dr Padin, as well as in private medical offices.

1976: WHO organized training courses in China and was active in systematization of the knowledge of acupuncture and TCM – a supportive element to our work.

1979: WHO specified, through the work of Dr R. N. Bameman, which persons are qualified to perform the practice of acupuncture. That document established as basic requirements, a knowledge of the basic sciences and status as specialized physicians or health care auxiliaries.

1980: During the 1980s, massive teaching courses for this type of practice were started among physiotherapists. At the same time, in several European countries these techniques were legalized and introduced into the field of physiotherapy. During this decade, more than 150 physiotherapists gained the knowledge to implement these therapeutic techniques through courses and training activities in different institutions, lectures, seminars, etc. Also in national hospitals, such as the Argerich Hospital, some treatments that included several techniques of TCM, such as digitopuncture and self-massage, were introduced in self-help meetings for patients suffering from asthma and allergies.

1985: During the Eighth Congress on Pain, held in Buenos Aires, Dr Sven Andersson gave lectures and conferences on acupuncture. It is through him that the Argentine physiotherapists learned that acupuncture had been officially recognized in Sweden for physiotherapists as well as for medical doctors.

1991: Supported by Dr Cova and Professor Decurgez, I started to introduce a postgraduate course on acupunctural reflexotherapy for graduates in physiotherapy.

1993: The course on acupunctural reflexotherapy was given for the first time in the Medical School of the University of Buenos Aires, being the only one officially recognized as valid. It has now been held for 3 consecutive years and has been completed already by 75 attendants.

1994: Within the Argentine Association of Physiotherapy, the Committee of Physiotherapists specializing in acupunctural reflexotherapy was formed, and will be part of the research area for reflexotherapy within the recently created Academia Argentina de Kinesiologia, which, at present, is being legally constituted.

1995: In November of this year, the second-level course on acupuncture, which was given by me at the Bemardo Houssay Hospital in the city of Vicente Lopez, will be completed. This course was sponsored by the College of

Physiotherapists of the Province of Buenos Aires.

References

Alltree J 1993 Physiotherapy and acupuncture: practice in UK. Complementary Therapies In Medicine 1(1): 34–41

Haker E 1993 Lateral epicondylalgia. Diagnosis, treatment, and evaluation. Critical Reviews in Physical and Rehabilitation Medicine 5(2): 129–154

List T 1992 Acupuncture in the treatment of patients with craniomandibular disorders. Theses. Swedish Dental Journal (suppl): 87

Thomas M 1995 Treatment of pain with acupuncture. Factors influencing outcome. Theses

Wiederstrorn E N 1993 Analgesic effects of somatic, afferent stimulation – a psychobiological perspective. Thesis

15

Advancing horizons: examples of approaches to three case studies

Jan Naslund, Charles Liggins, Diana Turnbull

This is an international book with contributions from physical therapists in many countries. Many case studies have been included with their contributions. In the first half of this chapter are included three detailed case studies from the 1995 WCPT Congress. In the second half are included many shorter case studies, illustrating individual approaches from around the world.

Three detailed case reports from the WCPT congress 1995: introduction

Eva Haker, Chairman of SALS, Sweden

After the 12th WCPT congress held in Washington DC in June/July 1995, IAAPT organized a postcongress course on "Acupuncture advancing horizons". During the 2 days, some physiotherapists were invited to comment and present their suggestions of how to treat three cases of varied pain history. The three cases were sent out 2 months in advance and were meant to represent nociceptive pain (with the nervous system intact), neurogenic pain (nervous system not intact) and referred pain. The physiotherapists were chosen because of their different approaches to acupuncture: Jan Naslund from Sweden, Diana Turnbull from New Zealand and Charles Liggins from South Africa. To some extent they all represent different ways of considering acupuncture and the intention was to enlighten these discussions and see where we landed. Unfortunately we do not know the final outcomes of the suggested treatments; however these

case reports make interesting reading and hopefully give some interesting new aspects of how, when and why to treat. In considering treatments, the following questions may be asked: What conclusions can be drawn? If you are combining several modes of treatments, how is it best to evaluate the results? Is there any scientific support for your method of choice, or is it just empirical?

Theoretical background

Jan Naslund

If you are planning acupuncture treatments for a patient with pain problems and want to have a Western biological base for your treatments, there are some important facts to which you should pay attention. First, you should try to find the tissue that is causing the pain and the segmental innervation of that tissue (Fields & Basbaum 1994). Second, you ought to define the type of pain, as to whether it is a nociceptive, neurogenic/neuropathic, idiopathic or psychogenic type of pain (Thomas 1995).

The biological/physiological explanation of the mechanisms of acupuncture relate to the different pain inhibition mechanisms within the human body. Such mechanisms could be local changes in the tissue (Lundeberg 1993), segmental reflexes (Melzack & Wall 1965) or central descending pain inhibitory pathways (Andersson 1993, Le Bars 1983). Local needles are important, especially for the local and segmental effects. These needles should cover the area of pain and are often located in trigger points

(Baldry 1993). The distal needles have a more general pain inhibitory effect (Le Bars 1983) and will extend the treatment effects (Andersson 1993). You may place the distal needles both segmentally (Baldry 1993) and extrasegmentally (Le Bars 1983). Distal needles are often placed in "strong" acupuncture points, often situated in motor points of muscles distal to the knee and/or the elbow.

Case 1

History

The patient is a 63-year-old woman, who for the last 10 years has been working in an office. Her husband is retired and the couple are house owners. She has been on the sick list for the last 9 months because of a dull aching pain in her neck and left shoulder.

Signs and symptoms

In addition to pain and stiffness in her neck and shoulder, she has experienced sensory dysfunction along the radial side of her left forearm for the last year (Fig. 15.1). X-rays reveal severe spondylosis in the cervical area and decreased intervertebral disc space between the fifth and sixth cervical vertebrae.

Jan Naslund

From the case history I think that this patient has got both a nociceptive type of pain in her neck and right shoulder region and also a neuropathic pain in her

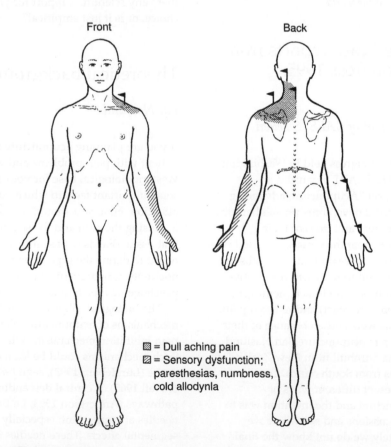

Fig. 15.1 *Case 1*.

left forearm. For this reason I will put my local needles in the area of pain in her neck and shoulder and also in her left forearm. If there is a disturbance in the sensory innervation of her left forearm, I will instead put needles in the contralateral forearm. I will choose the distal needles to be as segmental as possible, because one could not find good segmental points! I will also needle some extra segmental distal points. The needles in the left forearm will in this case be looked upon as both local and distal ones.

Treatment

■ *Points to be used –*
   Local points: GB-20, 21; GV-14, LI-4, 11 (LT)
   Distal points: LI-4 (RT), 10 (RT); ST-36 (LT)

Treatment parameters: duration: 20–30 min.
   Stimulation: start with manual stimulation both local and distal. If no or bad effect of treatment, try low frequency electroacupuncture or, in the area of neuropathic pain, high frequency electroacupuncture.
   Number of treatments: 10–15.
   As I am using acupuncture as a pain treatment in this case, I would add other types of treatments suitable for this patient such as medication, exercises, etc.

Charles Liggins

Physiotherapy examination
Subjective: as given on the case sheet
Objective:
Posture: check neck and the possibility of tight pectoral muscles, and weak rhomboids.
Active neck movements: C1–T3
Passive intervertebral movements:
Check: acromio-clavicular, shoulder and elbow joints and the scapular movements.
Test: upper Limb Tension tests
Neurological: sensation, reflexes and muscle power
Palpation: particularly for myofascial trigger points.

Treatment approach: mobilize joints involved; stretch muscles concerned (fascial release); postural re-education.

Acupuncture approach:

1. Empirical:

   ■ *Points to be used –*
      Local: GB-20, 21; LI-15; ST-14; SI-10; B-11; tender trigger points
      Distal: LI-4, 11; TE-5

2. If complex, consider sympathetic outflow approach: Sympathetic outflow controls blood circulation to the neck.
   Nerve cells in spinal cord at T4–9 (which service the upper limb) may cause symptoms in any part of the upper limb.
   Assuming pain, sensory and other symptoms are due to blood flow problems, needle Back Shu points (situated T4–sacrum). To relax sympathetic outflow activity, use superficial needling to appropriate acupoints associated with segmental levels. To stimulate sympathetic outflow activity use tonification needling (quick in and out), to appropriate acupoints associated with segmental levels.

Diana Turnbull

Signs and symptoms

- pain and stiffness neck and shoulder
- sensory dysfunction radial aspect left forearm for 12 months
- X-ray – severe spondylosis in cervical spine – decreased disc space in C5/6 vertebrae.

I feel this is a complex problem involving dysfunction in disc, nerve, ligament, bone and muscle. There is also the psycho-dynamics of the whole situation to consider.

Other pathologies that need to be excluded: rare disorders – spinal cord tumour, etc. – bone secondaries that may not readily show on X-ray in early stages.

Treatment approaches The following modalities would be suitable:

- acupuncture
- laser
- TENS
- physiotherapy modalities.

Points to note:
- patient must be given an explanation and choice of treatment options
- consent must be gained prior to treatment commencing.

Suggested treatment: acupuncture (or a combination of TENS and acupuncture) combined with other physiotherapy modalities as follows:

1. Acupuncture:
   I would begin with ear acupuncture using the following points:

   - Shenmen
   - cervical spine zone – especially the sympathetic chain–muscle zone
   - forearm points.

   I would acupuncture using $1/2''$ (25 mm) needles retaining them for 20–30 minutes, and may use a press needle or iron bead for prolonged stimulation. Depending on the patient's reactions and responses to treatment, I would also select from the following points for subsequent treatments:
   GB-20 Fengchi: Bilateral insertion for local pain and stiffness in the cervical spine. This point is a powerful local point on the Gall Bladder meridian, and also is in close proximity to the short muscle extensor of the cervical spine, plus major nerves and blood vessels for this region.
   GV-14 Dazhui: This point is useful for any local disorders of the neck or shoulders. It is also closely associated with the autonomic plexus at this level.
   C5/6 segment: To gain maximum relaxation of this segment, and local stimulation of the nerve and blood supply to the area the following points can be acupunctured:

   - Governor point between C5 and C6
   - EX-21 Huatuojiaji points 0.5 Cun lateral to the C5 spinous process (these relate closely to the facet joint)
   - B points lateral to the segment.

   ■ *Distal points* –
   LU-7: This point is excellent for cervical spondylosis, any stiffness or headache on the back of the head. It lies on the C6 dermatome. It is a Luo connecting point and one of the six important distal points for the back of the head and neck.
   SI-3: The main importance of this point is that it is the confluential point of the Governor meridian, and has special influence in spinal disorder.
   B-62: This point, used in conjunction with SI-3, makes up a confluential pair of points that can influence spinal disorders.
   GB-34: This point could also be used because of its influence on muscle and tendons.

   ■ *To increase energy level, the Five Element points* – KI-7 Metal point, Kidney; LU-5 Water point, Lung

   Or: Take care not to deplete her energy further but keeping needles to a minimum, reducing retention time and treating only once or twice a week.

2. Trigger points: This lady may have trigger points that need attention.
   I would use dry needling (with an acupuncture needle), laser or myofascial release techniques, e.g. spray, stretch and manual techniques, on the following: levator angulae scapulae, trapezius, supraspinatus, teres major and minor, local trigger points, infraspinatus, brachioradialis, scaleni and extensor carpi radialis longus.

3. Physiotherapy modalities:
   Any of the following that I thought were suitable for this patient:

TENS (in conjunction with acupuncture)	manual cervical mobilization
heat – hot packs, shortwave diathermy	soft tissue work – massage and myofascial release
specific home exercises – postural – mobility	stress management
drug therapy to assist	ergonomics at work/home

Time frame: I like to begin with ear acupuncture, as this will often improve patients without body acupuncture application. I would then use body acupuncture, using a maximum of 6 needles per session. Probable needle retention time: ear 20–30 min; body 10–15 min.

Acupuncture once/twice weekly.

Case 2

History

The patient is a 20-year-old female student with dull pain in the lower back and abdomen during her menstrual periods (Fig. 15.2). She has never been pregnant nor used contraceptive pills. Non-steroidal anti-inflammatory drugs (NSAIDS) gave insufficient relief.

Signs and symptoms

During the episodes of pain she also becomes nauseated. She has no problems at the time of ovulation.

Jan Naslund

From the case history, the description indicates that here is a patient with a cyclical nociceptive visceral pain. Needles will in this case be placed in somatic sites, both local and distal in segmental myotomes of the hypogastric and splanchnic nerves. In addition to these needles I will use SP-6, a point that in TCM is recognized to have specific effects in premenstrual treatment of dysmenorrhoea. SP-6 is located in the tibialis posterior muscle and stimulation here sets up activity in muscle afferents (T12, L1, 2 and S2, 3, 4), presumably effective at the synapses of uterine segmental innervation responsible for pain and autonomic activity.

This description goes also for the point SP-9. The point PE-6 is recommended for use for nausea. The

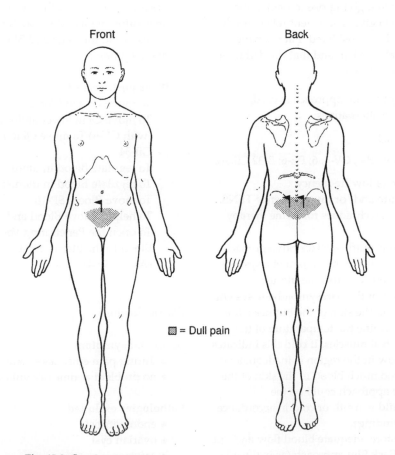

Front   Back

☒ = Dull pain

Fig. 15.2 *Case 2.*

effects have been tested in clinical research (Dundee J W 1991).

Treatment
- *Local points* – CV-4; B-32 (bilaterally)
- *Distal points* – SP-6, 9; PE-6.

Treatment parameters: duration 20–30 min.
Stimulation: manual.
Number of treatments: two treatments each month, approximately 7 days and 3 days prior to the presumed onset of the period, for 4–5 months.

This concept of treatment has been tested in clinical research (Thomas 1995).

Charles Liggins

Is this a case of a mechanical problem giving rise to referred pain to lower abdominal–uterus areas, or a gynaecological problem giving rise to pain in the back? As the NSAIDS give insufficient relief and the patient has nausea, it is considered that the patient has a gynaecological problem and that the definitive diagnosis is dysmenorrhoea.

Treatment The acupuncture approach is used, for which there are three alternatives:

1. Empirical approach:

   - *Points* – ST-36; SP-6; CV-4, 6; PE-6; B-32 Ciliao.

   Consider the use of low frequency electroacupuncture and/or low frequency TENS. Teach acupressure techniques for home therapy and prophylaxis.
2. Use of sympathetic outflow/Back Shu approach: Think sympathetic and parasympathetic systems. The parasympathetic controls the uterus; cutaneous reflexes of the parasympathetic system of this region are in the skin of the buttocks. It is necessary to determine the temperature of the skin over the gluteal muscles. If cold this indicates that the blood flow in the region is inadequate; if hot it indicates too much blood in the skin of the region. A simple approach could be the application of mild warmth or cold in accordance with the above findings.
   Explanation: Restore adequate blood flow and gut function, using Back Shu approach (as in Case 1).

3. TCM approach. Dysmenorrhoea is pain during and after menstruation. Pain may occur in lower abdomen and/or sacrum. Normal menstruation requires movement of Blood (Liver Qi and Liver Blood); however, stagnation is the key pathological feature of dysmenorrhoea. Pain during menstruation is due to Liver Blood stagnation, which can be due to emotional strain, overwork, chronic illness, excessive sexual activity, childbirth or invasion of Cold/Dampness.
The condition may be one of Excess due to stagnation of Qi and Blood, stagnation of Cold or Damp-Heat, or Deficiency, due to Qi and Blood Deficiency or Kidney and/or Liver Deficiency.
General principles:
1. Regulate Qi and Blood in the Penetrating and Directing vessels.
2. During period move Blood and stop pain.
Treatment: Consider the cause as one of stagnation of Qi and Blood; therefore it will be necessary to move Qi and Blood, eliminate stasis and stop pain.

- *Points to be used* –
  To move Qi and Blood and stop pain: LIV-3
  To move Qi in lower abdomen: CV-6
  (with CV-6) To move Qi in lower abdomen: GB-34
  To regulate Blood in uterus and stop pain: SP-8
  To regulate Blood in uterus: ST-29
  To move Blood: SP-10
  To help to move Blood and stop pain: SP-6
  To open the Penetrating Vessel and regulate Blood to the uterus: SP-4
  (As for SP-4): PE-6

Diana Turnbull

Signs and symptoms
- during pain episodes – nauseated
- no problem at time of ovulation

Pathologies excluded
- endometriosis
- ovarian cyst
- carcinoma

The diagnosis of this student is probably dysmenorrhoea. This condition is probably related to an imbalance of hormones resulting in altered levels of prostaglandins that increase spasm in the uterus.

Treatment options
1. Acupuncture.
2. Review drug therapy with the medical practitioner (the NSAID tried may not be the most suitable).
3. Use of supplements such as B vitamins and Oil of Evening Primrose (gamma linoleic acid).
4. Active exercise programme.

Points to note:
The patient is given an explanation and choice of treatment options. Consent is obtained prior to treatment.

1. Acupuncture treatment
   This needs to be divided into:

   • acupuncture when she has pain
   • acupuncture to alter the body's imbalance, which is done prior to menstruation, beginning usually at mid cycle.

   Acupuncture at time of pain: ear points I would use include HE-7 Shenmen and the uterus points. Press needles can be put in both or a needle threaded between these points. This has a strong relaxation effect on the uterus, reducing any spasm.

   ■ *Body points that could also be used –*
   For a strong analgesic effect on the body; indicated in painful menstruation: LI-4
   To effect directly the hormonal imbalance of the prostaglandins and therefore reduce the spasm of the uterus. (also an important tonification point and one of the six important distal points with specific action in the uterine area): Spleen SP-6
   For nausea and homeostatic/regulatory functions: Stomach ST-36
   Of particularly benefit for menstrual dysfunction: CV-4 or 6

   Mid cycle and just prior to menstruation: The best times to acupuncture these patients, as the aim of acupuncture is to regulate or bring back into balance the body dysfunction. Treatment will

need to continue for approximately 3 months to regulate hormones.

■ *Points that can be used –*
To regulate hormonal dysfunction: SP-6
For influence in menstrual dysfunction: CV-4 or 6
For homeostasis/regulation and nausea: ST-36 or SP-6
To regulate menstrual disorders: confluential points SP-4 and PE-6

For general tonification: CV-6; ST-36; SP-6
Time frame:

• ear acupuncture first
• add body acupuncture points
• retention time of needles: ear – semipermanent (3 days to 1 week); Body – 20 min
• daily at acute time
• weekly from mid cycle for 3 months' long term regulation of system.

2. Other treatment
   Exercise has been shown to help the symptoms of dysmenorrhoea. It would be useful to advise her to begin a regular exercise programme of walking/swimming.

Case 3

History

The patient is a 43-year-old cab driver who for the last 18 months has had pain in the lumbar and sacroiliac regions (Fig. 15.3). Because of suspected prostatitis, antibiotics were given but no improvement was seen. Specialists in orthopaedics were consulted but no indication for orthopaedic surgery found.

Signs and symptoms

The aching pain radiates to the lateral side of the right leg down to the knee and is worse in the early hours of the morning. Occasionally the pain is felt in the scrotal region and is accentuated when the bladder is full. No neurological abnormalities were found; muscles strength and reflexes were normal; no muscle atrophy or diminished sensibility was

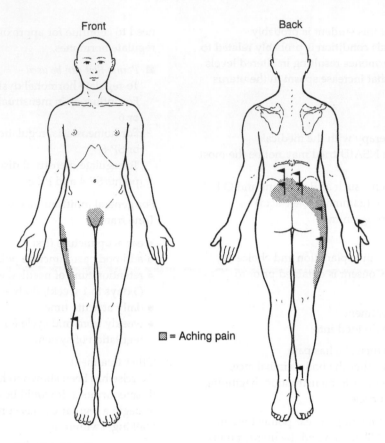

Fig. 15.3 *Case 3.*

found. The patient is HLA-B27 negative and X-rays of the thoracic lumbar and sacroiliac regions were normal, therefore ankylosing spondylitis is unlikely. Magnetic resonance imaging of the low back showed a slight protrusion of the disc between the 4th and 5th lumbar vertebrae, but there was no mechanical pressure on the nerve roots or the dura. No abnormalities were found at the level of the conus medullaris.

Jan Naslund

The case history reveals that this patient has got a nociceptive type of pain emerging from the muscles in the lower back and referred pain down the right leg. Local points will be chosen both in the low back region but also in the area of referred pain (Baldry 1993).

Treatment

- *Points to be used –*
  Local points: B-25, 27 (bilaterally); GB-30, 31
  Distal points: LI-4; ST-36; B-60
  Treatment parameters: duration 20–30 minutes.
  Stimulation: manual stimulation both local and distal.
  If no – or bad effects – try low frequency electroacupuncture or high frequency in the low back region.
  Number of treatments: 10–15.

Charles Liggins

Physiotherapy examination

Subjective: as given on data sheet.

Mechanical approach: symptoms in L5 distribution; if it is disc compression which affects the sino vertebral nerve, pain can cross the midline.

Objective: consider mechanics of the situation – the patient is a cab driver; therefore check posture, taking into consideration the possibility of: weak abdominal muscles/tight hamstrings and tight iliopsoas/weak gluteal muscles.

Check joints: vertebral, sacroiliac and hip. Check muscles around the area. Palpate for trigger points.

Treatment

Conventional approach: mobilization; emphasis on rotation; clear trigger points: use appropriate methods (see Chapter 7).

Acupuncture approach:

1. Empirical: Choose points from the Bladder and Gall Bladder channels, plus LIV-1 and 5 and GB-41 for the pain in the scrotal region.
2. Sympathetic outflow approach: Think T10 to L2/4: this controls blood outflow from waist down. The connective tissue involvement in the pain region is gross; connective tissue has a low density of blood vessels but high density of sensory nerve endings.

   With movement during the day the patient's pain is diminished; however, at rest (at night) the pain is maximized. Reason: at rest the blood pressure lowers and therefore blood flow is slowed down and nutrition to nerve cells lowered and these can become relatively anoxic, resulting in pain at rest.

   It should be noted that if blood flow slows to unacceptable levels in the spinal cord, reflex control of that very same system may be diminished.

   Scrotal pain is possibly from feedback to sensory nerve cells for that region.
   Treatment: Needle appropriate Back Shu points.

Diana Turnbull

Signs and symptoms

- aching pain radiates to lateral side right leg
- occasional scrotal pain – worse when full bladder
- worse in early hours morning
- no neurological abnormalities

- no muscle atrophy or diminished sensation
- muscle strength and reflexes normal
- HLA-B27 negative
- magnetic resonance imaging – slight protrusion of disc L4/5 vertebrae
- X-ray thoracic, lumbar and sacroiliac joints NAD (nothing abnormal detected)
- no abnormalities at level of conus medullaris

Other pathologies to be excluded

- bladder pathology
- prostate pathology i.e. negative genitourinary work-up
- Problem – no diagnosis.

Could be organ based – but shows no classic pain pattern for prostate, kidney or bladder.

Could be musculoskeletal – but does not fit dermatome, myotome or joint.

Points to note:

Patient given explanation, and choice of treatment options. Consent obtained.

Treatment

- acupuncture
- physiotherapy

1. Acupuncture approach: I would address both possible dysfunctions:

   - musculoskeletal LU-2/3, 4/5; plus local muscle trigger points
   - organ dysfunction – Urinary Bladder, Kidney, prostate.

I would begin with ear acupuncture, as this would also help me with my diagnosis.
Ear:

- look at organ zones – prostate – Bladder – Kidney
- musculoskeletal – lumbar spine zones – nerve – muscle – bone.

■ *Points to be used –*
   Local acupuncture points; points to affect the local segmental structures specifically; especially for musculoskeletal-based problems: Governor points GV-3, 4

Huatuojiaji points at GV-3, 4 levels
Also: Back Shu point for the Urinary Bladder (closely associated with the posterior rami of the first and second sacral nerves and the sympathetic ganglion that relates to the bladder): B-28
Treatment parameters: probable needle retention time because of chronicity – ear: 20–30 min (may use semipermanent 1–3 weeks); body: 15–20 min.
Treat one–two times per week.

2. Trigger points: if trigger points are active, these need to be dry needled (with acupuncture needles), treated with a laser and/or myofascial release techniques.
3. Possible muscle trigger points: quadratus lumborum, gluteus minimus and medius.
4. Other physiotherapy modalities: exercises, mobilizations and postural advice.

Acknowledgement

Charles Liggins is indebted to Roy Mitchell, Secretary of the Acupuncture Association of South African Society of Physiotherapy, for his contribution in respect of the autonomic nervous system approach to the management of the three cases.

References

Andersson S 1993 The functional background in acupuncture effects. Scandinavian Journal of Rehabilitation Medicine (suppl) 29: 31–60
Baldry P E 1993 Acupuncture, trigger points and musculoskeletal pain, 2nd edn. Churchill Livingstone, New York
Dundee J W 1991 Non-invasive stimulation of the P-6 Neiguan antiemetic acupuncture point in cancer chemotherapy. Journal of the Royal Society of Medicine 84: 210–212
Fields H L, Basbaum A L 1994 Central nervous system mechanisms of pain modulation. In: Wall P D, Melzack R (eds) Textbook of pain. Churchill Livingstone, New York, pp 243–257
Le Bars D, Dickinson A H, Besson J M 1983 Opiate analgesia and descending control systems. In: Bonica J J, Lindblom U, Iggo A (eds) Advances in pain research and therapy. Raven Press, New York, pp 341–372
Lundeberg T 1993 Peripheral effects of sensory nerve stimulation (*acupuncture) in inflammation and ischemia. Scandinavian Journal of Rehabilitation Medicine (suppl) 29: 61–86
Maciocia G 1989 The foundations of Chinese medicine. A comprehensive text for acupuncturists and herbalists. Churchill Livingstone, New York
Melzack R, Wall P D 1965 Pain mechanisms: a new theory. Science 150: 971–979
Thomas M 1995 Treatment of pain with acupuncture: factors influencing outcome. Thesis, Stockholm

16

Short case studies: a compendium

Ana Maria Carballo, Alan Clements, Sue Czartoryski, Val Hopwood, Sara Jeevanjee, Colette Lehody, Helen Madzokere, Val Marston, Passion Nhekairo-Musa, Kim Ong, Lorrene Soellner

Introduction

For the short case studies, contributors were asked only that the cases be set out clearly with easy explanations and obvious relevance to the international practice of physical therapy. Immediately it became apparent that while the general approach of physical therapists to their patients was very similar, the additional modality of acupuncture was being practised at very different levels and with profound differences in the underlying philosophies. Despite this, the most striking thing was the similarity in the points chosen.

Where acupuncture on its own would suffice it was used in that way, but where the cases were more complex the therapists did not hesitate to use all the modalities at their disposal. As has been also stated elsewhere, it is possible to obtain good results with very basic acupuncture and it is not necessary to know the finer points of traditional Chinese diagnosis to solve a simple pain problem. Some of the case studies that follow are indeed very simple and many practitioners have not felt the need to progress beyond these basic techniques, using acupuncture merely to augment their physiotherapy skills, perhaps treating postmanipulative tenderness or relaxing a patient before using stretches or manipulative procedures.

Please note that some of the terminology in these case histories has been retained as submitted, since professional titles and some terms in common usage will vary from country to country. We also acknowledge that not all our contributors speak English as their first language.

The case histories have been divided into three groups.

1. **Level I** Those at level one deal with simple pain relief. This is most often caused by channel blockage, preventing what TCM theory would consider to be the free flow of Qi or energy. The treatment usually involves use of local and distal points.
2. **Level II** The cases at this level have included other physical therapy, perhaps aimed at relief of swelling or inflammation. Homeostatic effects of points have been utilized in order to promote healing and it becomes necessary to understand a little more traditional acupuncture theory.
3. **Level III** These cases display a much more complex approach. Knowledge of TCM diagnosis and differentiation of syndromes enables the therapists to consider the balances within the whole body system and treat much more than the presenting symptoms. Due to the complex nature of many of these cases other physical therapy modalities have also been brought in.

Level I
Case 1

By Sue Czartoryski, UK

Female, aged 38 years
Arm pain – simple pain, level I
Basic acupuncture

A 38-year-old woman was referred for physiotherapy

after sustaining an injury at work approximately 7 weeks prior to assessment, when she swung round quickly and caught the back of her upper arm against a filing cabinet. She had had a great deal of pain in her arm ever since.

X-ray showed no bony injury. Drugs: ibuprofen.

Subjective history The pain was described as being all around the arm from the shoulder to the wrist but worse around the back and side of the arm. It was worse in the morning when the shoulder, elbow and hand were also stiff. Movement eased the pain a little initially but during the day any movement aggravated the pain. It was a constant, deep ache of varying degree.

Salient examination findings

- left elbow movements were approximately 80% of normal range and painful
- shoulder movements were approximately 75% of normal range and also painful
- cervical spine movements were full and pain free
- on palpation there was marked tenderness over the anterior aspect of the shoulder joint and over the common extensor origin of the forearm muscles

Physiotherapy treatment This patient was treated with interferential to the elbow joint, ultrasound to the common extensor origin and anterior aspect of the shoulder. She was also taught exercises. Tubigrip was applied to the elbow joint and a sling was to be used if the arm became very painful. After three sessions the patient was referred for acupuncture but the patient refused and continued with the physiotherapy for two more treatments.

She continued to make progress, her range of movement was improving but she still had pain from her shoulder to her wrist and eventually requested to try acupuncture. It seemed possible that the patient may have caught the radial nerve as it ran around the posterior aspect of the humerus in the radial sulcus, causing the pain she described and possibly causing an inflammatory process to be set up in the forearm extensors and brachioradialis. She had probably also strained the structures around the

anterior aspect of the shoulder joint as the head of the humerus would have been pushed in that direction with the blow. There was also increased tone in the deltoid muscle and pain on palpation of the upper fibres of trapezius.

- *Points used –*
  LI-4 Hegu, LI-11 Quchi, LI-15 Jianyu
  Points were selected on the Large Intestine channel since it ran through the area of pain: LI-4 Hegu is the distal point for the channel, also a calming point and a point for pain in the upper body. This is a good point to use for Painful Obstruction Syndrome of the arm or shoulder (Maciocia 1989). LI-11 Quchi is the local point at the elbow, and the He Sea point on the meridian; Qi is considered to gather at this point and therefore it is useful for promoting the flow of Qi along the meridian. It also benefits the sinews and joints and is useful to treat muscular problems in this area. LI-15 Jianyu is the local point for the shoulder. It benefits the sinews and stimulates the circulation of Qi in the channel.

The minimum of needles were used because the patient was nervous about the use of acupuncture. Deqi was obtained at all points and the needles were retained for 15 minutes. The interferential treatment was discontinued but the mobilizations remained unchanged, with glenohumeral glides and massage to the upper fibres of the trapezius and deltoid. Active exercises and stretches were continued at home.

At the next appointment the patient reported some improvement, with much less pain below the elbow. The other points were used as before with the addition of SI-12 Bingfeng as the muscles locally were found to be tender on palpation. This point is also indicated for aching in the upper limb. Deqi was obtained and described as tracking up into the neck. The needles were left in for 15 minutes.

The following week the patient reported feeling very much better. She had no pain below the elbow and much less pain in the upper arm. Shoulder movement was virtually full range. The same treatment was repeated.

The patient rang the following week to cancel her appointment as she had been pain free since her last visit and felt back to normal. It was agreed that she would contact the therapist within the next 2 weeks if the pain recurred. She did not contact the department again.

Case 2

By Val Hopwood, UK

Male, aged 63 years
OA Knee – simple pain, level I
Basic acupuncture

A 63-year-old builder was complaining of pain and swelling in his right knee joint for the last 2 weeks. This has been relieved by the application of heat, through the use of a hot water bottle or thick bandaging. The pain has reduced the range of movement in the joint, and standing, kneeling and climbing ladders have all become difficult. He was referred for physiotherapy treatment by his doctor.

Salient examination findings

- no change in skin colour
- swelling both suprapatellar and prepatellar
- knee flexion only 20°
- pain on weight bearing
- no ligamentous involvement

Treatment plan and goals To reduce pain and swelling in order to return to work.

■ *Points used –*
For knee pain: ST-35, Dubi; EX-42 Xiyan ("Eyes of the Knee")
Distal points: ST-44 Neiting; GB-43 Xiaxi

■ *Supplementary points –*
Ah Shi points or painful points around the knee

Method Needling to achieve Deqi, needles retained for 20–30 min.
Additional advice: The patient was taught graduated quadriceps exercises to stabilize the knee and advised to rest as much as possible until the pain had decreased.

Treatment course and outcome Six treatments over 3 weeks; pain much decreased, and patient returned to work.

Case 3

By Passion Nhekairo-Musa, Zimbabwe

Female, aged 30 years
Shoulder pain – simple pain
Basic acupuncture

A 30-year-old housewife, league squash player was complaining of severe pain in left shoulder that has been building up for a while. This was diagnosed as left rotator cuff syndrome.
Past medical history of two hydrocortisone injections with effects lasting up to 6 weeks.

Salient examination findings

- pain in elevation and abduction midrange; all other movements slightly painful
- no history of trauma
- X-ray shows no joint or bone abnormality
- trigger points in the trapezium, subscapularis, pectorals, quadratus lumborum, scalenae and sternocleidomastoid muscles on the left side
- main problems:
  1. Pain on lifting arm to play squash or reach a top shelf
  2. Inability to play squash

Goals

- To relieve pain
- To increase range of movement
- To return to competitive squash

Treatment

■ *Points used –*
For sedation: GV-20 Baihui
Ah Shi points in tender muscles
Local shoulder points: TE-14 Jianliao; LI-15 Jianyu
For analgesia: distal point: LI-4 Hegu
For homeostatic action: LI-11 Quchi
For the influence on muscles: GB-34 Yanglingquan

These points were stimulated by hand and the treatment of the Ah Shi points was done two or three at a time. Stretching of both shoulder and cervical muscles was taught.

The patient attended three times in the first week, twice in the second week and once a week for 4 weeks. She was discharged with the plan achieved. The patient has been symptom free for 4 months to date.

Case 4

By Helen Madzokere, Zimbabwe

Male, aged 42 years
Neuropraxia right leg – pain and oedema
Basic acupuncture

The patient was a 42-year-old railway track worker. He was suffering from post-traumatic neuropraxia of the right peroneal nerve and sympathetic dystrophy of the right leg. He had fractured the upper third right tibia and fibula 8 months previously.

Examination findings

- chronic pitting oedema right lower leg and foot
- paraesthesia on dorsum of right foot and anterior aspect of the leg
- mild foot drop; weak dorsiflexors and evertors, grade 2
- cold clammy foot and ankle
- reduced sensation to touch, pin prick and hot and cold
- trophic ulceration on the dorsum of the first web space
- constant severe burning pain in right foot; patient could not wear closed shoes

Goals

1. Reduce pain.
2. Reduce oedema.
3. Restore muscle function.
4. Re-educate gait.

■ *Points used –*
For sedation: GV-20 Baihui; ear Shenmen
For analgesia: ST-44 Neiting
The Influential point for muscles: GB-34 Yanglingquan
For their homeostatic properties: SP-6

Sanyinjiao; ST-36 Zusanli
Motor point of tibialis anterior muscle

Method and outcome The patient received three treatments per week for 3 weeks and electrical stimulation was applied to GB-34 and the tibialis anterior motor point at 10 Hz for 30 min at every visit. The other points were manually stimulated.

In addition, laser was applied to the ulcer, a footdrop splint was provided, and autoassisted and active exercises were given.

After 3 weeks of treatment there was considerable improvement. The oedema and ulcer were completely gone. There was minimal pain on wearing shoes and there was no footdrop. Muscle power was grade 4+. The patient was discharged with exercises to do at home.

Case 5

By Lorrene Soellner, Canada

Female, aged 43 years
Neck pain – simple pain
Basic acupuncture

A 43-year-old secretary was referred for acupuncture after having had neck pain continuously for 10 months. Physiotherapy (ultrasound, neck traction and exercises) had not helped, nor had chiropractic treatment. Traction had eased the pain temporarily. She had also been instructed in correct posture, and an ergonomically correct work station with frequent breaks to change position had been incorporated into her work. Numbness, primarily in the middle finger, had subsided.

Medications: thyroxin for a thyroid dysfunction had been taken for 3 years; Tylenol when the pain was acute.

Salient examination findings

- neck movements: extension – only 20° beyond neutral
rotation – full both directions
right lateral flexion – full
left lateral flexion – half range with pain

- shoulder movements – full range of motion bilaterally
- trigger points found in upper right trapezius at GB-21 and SI-10; pain radiated down the posterolateral aspect of the arm
- kyphotic at C7/T1
- X-rays showed narrowing of discs at most levels of cervical spine and bony spurs

Treatment goals – Pain relief

Treatment

- ■ *Points used –*
  (Area of kyphosis): GV-13, 14
  Areas of point tenderness experienced by patient: GB-21; SI-9, 10, 11

Patient felt slightly giddy after these needles so no more were inserted. The patient experienced increased pain following acupuncture but later the arm felt better for a day before the pain returned.

Subsequent: The same points were reused and LI-4 and LU-7 were added.

GB-39 was added after four treatments.

Treatments were given twice weekly for a total of 10 treatments. Pain down the arm subsided by the fifth treatment and the neck started to feel better than it had in the previous 10 months. At the completion of treatment neck extension was half of normal range, left side flexion was nearly full range except for a small area of minor discomfort near the right gall bladder at the end of the range. No Tylenol was needed.

Case 6

By Colette Lehodey, Canada

Female, aged 44 years
Shoulder pain – painful obstruction
Basic acupuncture, complicated by fever

A 44-year-old civil servant was referred for pain in the left shoulder girdle for 2 months and was not able to tolerate anti-inflammatory medications. She had had similar problems 2 years ago. The cause of the shoulder pain was unknown but the patient was noted to be experiencing intermittent fevers at the same time although the white cell count was not markedly elevated.

Salient examination findings

- full range of motion in neck and right shoulder
- full passive left shoulder flexion
- 15° active left shoulder movement due to pain
- full passive abduction
- passive extension in the horizontal plane produced pain
- pain was felt over the long head of biceps
- external passive rotation produced pain in the same area

Treatment plan Provided with a sling to rest when working.

- ■ *Points used –*
  Ear points, shoulder joint and muscles bilaterally
  Neck: local point between C6 and C7 on the GV channel
  For pain in opposite shoulder: ST-38 Tiaokou "experience point" (right)
  Influential point for muscles and tendons: GB-34 Yanglingquan (bilaterally)
  Local points for the shoulder: TE-14; LI-15 (left)
  For pain in upper limb: LI-4 Hegu; Extra point near biceps tendon
  To influence biceps muscle: LU-3, 4, 5

Outcome Twelve hours after the first treatment the patient had full range of shoulder flexion activity. Extension in the horizontal plane was still painful, however. Treatment was given twice weekly. After the fourth treatment the fever increased, there was a headache, a painful left knee and a new pain in the right shoulder. ST-36 Zusanli was added bilaterally for its homeostatic effect in endocrine and metabolic disorders. Other points remained the same.

Intermittent fever persisted until the sixth treatment but then subsided (the doctor was investigating this). The anterior shoulder pain was much improved but a tender point developed in the supraspinatus muscle. SI-16 was added to the points.

Static-resisted external rotation with a stretch band was started at treatment six. By treatment seven the arm was nearly normal, only a slight twinge over the left biceps tendon at the extreme range of shoulder flexion and anterior range in the horizontal plane. The patient was discharged but continued resisted exercises.

Case 7

By Alan Clements, New Zealand PAPMA

Female, aged 47 years
Arm and shoulder pain – complex history, simple pain treatment
Basic acupuncture

A 47-year-old married woman presented with a painful right shoulder (throughout the whole glenohumeral joint) and referred pain down to the right hand. One year ago a car boot lid fell on to her right shoulder, elbow and face while loading groceries into the car boot. Her occupation was as a clinical forensic psychologist. Conservative physiotherapy treatment had no benefit.

Three months later, the patient fell down a flight of steps and landed on her elbow. This also resulted in coccydynia and an admission to an intensive care unit for a respiratory arrest, possibly owing to the shock of the fall. A portacath inserted due to five previous arrests (two respiratory and three cardiac). The patient now carries her own portacath needles and adrenaline.

Past medical history included:

hysterectomy 1982; asthma 1982, after Hong Kong flu; full acute attacks with hospital admission; hiatus Hernia operation (not successful) – reoperated later, nerves to stomach cut resulting in pain plus dumping syndrome; after stomach operation developed photobazoa (a live slug growing and living in the gut); a very unusual condition, presumably cured; cholecystectomy 1989.

Medication: Pulmicort 400 mg – asthma; atrovent; prednisone 20–60 mg; Duovent; Nuelin 200 mg; omeprazole 20 mg; Ventolin 8 mg; Rhinocort; Multivite six; Slow K as needed; quinine sulphate – cramps; Pevaryl – antifungal; Kliogest – postmenopausal osteoporosis.

Summary:

A severe asthmatic who requires continuous prednisone, 20–80 mg per day, as well as high dose inhaled steroids, Rhinocort for her nose and a Ventolin inhaler. Operations include a Nissan fundiplication – photobazoa. Additional problems include steroid-induced osteoporosis and mild obesity, von Willebrand's disease and an allergy to penicillin and tetracycline. History of numerous hospital admissions for severe asthma attacks, respiratory arrests and cardiac arrests.

Examination findings

- X-ray, leaking of calcium from humerus, generalized osteoporosis
- solid lady complaining of constant unremitting pain from glenohumeral joint down to fingers, worse at night; sleeping 2–3 h maximum

Observations

- visible decrease in muscle bulk around shoulder joint, particularly deltoid
- active movements:
  flexion/elevation – 90° (positive throughout range)
  internal/external rotation – half positive
- passive movements – same as active, pain at end of range of movement
- resisted movements – all positive on attempted resisted tests
- palpation – no specific tender points on palpation
- special tests – apprehensive test (positive – unable to take test in full range)
  – impingement test (positive – unable to take test in full range)

Pathology Chronic tendinitis secondary to osteoporotic changes in the glenohumeral joint and the humerus.

Goals

1. To decrease pain.
2. To increase active range of movement.
3. To restore activities of daily living and normal function.
4. To increase muscle bulk and strength.
5. To re-educate with regard to self-care.
6. To re-educate with regard to work station design.

Treatment plan Informed consent obtained. 1″ (25 mm) 34 gauge sterilized disposable needles used.

- ■ *Points used –*
  Autonomic point; Yuan primary point – best analgesic point in body: LI-4 Hegu (right)
  Distal point for shoulder; He Sea point – homeostatic point for body: LI-11 Quchi (right)
  Alarm point for Gall Bladder and also beyond glenohumeral joint: GB-21 Jianjing (right)
  Influential point for tendons; He Sea point: GB-34 Yanglingquan
  To tranquilize and sedate, and for insomnia; Controlling point for all channels and points: GV-20 Baihui

Treatment course
Treatment 1: needles inserted in following order:
R LI-11/GB-21/GB-34; L/R LI-4; GV-20
Stimulation of needles to achieve Qi in the following order:
LI-4, 11; GB-21, 34; no stimulation to GV-20
Immediately after treatment, range of movement increased to full and pain decreased to 50%. No exercise to be done other than normal activities.
Treatment 2: reassessment – slight catch end of range of movement of all movements.
Treatment 3: no pain. Range of movement full – slight ache returning.
(Two weeks later – been away on a course) – sleeping through the night with 2–3 waking periods due to toiletting only.
Treatment 4: as above with manual stimulation of LI-11 only.

Outcomes This lady returned for acupuncture for other problems (e.g. pain in her abdominal scar) but has not returned for treatment for her right shoulder in any way. She still has full, pain-free range of movement.

Case 8

By Kim Ong, UK

Female, aged 45 years
Trigeminal neuralgia – simple pain relief, level I
Basic acupuncture, electroacupuncture added

A woman aged 45 presented with chronic right trigeminal neuralgia of the mandibular branch. The condition had lasted for 4 months. Two years previously a phenol nerve block at the origin of the maxillary branch had been performed. This alleviated the pain but the patient suffered from nausea and vomiting for 6 months. She was offered another nerve block and refused. As a last resort she decided to try acupuncture.

Salient examination findings

- patient very anxious and angry that the pain had returned
- difficulty masticating ordinary food; semi-liquid was better
- acute spasms preventing speech
- continuous dull ache in the mandibular area exacerbated by cold and wind; warmth alleviated the pain a little
- pain worse early in the morning on her way to work
- sleeping well, pain mostly during the day
- taking Tagamet to relieve the pain; drowsy due to high doses

Treatment goals

1. To alleviate the anxiety.
2. To diminish pain to allow a normal lifestyle.
3. To alleviate the spasms, which were affecting her speech.

Treatment Local points in the area were needled and stimulated with electroacupuncture, 100 Hz constant for 20 min.

- ■ *Points used –*
  ST-4 Dicang, ST-5 Daying, ST-6 Jiache; CV-24 Chengjiang
  Distal point on the Stomach meridian: ST-36 Zusanli
  For pain (particularly leg pain): ST-44 Neiting
  General anaesthetic point but distal to the area of pain and with a particular effect on the lower jaw: LI-4 Hegu

Treatment course Treated twice weekly for the first 2 weeks and once weekly for the next 4 weeks.

Outcome The patient had relief from pain. The paroxysmal spasms disappeared. Her speech become more normal and she could chew food more easily. On review a year later she had acute pain on waking but two further treatments alleviated her symptoms. She has returned for one more treatment in the past year and keeps in touh by telephone.

Case 9

By Kim Ong, UK

Female, aged 36 years
Acute shoulder pain – basic pain relief, level I
Mixture of acupuncture and acupressure

A 36-year-old woman presented with an acute right shoulder. She had injured her arm while leading a horse through a gate, resulting in a jerking movement to the shoulder. She was referred by a physiotherapist who was already treating this woman for neck problems. The physiotherapist felt that acupuncture might be helpful for this patient owing to her anxious personality.

Salient examination findings

- excruciating pain and patient hysterical
- patient too distressed by pain to be able to manage any movement of arm, wrist or fingers
- previous physiotherapist had eliminated possibility of a fracture or dislocation
- no further examination as possible or appropriate at this stage

Treatment goals

1. To eliminate anxiety and calm patient down.
2. To diminish pain.
3. To increase range of arm movement.

Treatment course Day 1: The patient was seated so that her right elbow and forearm were resting on a pillow on the therapist's knee. Gentle acupressure and massage were given, focusing on the Stomach meridian from ST-36 to ST-38. While the massage was being done the therapist was moving her knee. Gradually the patient's arm was moved more into abduction by this method. By the end of this session she was able to move her fingers, wrist and elbow and had 25% more movement in her shoulder. Gentle home exercises were encouraged.

Days 2, 3 and 4: Daily treatment was given. Acupuncture was given to ST-38 Tiaokou on the Right leg, using 1.5" needle. Also needled were LI-11 Quchi, LI-4 Hegu and LI-15 Jianyu.

Treatment continued twice weekly for 2 more weeks. Range of movement was almost full at the end of this period. Lateral rotation was still slightly painful and limited. The patient was advised to try and lead the horse with her left arm.

Discussion This was an acute traumatic shoulder that was treated the day after injury. It was necessary to placate the patient before any mechanical treatment could be given. Fortunately ST-38 is a good point for painful shoulders so acupressure could be given on this point. Here, the placebo response is very important. Good results were achieved by talking to the patient and moving her arm very gently while explaining that this point was a miraculous point for painful shoulders. Another factor that may have assisted in the speed of recovery is that this treatment could be given very soon after the injury.

Level II

These cases are slightly more complicated, more TCM theory is used and more physiotherapy modalities have been brought in.

Case 1

By Ana Maria Carballo, Argentina

Male, aged 45 years
IMS syndrome knee – simple channel blockage, level II
Basic acupuncture with TCM theory

A male patient, a civil engineer 45 years old, was referred from traumatology with a diagnosis of internal meniscal syndrome and tenosynovitis in the right knee (Fig. 15.4). Sports practised were Tai Chi

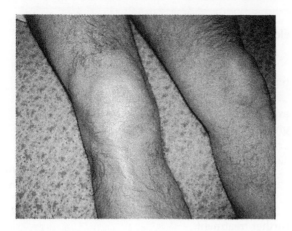

Fig. 15.4 *Internal meniscal syndrome and tenosinovitus in right knee.*

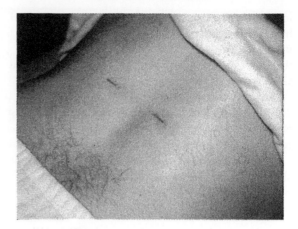

Fig. 15.5 *First session, selected points.*

Chuan. X-rays showed nothing abnormal. Pain was of 2 months duration. He had been given physiotherapy, short wave, laser and massage for 10 sessions. There was no progress after 3 weeks, and he was referred to acupuncture.

Previous history included knee pain 3 years earlier, and difficulty with flexion after Tai Chi Chuan exercises. The problem resolved with acupuncture treatment. There was a previous history to duodenal ulcers (from acute emotional stress). The ulcers were cured but there was residual gastritis problem, eye blinking, nausea, dizziness and spontaneous stomach pain. Acupuncture has resolved these symptoms, recurring only when under stress.

Salient examination findings

- pain in right knee with an increase in synovial liquid, particularly produced after having his leg in a half-lotus position
- pain worst when climbing stairs
- swelling, right suprapatellar bursitis (see erythema in Fig. 15.4); some local heat
- atrophy of the quadriceps muscle
- knee flexion only 90°
- no mechanical restriction, movement limited by pain

TCM differentiation According to Eight Principles:

- External, related to musculoskeletal aspects

- no alteration of internal defences noted
- Yang: pain increases with heat and exercise; subacute pain that grows with movements; increase of the local temperature.

According to the channels involved:

- those crossing the area are the Bladder, Spleen and the Stomach meridians.

According to the nerve roots: the following dermatomes are involved: L4, L5 and S2.

Treatment and rationale for point selection First session:

- ■ *Points used –*
  Back Shu point for Spleen, influences excess fluid in the knee spaces, raises Qi: B-20 Pishu (Bilat)
  To eliminate local heat; also local point for knee: B-40 Weizhong (right)
  Water point of Triple Burner: B-39 Weiyang (right)
  To achieve energy balance: CV-6 Qihai
  Psychophysical point: GV-20 Baihui

Simple needling technique; duration 20 min.
Auriculotherapy: right ear – 0 Point (zero); suprarenal point; knee point 1.

This was combined with physiotherapeutic treatment and complementary treatment to be carried out at home as follows: indirect ice (with an icebag) twice a day, for 40 min. Repeat in the next 48 hours. Some rest was indicated, putting a pillow under the popliteal cavity to decrease the strain on the knee. The patient was advised to suspend his Tai Chi Chuan exercises.

Second session (48 h later): Pain decreased by 20%. An increase in mobility has been produced by a 50% decrease in heat and swelling. Acupuncture repeated, no further ice treatment.

Third session: No pain. Knee returned to normal size and shape (see Fig. 15.6). No swelling, no palpable heat in the joint.

■ *Points used –*
Local point with an effect on the Qi and Blood: ST-35 Dubi (right)
Influential point for muscles and tendons: GB-34 Yanglingquan
Specific points for knee pain: EX-42 Xiyan, EX-41 Heding; GV-20 Baihui

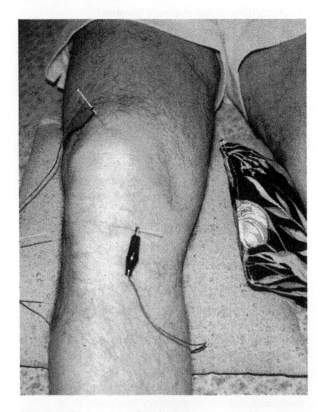

Fig. 15.6 *Third session, selected points.*

Technique: simple acupuncture combined with electroacupuncture (Fig. 15.6).
Duration: 20 minutes.
Auriculotherapy: right ear; the same points were repeated.

The patient was able to resume Tai Chi Chuan exercises. Three more acupuncture sessions were given with intervals of 4 days.

■ *Points used –*
Local point, effects Qi and Blood: ST-36 Zusanli
Local point, effects swelling: SP-9 Yinlingquan

The pain disappeared and the patient needed no further treatment.

Case 2

By Ana Maria Carballo, Argentina

Male, aged 15 years
Acute torticollis – fairly simple channel blockage, level II
Basic acupuncture, with TCM theory

A 15-year-old male student was referred from the paediatric orthopedist with what was defined as psychosomatic spasm, occurring after the news that one of his dogs was to be given away. The condition was acute, having begun only 24 hours previously.

Salient examination findings

- subjectively, patient reports a sharp pain when the neck is actively moved; pain is slightly eased when rotated to the left with lateral inclination
- history of previous incident at 7 years old, due to exam tension
- until age of 6 several episodes of otitis
- no history of scoliosis
- suspicion of hypermobility in joints

Objective physical examination:

- right shoulder slightly raised, head tilted laterally to the left
- right axilliary angle (between arm, armpit and rib cage) decreased
- bilateral differences (Figure 15.7)

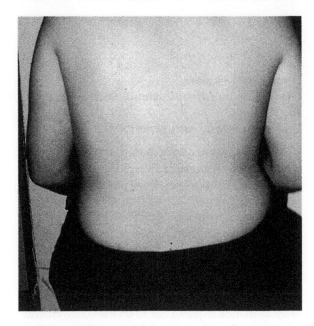

Fig. 15.7 *Acute torticollis: physical assessment first session.*

- left extension, inclination and rotation of spinal column severely limited
- on palpation, increased tone in sternocleidomastoid and trapezius
- external aspect; reddish face, wide variations in body temperature.

Psychological characteristics:

- extroverted, good at relating to people
- cautious, careful to avoid falling
- intelligent and physically active.

TCM differentiation Two methods were used to differentiate the various syndromes, one based on the theory of Eight Principles and the other on the theory of the channels (Conghuo 1992).

Eight Principles:

- External, related to musculoskeletal aspects, no alteration of internal defence system observed
- Yang: according to the localization and the characteristics of the pathology: acute and continuous pain, increasing with movement and alleviated by application of cold. Generalized Heat.

Theory of channels:

- according to the localization and the characteristics of the symptoms and signs, the following channels and meridians are involved: Small Intestine, Bladder, Governor Vessel.
- according to the nerve roots, the following dermatomes are involved: C2, C4, D1, D2.

Treatment and rationale for point selection
First session (Fig. 15.8):

■ *Points used* –
Point of confluence that acts on GV channel; distal point indicated for cases of torticollis and stiffness: SI-3 Houxi (left)
Specific distal point for neck pain: EX-31 Luozhen (left)

Technique: TENS was used. Flat electrodes were used on the above points; frequency applied was 90 Hz plus modulation. The intensity was according to the tolerance of the patient, but below the limit of contaction. Duration: 30 min.

■ *Points used* –
Meeting point of the Yang meridians, influence on dorsal spine: GV-20 Baihui
Important action on mental activities; Source point of meridian: H-3 Shaohai (bilaterally)
Specific distal point for neck pain: B-60 Kunlun (bilaterally)

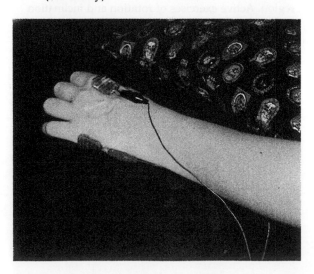

Fig. 15.8 *First session selected points for TENS.*

Simple needling, duration 30 min, combined with physiotherapy mobilization. Cryotherapy (massage with ice for 8 min) on the left shoulder, concentrating on the most painful points, which were, SI-9 Jianzhen; SI-14 Jianwaishu; TE-15 Tianliao.

A foam rubber collar was added in case the pain did not subside.

Second session (48 h later) (Fig. 15.9):

Pain had improved by 70%. A slight elevation of the shoulder was observed and the head was still slightly tilted to the left. The axilliary angles were equal. Mobility of the neck improved although there is still a slight pain when extending the neck.

Left lateral rotation and inclination of the head is still only 50% but the affected muscles have markedly decreased in tone.

- the TENS treatment was repeated for 30 min
- further TENS treatment was applied to SI-14 Jianwaishu and TE-15 Jianliao on the opposite side; frequency 30 Hz; duration 15 min
- needling to GV-20 Baihui and H-3 Shaohai, 30 min
- physiotherapy mobilization was interspersed

Third session (72 h after first treatment):

No specific symptoms were observed. As a support, to finish the treatment a simple puncture on point GV-20 Baihui was applied while patient was in the office while Tui-na (a type of Chinese massage) was carried out on the neck, shoulder and dorsal region. Active exercises of rotation and inclination with flexion to right and left were added.

Further checks were carried out after 3 and 7 days without observing any symptoms.

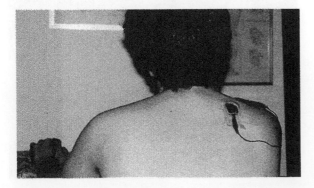

Fig. 15.9 *Second session: selected points for TENS.*

Case 3

By Colette Lehodey, Canada

Female, aged 44 years
Low back pain – simple, painful obstruction, level II
Basic acupuncture, with some TCM theory

A 44-year-old woman self-employed manufacturer of artificial trees presented to the clinic for a trial of acupuncture. She had sustained a back injury in a rear end automobile collision 5 months previously. Her chief complaint was right low back pain, which she described as burning and sharp in quality and radiating up the lower back, down into the right buttock and around the front of the hip. The pain was constant and would increase in intensity when she did too much reaching, bending or turning. Her work demands required her to do these movements especially when she was working on a big project. She was frustrated by the inability to carry out her work effectively and was concerned with the success of her business.

Salient examination findings

- limited lumbar flexion, right side bending more than extension
- joint dysfunction at L4/5; L5/S1
- myotomes, dermatomes and reflexes were normal
- muscle spasm and facilitation noted on left paravertebral muscles and skin
- all her other systems were working well except her mood was depressed and frustrated
- she had sustained a thoracic and cervical spine extension injury, which had resolved with an active physical therapy programme
- tongue signs: redness on the tip; pulse: wiry

Treatment plan and goals The patient's goal was to reduce and/or eliminate the low back pain so that she could carry out her daily work activities with less pain. To achieve this the following treatment plan was instituted:

- resolve the joint dysfunction with muscle energy techniques and specific traction at L4/5 and L5/S1

- strengthen the low back with specific stability drills and by reinforcing the Kidney
- remove obstruction from the Urinary Bladder meridian to reduce muscle spasm and pain
- disperse signs of Heat in the channel (burning pain)

■ *Points used –*
To tonify the Kidney, nourish Kidney Essence and strengthen the lower back (Kidneys are said to rule the lower back and therefore tonification points are used in chronic backache): B-23 Shenshu
To relax the low back muscles and remove obstruction from the Urinary Bladder channel (for bilateral or unilateral backache): B-40 Weizhong
To strengthen the back, clear inflammation from the back and relax the low back muscles and remove the obstruction from the Bladder channel: B-60 Kunlun
To nourish Congenital Qi; strengthen the lower back, tonify Kidney Yang and benefit Essence: GV-4 Mingmen
To lift spirits and clear mind: GV-20 Baihui

Congenital Qi is related to the person's basic vitality and constitution; Mingmen (GV-4) strengthens Congenital Qi and is therefore very useful for chronic weakness both on the physical and on the mental level. Also if the Essence is strong and flourishing the person will be happy and positive. This lady had demonstrated feelings of depression and lack of initiative since her accident and this was unusual for her, therefore B-23 and GV-4 were used for their effect on her mind.

■ *Supplementary points –*
To benefit the back (especially good for low back ache on the sacrum or just above it i.e. lumbosacral region whether bilateral or on the midline): EX-25 Shiqizhu
To strengthen the lower back, reduce muscle spasm: B-25 Dachangshu
To reduce pain radiating to the buttock: B-54 Zhibian

■ *Ear points –*
KOA: Kidney, adrenal, occiput; an auricular point combination used to reduce

inflammation and pain
Shenmen: used for relaxation, to calm the mind and relieve pain

Method Manual stimulation to achieve Deqi, retention of needles for 20–30 min.

Treatment course and outcome The woman received treatments twice weekly for 1 month then four treatments in the following month, three the following month and finally she is now requiring a treatment only once every 3 weeks. She regained full range of motion in the lumbar spine with some occasional difficulties with stiffness in right sidebending. She has been able to return to working on several projects requiring moderately heavy work. She does have some difficulties with prolonged sitting and with sustained flexion. I suspect that there was injury to the intervertebral disc and zygapophyseal joints from the motor vehicle accident. She had to make significant business decisions and has found this period in her life particularly stressful owing to her injury. She has found significant relief with acupuncture that is long lasting and enables her to carry out her work. She found the acupuncture especially helpful in regaining a feeling of control in her life. She continues to require treatments on an "as necessary" basis.

Case 4

By Val Marston, UK

Female, aged 59 years
Chronic low back pain – painful obstruction of channels, level II
Basic acupuncture using TCM theory

A housewife of 59 presented with chronic low back pain; symptoms started 15 years previously, and she is now experiencing difficulty with housework and leisure activities, painting and piano playing owing to the pain. Symptoms have included acute attacks of left sciatica and more chronic localized low back pain. She was originally treated by rest and encouraged to take up swimming. There was nothing else of relevance in the medical history.

Salient examination findings

- two pains apparent: pain 1, that radiating from her lumbar spine into her left buttock, was almost constant; this was described as a deep pain; pain 2 was described as a surface pain
- both pains were static and she was sometimes disturbed by symptoms during the night; first thing in the morning her back ached but this eased with movement although the deeper pain remained
- aggravating factors were bending forwards and coughing and sneezing
- the deeper pain was of the same intensity throughout the day
- the patient had no pins and needles, numbness or muscle weakness
- on a Visual Analogue Pain Scale, where 0 = no pain and 10 = maximum pain, pain 1 registered at 4–5 and pain 2 as 7
- X-rays showed only a slight scoliosis of the lumbar spine concave to the right
- range of movement: extension – pain free, reasonable range
  flexion – pulled in pain 2 area, fingertips to base of patella
  left side flexion – fingertips 2/3 down thigh
  right side flexion – as above
  rotation – pain free, good range of movement
  neck flexion – increases both pains
- straight leg raise: right leg, pain free to 80°
  left leg, increased pain on return to horizontal, 75°
- sensation was normal on both legs
- no muscle weakness
- reflexes: the left ankle was slightly decreased, otherwise normal

Impression: Probable disc problem in the past that has left her lumbar spine vulnerable to any aggravation, to give further inflammation, with consequent irritation of the nerve roots, particularly on the left side; the Right-sided pain seemed to be of more muscular origin.

Treatment plan and goals

- maintenance of muscle strength and stability of lumbar spine
- referred to back school and hydrotherapy

Returned for reassessment after two hydrotherapy treatments, pain 1 aggravated:

- range of movement, flexion now pain free, other problems as before

TCM diagnosis

Pulses: all weak and forceless, especially the Pericardium and Triple Burner. Rate generally slow.
Tongue: wide and toothmarked with a thin yellow coating over the LI and SI areas.
Time of day: her symptoms were the same at all times of the day and were not affected by cold, heat or damp.
Channels: symptoms located over Urinary and Gall Bladder channels.

Impressions: The slow pulse indicated a Yin condition. All the pulses were weak indicating Deficiency of Qi and Blood. The weakness of the Pericardium pulse indicated a Deficiency of Kidney Yang. The tongue was toothmarked indicating Deficiency of Spleen Qi. The yellow coating of the tongue indicated some Heat but did not seem to fit into the pattern of the other findings.

Diagnosis: Kidney Deficiency of both Yin and Yang, a Cold, Empty, Internal condition. This would fit with the pattern of her pain, worse on movement, easier on rest.

■ *Points used –*

B-25 Dachangshu, B-23 Shenshu; GB-30 Huantiao; B-40 Weizhong; Ah Shi points (all on the left side)
Moxa to B-25 Dachangshu

After five treatments the patient was reassessed. Both pain 1 and pain 2 were now at grade 2 on the pain scale, although pain 2 occasionally reached grade 4. The patient could do more without aggravating her symptoms.

Range of movement was the same. The back school was found to be very informative.

Outcome The pain symptoms had decreased by 50% at the end of the course of treatment. Considering that she had had problems with low back pain for 15 years, this was a good result. Her improvement in movement range was not sustained; the input on back care was felt to be very valuable, since much of the advice had been new to her and she had often aggravated the symptoms by incautious activity.

Case 5

By Sara Jeevanjee, UK

Male, aged 50 years
Chronic low back pain – painful obstruction and stagnation, level II
Combination of acupuncture and related techniques

A carpenter, 50 years old, presented with a 14-year history of back pain and deviation to the right with radiation of pain into the left buttock. He had had frequent treatment by chiropractors throughout this period. The back was unstable, with three to four attacks per year, affecting his job. Complete relief of main symptoms of stiffness and central ache was never achieved in spite of treatment.

Salient examination findings

- deviation to the right, pain in left sacroiliac joint
- lumbar movements were all very stiff and painful
- "light" pain was also felt in posterior aspect of lower limbs
- pain worse in the morning, gradual improvement with movement
- pain relieved by application of heat
- symptoms were caused by job (constant sawing in semiflexed position)
- some recent thoracic pain

TCM differentiation

- stagnation of Qi and Blood in the area
- Kidney Deficiency
- invasion of External Cold and Damp

Treatment goals
TCM: resolve stagnation of Qi and Blood, tonify Kidneys and expel Cold and Damp.

Physiotherapy: correct deviation, resolve stiffness with mobilization and strengthen the back muscles with exercises. Teach correct lifting and bending techniques.

■ *Points used –*

GV-26 Renzhong; TE-3 Zhongzhu
The first needle was inserted with the patient in standing position. Point GV-26 Renzhong chosen because the pain starts from the midline and spreads out. The patient was instructed to walk up and down the room for about 5 min. McKenzie's correction of deviation procedure was carried out in front of a mirror so that the patient could observe the correction. Within 10 min of needle insertion the deviation was corrected and the range of the lumbar movements was increased.
On correction, stiffness was observed in the left haunch area only so point TE-3 hand Zhongzhu was inserted in the left hand only. Correction procedure was carried out. The patient was instructed to walk up and down the room, stopping at intervals to carry out pelvic tilting. After 10 min of self-mobilization, the correction procedure was repeated. Stiffness had considerably decreased in the left haunch area.
SNAGS were also carried out in standing position (total treatment time 30 min). Auricular acupuncture was used and seeds were placed on Shenmen, lumbar, Kidney and Urinary Bladder points. The patient was instructed to stimulate these three to four times a day, pressing each point about 30–40 times.

No examination or treatment procedures were carried out in lying positions as experience has shown that patients with the above symptoms react adversely to immobility for 10–20 min.

The patient was advised not to go back to work. Instructions were given for self-correction procedures and the patient was advised to use hot compresses.

Subsequent treatment: Slight deviation was present. All movements had increased in range; pain had decreased. Bilateral "light" ache in lower limbs had been alleviated. Patient complained of a feeling of stiffness in the thoracolumbar region and a central ache.

■ *Points used –*
Points to open the Governing Vessel (or Du
Mai) in men (the reverse is used for women):
SI-3 Houxi (left); B-62 Shenmai (right)
To open the Governing Vessel and remove
obstruction from it, strengthening the Kidneys
and the spine, expel Wind, calm the mind,
relieve spasm and straighten the spine. (An
excellent treatment for chronic backache from
Kidney Deficiency. This combination is
effective only if the pain stems from the
midline): H-7 Shenmen (right); SP-3 Taibai
(left)
To tonify Kidney Yang and strengthen the
back. (Moxabustion was applied to this point
for 10 minutes): GV-4 Mingmen

The needles were retained for 20 min and cupping
was carried out on the thoracolumbar region after
the needles were removed. It was noted that the
feeling of stiffness was still present so treatment to
GV-26 Renzhong was repeated with the walking for
10 min. The stiffness decreased.

Two days later, very slight deviation was noted on
examination. Patient's overriding symptoms were of
feeling of stiffness in the lumbar spine and lower
thoracic region. Dr Gunn's needling technique was
carried out in lumbar and lower thoracic region on
the erector spinae, iliocortalio, longissimus, spinalis
and hamstring muscles. This produced a
considerable decrease in stiffness. The patient was
very anxious to return to work as soon as possible.

GV-26 Renzhong and TB-3 hand Zhongzhu were
needled only. Sustained natural apophyseal glides
(SNAGS) and pelvic tilting were also carried out for
10 min. Bilateral sacroiliac mobilizations were also
done. Advice given was as previous treatment.

All movements had increased range and the pain
was eliminated.

After a further 5 days: the patient had returned to
work successfully. No pain or ache remained but still
slight stiffness in lumbar region, which felt tight.

Dr Gunn's needling technique was carried out on
the shortened spinal muscles. This increased flexion
range and decreased stiffness.

■ *Points used –*
Influential point for bone: B-11 Dashu
To strengthen the back: B-23 Shenshu

Influential point for muscles and tendons: GB-
34 Yanglingquan
Important distal point for chronic backache: B-
60 Kunlun
Moxa was given to B-23 and to the lumbar
region generally

Needles were retained for 20 min and cupping on
lumbar and lower thoracic region for 10 min. On
reassessment, there was no pain and all movements
except flexion were full in range. Patient was advised
to swim on a regular basis.

After another 10 days: the patient returned for
one more treatment as he was going on holiday and
wanted to feel 100% fit. The only symptoms were
slight stiffness in the lumbar movements and
thoracolumbar region.

Final treatment: Dr Gunn's needling on left
lumbar muscles.

The same points were used as the previous
treatment, given with cupping for 20 min. On
reassessment all stiffness had been alleviated and
according to the patient he had "never felt better".

Outcome Considering the long history of pain and
stiffness I feel that a combined treatment of
acupuncture and mobilizations has aided in a
speedier recovery and hope the recurrent attacks will
be fewer.

Level III

These are complex cases given careful and detailed
TCM diagnosis and varied treatments.

Case 1

By Colette Lehodey, Canada

Male, aged 50 years
**Multiple sclerosis – deficiency of Qi with empty
heat, level III**
**Complex case, using TCM diagnosis and
differentiation of syndromes.**

A man of 50 years with multiple sclerosis presented
to the clinic with chief complaints of fatigue,

headaches, reduced concentration and problems with balance and coordination.

History He had a 2-year history of transient numbness in both legs and left hand and arm numbness. Also, he had a sensation of a cap on his head associated with a fuzzy-headed feeling. He had recently been diagnosed with MS after having undergone numerous investigations including magnetic resonance imaging, computerized tomography and evoked potentials. He had had previous physical therapy for neck strain and low back pain. He had a history of spastic bowel.

Medications: Elavil 10 mg p.r.n.

Allergies: penicillin

Family history of MS: two cousins and an uncle with MS.

Social history: designer of lay-out for a local newspaper; married.

Salient examination findings

- weakness of left leg muscles, namely hip extensors, quadriceps and tibialis anterior (3+/5)
- reduced balance reactions in standing, kneeling and half-kneel standing
- able to carry out activities of daily living including work, but finding fatigue interferes with concentration and ability to handle late night shifts
- heel-shin test revealed moderate ataxia on the left
- gait: slow and deliberate with foot slapping on heel strike on the left
- mood: normally good natured but irritable of late especially when fatigued
- tongue signs: thick on sides with toothmarks; deep red with yellow coating (smoker)
- pulse: deep Kidney positions; Empty on Liver and Spleen; soft Heart and Lung
- differentiation of syndrome: Deficiency of Qi with Empty Heat

Treatment plan and goals

- reduce fatigue with acupuncture and education with regard to energy conservation

- control headaches by reducing fatigue with acupuncture
- improve or maintain strength in the lower extremities and trunk with a home exercise programme
- maintain or improve standing balance with stability drills and home exercise

Principles of treatment according to TCM

- tonify Qi
- tonify Kidney Qi and Essence
- tonify Stomach/Spleen Qi to support transformation and transportation functions of the spleen, to support the muscles
- send clear Yang to the head
- tonify Yang

General rationale according to the theory of Zang Fu organs: MS is a disease of the nervous system whereby sclerotic plaques are formed on the spinal cord tracts and brain. There is some evidence to support an autoimmune disorder. There can be a hereditary component. In TCM this involves the Kidney and especially the Essence of the Kidney. The essence of the Kidney produces Marrow. In Chinese medicine the Marrow is said to generate the spinal cord and fills up the brain. Therefore the Kidney in TCM has a physiological relationship with the central nervous system. Consequently it is important to tonify the Kidney in the treatment of MS.

■ *Points used –*
Initial:
Meeting place of all Yang channels, which carries clear Yang to the head; to clear the mind, lift the spirits and tonify Yang: GV-20 Baihui
To tonify the kidneys, benefit Congenital Qi, tonify Qi and Blood: CV-4 Guanyuan
To tonify Qi and Yang, tonify Congenital Qi: CV-6 Qihai
To tonify stomach and spleen, raise the clear Yang energies towards the head and reduce the patient's fuzziness in the head: CV-12 Zhongwan
To benefit the stomach and spleen and therefore used for the above reason, tonifies Qi and Blood: ST-36 Zusanli

To calm the mind and allay irritability: SP-6 Sanyinjiao
Moxa to CV-4, 6 and 12 at home

This prescription was used for the first eight treatments spanning 3 months. At this point the patient's headaches and fuzziness in the head were subsiding but he still had symptoms of fatigue and therefore the following points were selected:

■ *Points used –*
Source point, used to tonify Qi: KI-3 Taixi
To tonify Kidney Yin: KI-10 Yingu
To tonify Kidney Yang, nourish Congenital Qi, benefit Essence and warm the Gate of Vitality: GV-4 Mingmen
To tonify the kidneys and nourish the Kidney Essence, benefit Marrow: B-23 Shenshu
To reinforce effect of tonifying kidneys and also as this segmental level benefit the lower extremities: EX-21 Huatuojiaji at L2/L3
To nourish Blood: B-20 Pishu
To transport clear Yang upwards to the head, clear the mind and stimulate the brain: GV-14 Dazhui

The chronic nature of this condition leads to deficiency of Spleen Qi. If you can invigorate the transportation and transformation functions of the Spleen (e.g. B-20) then this will assist in reinforcing Qi and provide nourishment for the nervous and muscular systems.

Method Retention of needles for 30 minutes, tonification method.

Treatment course and outcome The man's initial response was a reduction in the headaches, improved concentration and a general reduction of fatigue but this was not long lasting. Consequently the second set of points was used and the use of moxibustion on GV-4 and B-23 or CV-4, 6 was prescribed on alternate days at home. During that period of time the man made significant gains in that there was no recurrence of headaches. There was an increase in tone in his lower extremities and after treatment the patient had reduced ataxia on the heel–shin test. The patient continues to require treatment at 2 to 3 week intervals to remain

headache free. He has found the home exercise programme very useful in maintaining strength and a way in which to monitor his fatigue level. He has found his work to be more enjoyable as a consequence of improved memory and concentration.

Case 2

By Colette Lehodey, Canada

Male, aged 37 years
Neck pain – channel obstruction, level III
Integrated TCM and physiotherapy

A normal consequence of aging is the development of degenerative changes in the cervical spine. These changes involve the intervertebral disc as well as the facet joints. Some individuals may experience pain as the aging process of the spine evolves. Symptoms are normally a manifestation of encroachment on local neural structures.

In TCM neck pain and stiffness can be a consequence of what is known as a Bi Syndrome. This is characterized by obstruction of Qi and Blood in the meridians and collaterals owing to the invasion of pathogenic Wind, Cold and Damp. Signs of this condition are soreness, pain, numbness and heaviness of limbs and joints and limitation of movement. The following case is an example of an integrated approach to a degenerative disorder of the spine.

A 37-year-old male graduate student presented with a four month history of neck pain, right arm numbness, weakness and pain. He was seeking pain relief with acupuncture. He had sustained a neck injury while playing baseball 4 months previously and had received 4 weeks of physical therapy and a course of ibuprofen (NSAID) with minimal relief.

Past medical history Right neck and shoulder pain resolved previously with physical therapy.
Medications: ibuprofen.
Allergies: Wasp stings.
General health: lactose intolerance.
X-rays/computerized tomography scan results: bone spur and disc protrusion at C5/6.

Consultations: neurosurgeon who recommended continuing course of ibuprofen and observation. Surgery if no resolution.

Salient examination findings

- limited and painful cervical spine flexion, extension and right rotation
- wasting of deltoid and supraspinatus
- weak biceps, numbness C5 dermatome, hyperaesthesia C6, bilateral hyporeflexia C5–7
- throbbing pain down arm to elbow and sensation of numbness in forearm, thumb and index finger
- sleep disturbed, mood irritable, headache
- tongue: red with light yellow coating in centre
- pulse: Shi pulse, Liver position, Kidney weak

Diagnosis and differentiation of syndrome
Western: cervical radiculopathy due to C5/6 disc protrusion.
TCM: Painful Obstruction Syndrome due to Wind, leading to Blood and Qi stagnation in the Yangming meridian of the hand.

Treatment goals

- instruct patient in neck care, ergonomics, posture, sleeping positions and active exercise; also flexibility, strength and aerobic exercises
- disperse Wind, remove obstruction from the channel, calm the mind and eliminate the headache

■ *Points used* –
Distal point for Painful Obstruction Syndrome, harmonizes the ascending of Yang and the descending of Yin to resolve the headache: LI-4 Hegu
To clear heat, expel Exterior Wind and benefit the joints and sinews: LI-11 Quchi
To remove obstructions from the channel: LI-10 Shousanli
To regenerate, benefit the sinews and remove obstruction from the channel: SI-6 Yanglao
Ear points: kidney, occiput and adrenal, anti-inflammation point combination

Method Dispersing technique on LI-4, 11 and 10. Tonifying to SI-6.

Ear points were treated with electroacupuncture on dense disperse mode for 20 min.

Outcome

- the patient received four treatments
- there was complete resolution of pain, parasthesia, headache and restoration of sleep
- a 6 month follow-up showed a restoration of reflexes, strength and muscle bulk
- the patient had returned to exercising three times weekly and was back to playing slow pitch; he was avoiding activities that might aggravate his neck, like diving for grounders
- results demonstrate the benefits of an integrated approach in the management of cervical radiculopathy
- results support published articles that studied a combination of physical therapy and acupuncture
- use of TCM evaluation and differentiation of syndromes is an invaluable tool in the management of neck pain

Case 3

By Sara Jeevanjee, UK

Female, aged 85 years
Generalized OA – holistic pain treatment, level III
Traditional acupuncture mixed with physical therapy

A woman, aged 85, presented with generalized osteoarthritis dating back 20 years. She had been suffering with severe knee pain for the past 6 weeks, the knee joint injected with hydrocortisone 3 weeks previously; this increased the pain. She had been using a walking stick for years because of poor balance.

Salient examination findings

- all knee movements very painful
  flexion – restricted by pain
  extension – painful in joint and over medial aspect
- knee swollen and hot to touch
- medial aspect very tender to touch

- difficulty experienced in walking and unable to weight bear on right leg
- unable to sleep owing to the pain
- patient very distressed

TCM differentiation

Hot Painful Obstruction Syndrome due to:

- local stagnation of Qi and Blood
- invasion of Wind and Damp
- Kidney Yin Deficiency

Treatment goals

- remove obstruction from the channel
- resolve Dampness and expel Wind
- tonify the Kidneys

Physiotherapy treatment:

- mobilize knee joint
- strengthen knee muscles
- possible use of interferential current.

■ *Points used –*
  To move Blood in the knee: SP-10 Xuehai
  To regulate muscles and tendons and clear Damp-Heat: GB-34 Yanglingquan
  To resolve Damp-Heat: SP-9 Yinlingquan
  Distal point for arthritis in lower limb, also to resolve Damp-Heat: ST-44 Neiting
  Distal point: GB-43 Xiaxi
  Ah Shi points on the medial aspect of the knee were used. Technique: needle inserted, Deqi obtained, then needle withdrawn.
  To resolve Damp-Heat, technique as above:
  B-40 Weizhong

Treatment Needles were retained for 2 min. On assessment she was very much improved after the first treatment, and able to flex knee without eliciting pain. Extension mobilizations were less painful. Heat and tenderness decreased in knee joint and on the medial aspect.

Second treatment: The patient felt better in herself. Severity of pain and swelling had decreased. The knee was still hot and tender on palpation. Pain was present at night. The improvement in knee

flexion was retained. Pain was present on the femur and tibial aspect during extension mobilizations.

Auricular acupuncture added: Ear Shenmen and knee points were needled. Within 10 min the pain and tenderness decreased.

■ *Body points used –*
  To relieve pain and clear heat: LI-4 Hegu (bilaterally)
  Distal points: ST-44 Neiting; GB-Xiaxi

The above points were left in situ for 10 min then the two "Eyes of the Knee", Dubi and Xiyan, were inserted for 10 min. B-40 Weizhong was inserted as before, just long enough to obtain Deqi.

On assessment she was very much improved. The burning and heat sensation were decreased. Flexion and extension are now both less painful.

Third and last treatment: The patient was now much better, with swelling, heat and burning now gone. In her words patient felt "rested". Sleep had improved. On palpation pain was felt on one point on the inferior medial aspect of the patella. Gait had improved; she was no longer limping.

A squeeze technique (Brian Mulligan) was carried out on the knee; pain decreased on the medial aspect and on extension.

The same points were used as in the first treatment: 20 min needling.

Interferential currents, 90–130 Hz, were given for 20 min (bipolar method with electrodes on medial and lateral aspects).

On assessment, pain and tenderness were quite gone. The patient was delighted as she was now able to go on holiday, something which had not seemed likely a week ago.

She was instructed to carry out static quadriceps exercises daily.

Outcome Relief of symptoms were obtained very rapidly with acupuncture. Besides pain relief the patient's general well-being also improved; she felt happier with life. If treatment were to continue then tonification points would be added in order to nourish Yin and Blood.

■ *Points – ST-36 Zusanli; SP-6 Sanyinjiao; B-20 Pishu, B-23 Shenshu*

Acknowledgements

Many thanks to the following contributors for the many and varied case histories in this chapter. Editorial changes have only had to be minimal.

Argentina: Ana Maria Carballo.
Canada: Colette Lehodey, Lorrene Soellner.
New Zealand: Alan Clements.
UK: Sara Jeevanjee, Kim Ong, Val Hopwood, Sue Czartoryski, Val Marston.
Zimbabwe: Helen Madzokere, Passion Nhekairo-Musa.

Further reading

Most contributors to this section had included references but since very few alluded to them in the text they are listed here. It is interesting to see the range of books and papers consulted and we are pleased to be able to include several in Spanish, thanks to Ana Carballo.

Anon 1992 101 enfermedades tratadas con acupuntura y moxibustion (101 illnesses treated with acupuncture and moxibustion). Ediciones en Lenguas Extranjeras, Beijing

Anon 1992 Fundamentos de acupuntura y moxibustion China (Essentials of Chinese acupuncture and moxibustion). Ediciones en Lenguas Extranjeras, Beijing

Barraquer Bordas L 1978 Neurologia fundamental (Fundamental neurology). Ediciones Toray, Barcelona

Bogduk N 1984 Neck pain. Australian Family Physician 13(1): 26–30

Borsarello J 1979 Acupuntura y occidente (Acupuncture and the West). Hachette, Buenos Aires, Argentina

Bossy J 1990 Atlas anatomico de los puntos de acupuntura (Anatomical atlas of acupuncture points). Masson, Barcelona

Bossy J 1985 Bases neurobiologicas de las reflexoterapias. (Neurobiological basis of reflex therapy). Masson, Barcelona

Bossy J , Prat-Pradal Dr, Taillander, J 1987 Los microsistemas de la acupuntura (Acupuncture microsystems). Masson, Barcelona

Cailliet R 1971 Sindromes dolorosos (Painful syndromes). Ediciones el Manual Moderno, Mexico DF

Carballo A M 1992 Digitopuntura (Acupressure). Editorial Kier, Buenos Aires

Carballo F 1971 Acupuntura China (Chinese acupuncture). Editorial Kier, Buenos Aires

Carballo F 1981 Acupuntura y auriculoterapia (Acupuncture and auriculotherapy). Editorial Kier, Buenos Aires

Conghuo T, 1992 Beijing

Dethlefsen T, Dahlke R 1991 La enfermedad como camino (Krankheit als Weg). Plaza y Janes, Barcelona

Guillaume M J de Tymowski, Fiévet Izard M 1979 La acupuntura (Acupuncture). EDAF, Madrid

Gunn C C 1989 Treating myofascial pain. University of Washington, Washington USA

Heller J G 1992 The syndromes of degenerative cervical disease. Orthopaedic Clinics of the North America 23(3): 381–394

Junying G, Zhihong S 1991 Acupuncture and moxibustion, practical Chinese medicine and pharmacology. New World Press, Beijing

Loy T T 1983 Treatment of cervical spondylosis – electro-acupuncture versus physiotherapy. Medical Journal of Australia July 9: 32–34

Requena Y 1987 Perfeccionamiento en acupuntura Las mil y una Ediciones, Madrid

Tan Jackson C, Nordin M 1992 Role of physical therapy in the treatment of cervical disk disease. Orthopedic Clinics of North America 23(3): 435–448

Villaverde J R 1993 Kinesiologia aplicada en acupuntura. Mandala Ediciones, Madrid

Xinnong C 1987 Chinese acupuncture and moxibustion. Foreign Languages Press, Beijing

Appendices

Appendices

Appendix One:
Further reading

Maureen Lovesey and Tanya Macracken

This chapter contains some brief summaries of books that readers may find of interest and useful for further study.

Acupuncture in Clinical Practice, 1994, Nadia Ellis
Chapman & Hall, London, UK

The book is divided into three sections: (1) the basic concepts of TCM, (2) concepts of Western acupuncture, (3) the synthesis of Western medicine and TCM in treating conditions met in clinical practice. The first and second sections contain a comprehensive overview of TCM and Western concepts of acupuncture. The third section includes many of the problems met by physiotherapists and includes a variety of case studies.

The book contains a wealth of information and provides a helpful quick reference for those with training in acupuncture, particularly TCM. Non-practitioners might find there was too much information to take in.

The Foundations of Chinese Medicine, 1989, Giovanni Maciocia
Churchill Livingstone, Edinburgh, UK

The book gives a full description of TCM including Yin and Yang, Five Elements, Qi and Vital Substances. The Organs, their functions and problems are well covered. The book also includes the causes of disease, diagnosis and principles of treatment, including case histories and finishes with a description of the channels and main points, their location and function.

This book will be of interest to those wishing to learn more about TCM.

The Practice of Chinese Medicine, 1994, Giovanni Maciocia
Churchill Livingstone, Edinburgh, UK

This book is intended as a companion to the Foundations of Chinese medicine. It describes 34 commonly treated conditions including low back pain, headaches, asthma, ME and strokes amongst others.

Each chapter starts with a detailed description of the problem from a TCM point of view; many of the chapters also include Western differential diagnosis. Treatments include suggested acupuncture points and the rationale for their use and herbal medicine. Each section includes some case histories and in the front there are a number of colour plates showing the tongues of some of these patients.

There are five appendices: the first describes some combination of points and includes case histories; the second and third identify patterns according to the six stages and four levels and the last two are on herbal prescriptions and patent remedies.

The author puts forward a new theory on allergic asthma and rhinitus and ME based partly on his clinical experience. The book is well written by a very experienced acupuncturist and will be of value to those with an interest in TCM.

Acupuncture, Trigger Points and Musculoskeletal Pain, 1989, P E Baldry
Churchill Livingstone, Edinburgh, UK

The book is divided into three sections. The first section is on acupuncture, an historical review. This includes chapters on TCM, how acupuncture spread to the West and the practice of acupuncture in the

West during the 19th century. The second section describes the principles of trigger point acupuncture. This section includes the description of trigger points, their activation and deactivation, the neurophysiology of pain and the effects and evaluation of acupuncture. The last part contains comprehensive descriptions and illustrations of trigger points around the body.

The book is well written and contains helpful information on scientific basis. It is essential reading for anyone wishing to use trigger point acupuncture.

Tongue Diagnosis in Chinese Medicine, 1987, Giovanni Maciocia
Eastland Press, Seattle, USA

This book gives an excellent description of tongues from a TCM point of view. It starts with a history of tongue diagnosis and is followed by how to examine the tongue. It then moves on to describe the relationships of various organs to the tongue and gives details of shape, colour, coating, etc. of the tongue. The last section gives histories of 40 cases vividly illustrated by colour photos.

The book is essential reading for anyone wanting to learn more about tongue diagnosis.

The Vital Meridian, 1991, Alan Bensoussan
Churchill Livingstone, Edinburgh, UK

This book makes a very good attempt to bridge the gap between TCM and the scientific basis of acupuncture. At the beginning of the book the author makes some observations about the difficulties for Western personnel in understanding TCM and about doing research into acupuncture. He describes some of the comparatively recent developments in acupuncture such as auricular therapy, anaesthesia and scalp acupuncture and mentions some of the good points of both Western and Eastern medicine. The author goes on to describe the physiological effects of acupuncture and the biomagnetic properties of the channels and points. Then in a chapter entitled "Paradigms of the biomedical action of acupuncture" he describes some of the hypotheses that have been put forward on the way in which acupuncture may work and then describes the role of the CNS in acupuncture.

This book will appeal to those who are looking for links between East and West and who enjoy a philosophical discussion.

The Principles and Practice of Moxibustion, 1981, Roger Newman Turner and Royston Low
Thorsons, London, UK

This is a comprehensive book devoted to the use of moxibustion and as well as the more conventional techniques includes Japanese methods, formulae and even how to grow, dry and prepare your own moxa.

The book is a small specialist book which will suit the therapist wishing to make full use of this method.

The Acupuncture Treatment of Pain, 1976 and 1983, Leon Chaitow
Thorsons, London, UK

This book gives very basic descriptions of acupuncture, how to use it and how it works. This is followed by a large section on formulae. The points suggested are described according to their anatomical position and angle of needle insertion is included. The points are well illustrated with line drawings of skeletal and ear locations. The following sections follow a similar vein, covering addictions and anaesthesia, and even open heart surgery!

This book will appeal to anyone who likes to work from formulae although it is probably worth buying for the line drawings and description of points.

Basics of Acupuncture, 1991 (2nd edn), Gabriel Stux and Bruce Pomeranz
Springer-Verlag, Berlin, Germany

This is an excellent and handy guide to acupuncture condensed from the Acupuncture textbook and atlas by the same authors. The authors produced this small paperback to combine practicality with an affordable price. It is written in a format combining Western science and medicine with traditional Chinese concepts. Chapters include the scientific basis of acupuncture, current research, theory and philosophy of traditional Chinese medicine, a comprehensive description of channels and most important acupuncture points. Each channel was summarized into a quick reference guide; for example: Lung Channel Lu.

A third of the book incorporates treatment based on Western methods of diagnosis (locomotor, respiratory, cardiovascular, gastroenterological disorders, etc.).

An excellent inexpensive handbook.

Chinese Acupuncture and Moxibustion, 1990 (2nd edn), anon
Foreign Languages Press, Beijing, China

This book was compiled as the textbook for advanced training and research courses in acupuncture in China (Beijing, Shanghai, and Nanjing training centres). It is based upon Essentials of Chinese acupuncture, is very comprehensive and entails 18 chapters and two supplementary sections. Chapters include theory and philosophy of TCM, a description of the 12 regular meridians, eight extra meridians, 12 divergent meridians, 15 collaterals, two muscle meridians, 12 cutaneous regions, acupoints of the 14 meridians and extra points (includes colour photographs and good diagrams), diagnostic methods emphasizing pulse and tongue diagnoses, differentiation of syndromes, acupuncture techniques and treatment principles, moxibustion and, lastly, clinical management of 63 kinds of diseases in internal medicine, gynaecology, paediatrics, surgery and ear, nose and throat. Supplementary sections include ear acupuncture therapy and acupuncture analgesia. Each disease is described in Western terminology, followed by the aetiology and pathogenesis, differentiation and treatment described in Chinese concepts. The rationale for each point selected is discussed including remarks regarding Western diagnosis and intervention. A complete, exhaustive textbook.

Anatomical Atlas of Chinese Acupuncture Points, 1988 (2nd edn), anon
Shandong Science and Technology Press, Shandong, China

There are 100 illustrative plates and pictures including 77 coloured ones. This text emphasizes 231 common points with their relationship to surface, superficial (between skin and deep fascia) and deep anatomical structures. Certain points are shown in dissected sectional drawings. Each point is explained in terms of location, acupuncture manipulation (le. perpendicular 1 Cun; with notes of precaution for points with vital structures underneath), anatomy and indications. This atlas provides an excellent visual aid to the novice.

Essentials of Contemporary Chinese Acupuncturists' Clinical Experiences, 1989, anon
Foreign Languages Press, Beijing, China

This book is predicated upon the premise that clinical experiences are essential for the understanding and practice of the science of acupuncture and moxibustion, important components of TCM. It consists of 69 articles written by a professor, an associate professor, or a research fellow on the topic of their various clinical specialty. Each article includes a mini curriculum vitae of the author followed by theory, the technique and case histories. There are 293 case histories predominantly outlined in the following format: complaints, prescription, treatment procedure and explanation. A wealth of clinical knowledge.

The Web That Has No Weaver, 1983 (reprinted paperback 1990), Ted J Kaptchuk MD
Congdon & Weed, London, UK

The author has written this book in the form of a commentary to a Western reader on the art and science of Chinese medicine. Throughout the book, Eastern and Western medicine are integrated in clinical sketches explaining diagnosis and treatment. Chapters include explanation of Yin and Yang, fundamental substances (Qi, Blood, Jing, Shen, Fluids), organs, meridians, External and Internal influences, examination and patterns of disharmony. Appendices are excellent, especially the comprehensive list describing the pulses, and Chinese patterns versus common Western diagnosis and complaints. It does not refer to any acupuncture points. It is an enjoyable book to read and a good book to lend to patients.

Acupressure Techniques – a Self Help Guide Home Treatment for a Wide Range of Conditions, 1988, Julian Kenyon
Healing Arts Press, USA

This fully illustrated guide designed for home use depicts how to use acupressure in the effective treatment of a wide range of Western disorders. The manual emphasizes the importance of deep finger massage on all charts accompanying each condition. There is a very brief description of acupuncture followed by the illustrated treatment of the following: painful disorders, ear, nose and throat problems, heart and circulatory disorders, abdominal problems, skin disorders, chest diseases, genitourinary problems and sports injuries.

This book is simple to use; one does not need previous knowledge of anatomy or acupuncture.

Illustrations of Acupuncture Points
Medicine & Health Publications

Consists of three large oblong charts of acupuncture points depicting a human body in anterior, posterior and lateral views; it includes points on the ear, hand and foot. Quick and handy reference charts to hang on your office wall.

The Science of Acupuncture Therapy, 1987 (2nd edn), J Wong and R Cheng
Kola Mayland Co, Hong Kong

This book is based on the neuroanatomical approach to acupuncture. It discusses the neurophysiology of pain, endorphins, acupuncture analgesia, analysis of acupuncture points, electroacupuncture and TENS. The authors propose that in clinical practice one should choose the acupuncture point that is relevant and specific to the underlying pathological condition. Therefore, the rest of the book describes treatment of headaches, disorders of the neck, lower back, upper and lower limb in a fashion that complements a Western practice in orthopaedics. Formulae of acupuncture points are given to correspond to Western musculoskeletal conditions.

Simple, inexpensive, gives a scientific basis for acupuncture. The Acupuncture Foundation of Canada's initial teachings were developed by one of the authors.

Insights of a Senior Acupuncturist, 1992, Miriam Lee
Blue Poppy Press, Boulder, Colorado, USA

A good book for those with some experience of TCM. It is subtitled, "One combination of points can treat many diseases". It could simplify many of the syndrome prescriptions for a busy therapist. It is

well worth reading for the experienced insights in the title.

Single-case research designs, 1982, Alan E Kazdin
Oxford University Press, Oxford

Since most of the research possible for physiotherapists just starting to use acupuncture will take the form of single case studies it is well worth reading a book on how to do it properly. This is the definitive work and could be very useful to those aiming to include this new modality into their practice.

Acupuncture Patterns and Practice, 1993, Li Xuemei and Zhao Jingyi
Eastland Press, Seattle, USA

A really good book for clarifying the process of syndrome differentiation. Gives many helpful flowcharts to organize thinking. A good Western approach to the Chinese logic process. The only drawback is that it only deals with a limited number of diagnostic categories, i.e. Cold, cough, dizziness, headache, Painful Obstruction, low back pain, windstroke, insomnia and palpitations.

Acupuncture Treatment of Internal Disease, 1985, George T. Lewith
Thorsons Press, London, UK

Similar in format to the book by Leon Chaitow on the treatment of musculoskeletal pain. Very good diagrams and clear summaries of the reasons for point selection. Formulae rather than deep reasoning but a good book to keep by you in the clinic.

Sticking to the Point, 1989, Bob Flaws
Blue Poppy Press, Boulder, Colorado, USA

Another book to help with putting together an effective prescription. Very little text but gives good lists of actions of specific points. Useful for the clinical setting.

Acupuncture Case Histories from China, 1994 (1st English edn), Zhang Dengbu
Churchill Livingstone, New York

Subtitled "A digest of difficult and complicated case histories" it is exactly that. I think it makes wonderful light reading and can in fact often offer new ways of looking at a tricky problem.

Between Heaven and Earth — a Guide to Chinese Medicine, 1991 (2nd edn), Harriet Beinfield and Efrem Korngold
Ballantine Books, Random House, New York, USA

This book guides the reader throughout the Chinese view of health and medicine and attempts to demystify the Chinese therapeutic techniques of acupuncture, herbology and nutrition. Throughout the book the use of metaphoric imagery helps to explain the difference between the Eastern and Western approaches to health and healing. It gives a balanced appreciation of both.

The initial section of the book consists of theory of TCM. The second section deals with Five Element theory, in particular how personality and emotions can predispose one to certain illness patterns and influence the process of healing. The final section gives a beginner's introduction to herbology and guides to foods as medicine.

This is an excellent overview of the various aspects of Chinese medicine for the intelligent questioning lay person and a good book for the beginning student. It is also a useful reference for practitioners in Five Element theory.

Appendix Two:
List of equivalent alphabetical codes of meridian names

	Meridian	Standard code*		Other alphabetic codes used[†]
1.	Lung meridian	L	I	F LU Lu P
2.	Large Intestine meridian	LI	II	CO Co Dch DI Di GI IC IG Li
3.	Stomach meridian	S	III	E Est M Ma ST St V W
4.	Spleen meridian	Sp	IV	B BP LP MP P RP RT Rt SP
5.	Heart meridian	H	V	C HE He HT Ht X
6.	Small Intestine meridian	SI	VI	Dii ID IG IT Si Xch
7.	Bladder meridian	B	VII	BL B1 PG UB V VU
8.	Kidney meridian	K	VIII	KI Ki N NI Ni R RN Rn Sh
9.	Pericardium meridian	P	IX	CS CX ECs EH HC Hc KS MC MdH PC Pe XB
10.	Triple Burner/Energizer meridian	TE	X	DE T TB TH TR TW SC SJ 3E 3H
11.	Gallbladder meridian	G	XI	D GB Go VB VF
12.	Liver meridian	Liv	XII	F G H LE Le LIV LV Lv
13.	Governor Vessel meridian	GV	XIII	DM DU Du GG Go Gv LG Lg T TM VG Vg
14.	Conception Vessel meridian	CV	XIV	Co Cv J JM KG Kg REN Ren RM VC Vc

* This is part of the alphameric code element of the standard acupuncture nomenclature proposed by the WHO Regional Working Group on the Standardization of Acupuncture Nomenclature.

† Some of the alphabetic codes shown here have already been discarded but may still have been used in older documents. They have therefore been included in this list.

Appendix Three: Self-study questions

Chapter 1 Introduction to TCM theory

1. How could you explain the concept of Qi?
2. What additional functions does the Heart have in Chinese medical theory?
3. Name the external pathogens that can affect the body.
4. Explain the difference between Yin and Yang.

Chapter 2 Physiological mechanisms in acupuncture

1. Explain why acupuncture and sensory stimulation can be used as synonyms.
2. Describe the different mechanisms that may contribute to the pain-relieving effect of acupuncture.
3. Explain why acupuncture is more effective in nociceptive than in neuropathic pain.
4. Sensory stimulation has been shown to increase the circulation in ischaemic tissue. Which are the mechanisms in this action?
5. The effect of acupuncture on asthmatic patients has been investigated repeatedly. Still, it is argued that positive effects are unproven scientifically. Discuss the requirements that must be fulfilled in a scientific study.

Chapter 3 Basic points

1. Which point is influential for muscles and tendons?
2. Which is the most powerful analgesic point?
3. Name two extra or non-meridial points.
4. Which combination of two points might lower blood pressure?

Chapter 4 Safe practice and needle techniques

1. List the contraindications to acupuncture.
2. Name three states, (problems, conditions or drugs) excluding pregnancy, where extra care must be taken when needling and why?
3. What should you do if a patient faints or feels dizzy?
4. Which points are contraindicated in pregnancy?

Chapter 5 Assessment procedures

1. What factors should you consider when making an assessment?
2. How would you plan a treatment programme for a patient with:
   (a) sciatica?
   (b) colles fracture?
3. What bench marks could you use for monitoring treatment?

Chapter 6 Introduction to acupressure

1. Name three methods of giving acupressure.
2. Name three acupoints that are particularly useful for acupressure.
3. Describe the possible uses of the above points.
4. Suggest points to treat a frontal headache.
5. Who might find acupressure useful?

Chapter 7 Trigger point therapy

1. Define the terms "myofascial syndrome" and "myofascial trigger point".
2. What types of trigger point are described by Travell?
3. What are the differences between an active trigger point and a latent trigger point?
4. According to Kawakita and coworkers, where is the myofascial trigger point situated?
5. List the factors that can perpetuate the presence of trigger points.
6. What are the three methods of diagnostic palpation described by Travell?
7. Which methods of physical therapy are useful in the management of myofascial trigger points?
8. What are the suggested physiological mechanisms for the action of dry needling of myofascial points?

Chapter 8 Moxibustion and cupping

1. What is the difference between using moxa and needles?
2. Is moxibustion always tonifying because of the heating effect?
3. In some cases moxibustion can have too strong an effect and is therefore contraindicated – explain.
4. Cupping and moxibustion are both heating in effect. What is the physiological difference between the two treatments?

5. Would you use moxibustion on:
   (a) An elderly diabetic patient with osteoarthritic knees?
   (b) A hypersensitive patient?

Chapter 9 TENS

1. Before modern TENS units became available, what were the sources of electrical currents for pain management?
2. What are the four TENS modes?
3. Name two electrode placement sites and give their rationale.
4. What group of nerve fibres are stimulated by high frequency/low intensity TENS?
5. How does burst train TENS differ from low frequency/high intensity TENS?

Chapter 10 Acupuncture for the treatment of pain

1. Explain Melzack & Wall's gate control theory.
2. How are the different types of pain classified in terms of their aetiology?
3. Explain the different modes of stimulation used, and the differences between them.
4. What different factors do you need to take into account when designing research studies?

Chapter 11 Laser acupuncture

1. What are the units of:
   (a) radiant/power output?
   (b) pulse repetition rate?
   (c) dosage?
2. What are recommended dosages for initiating laser acupuncture treatments?
3. What are the contraindications for laser acupuncture treatments?
4. What are the indications for laser acupuncture treatment?

Chapter 12 Ear acupuncture

1. How did the system of ear acupuncture develop over time?

2. Describe the main indicators of ear pathology.
3. Explain how the ear is classified:
   (a) according to contour;
   (b) according to histology;
   (c) according to the "inverted fetus" concept.
4. What is the basic procedure for ear acupuncture?

Index

Printed and bound by CPI Group (UK) Ltd, Croydon, CR0 4YY

03/10/2024

01040360-0004